The Injury Fact Book

The Injury Fact Book

Susan P. Baker
The Johns Hopkins University

Brian O'Neill
Insurance Institute for Highway Safety

Ronald S. Karpf
Insurance Institute for Highway Safety

Lexington Books
D.C. Heath and Company
Lexington, Massachusetts
Toronto

Library of Congress Cataloging in Publication Data

Baker, Susan P.
The injury fact book.

Includes bibliographies and index.
1. Wounds and injuries—United States–Statistics.
2. Accidents—United States—Statistics. 3. Mortality—
United States—Statistics. 4. United States—Statistics,
Vital. 5. United States—Statistics, Medical.
I. O'Neill, Brian, 1940– . II. Karpf, Ronald.
III. Title. [DNLM: 1. Wounds and injuries.
WO 700 B1675i]
RD93.8B34 1984 362.1'971'00973 82–49194
ISBN 0–669–06426–2

Sixth printing, December 1987

Published simultaneously in Canada

Printed in the United States of America on acid-free paper

International Standard Book No.: 0–699–06426–2

Library of Congress Catalog Card No.: 82–49194

In memory of
William Haddon, Jr., M.D.
1926–1985

Contents

Figures

Tables

Abbreviations

BAC blood alcohol concentration
CO carbon monoxide
FARS Fatal Accident Reporting System
ICD International Classification of Diseases
IIP Industrial Index of Production
NASS National Accident Sampling System
NCHS National Center for Health Statistics
NEISS National Electronic Injury Surveillance System
NHIS National Health Interview Survey
NHTSA National Highway Traffic Safety Administration
NPTS Nationwide Personal Transportation Study
OSHA Occupational Safety and Health Administration
PFD personal flotation device
SIDS sudden infant death syndrome
SMSA Standard Metropolitan Statistical Area

Foreword

Injuries are the leading cause of death in the United States from the first year of life to age 44. An incalculable cause of human suffering, injuries are also a major source of medical costs and losses to the economy. Yet the subject is largely unknown territory, even to professionals concerned with impairments to the health of the American people and ways in which the quality of life in the United States can be improved. Only rarely do colleges or universities teach the scientific aspects of injuries — except with respect to the treatment of the injured.

This is not because of lack of knowledge. Since about 1940, what is now termed "injury control" has evolved rapidly from the prescientific folklore that still dominates much popular thinking about the causes, prevention, and amelioration of injuries to a mature scientific field with sophisticated research methods, a practical theoretical base, an extensive body of empirical knowledge, and increasing examples of the successful control of the human damage.

In these respects, injuries and their prevention are the last of the great human plagues to be the subject of scientific inquiry and understanding. But, unlike the situation in the case of the infectious, cardiovascular, and neoplastic diseases, until the preparation of this book there has been no body of truly competent, comprehensive information giving, so to speak, the statistical lay of the land in the case of the many kinds of injuries.

Most of the basic analyses had never even been done before the authors meticulously performed them using a variety of governmental and other sources. Analyzed by cause, age, sex, race, socioeconomic status, urbanization, geography, time, and other variables, the results of this book, together with those the authors have drawn from other works, will constitute the indispensable statistical reference on injuries for years to come. The book will also undoubtedly be the source to which graduate students and others turn for injury research information, since the reasons for many of the trauma distributions it documents are, as yet, only poorly understood.

Since in many respects the authors have broken entirely new ground, many of the results they report will surprise, and in some cases shock, even specialists in the field. For example:

> Death rates from drowning are higher at ages one and two than at any other age, and remain high throughout the preschool period.
>
> State death rates from motor vehicle crashes correlate closely with death rates in the same states from other unintentional injuries.

The death rate per freight ton-mile varies a thousandfold, depending on the transportation mode employed. The lowest death rates are for freight moved by pipeline and marine transport, the highest for freight moved by highway.

Firearm suicide rates decrease and non-firearm suicide rates increase with increased socioeconomic status.

Per capita, Asians have by far the lowest motor vehicle death rates. Native Americans have by far the highest.

During World War II, more than 20,000 U.S. military personnel died in plane crashes in the continental United States.

With only four known exceptions, all male injury death rates greatly exceed those of females. The exceptions are deaths from falls on the same level (the rates for which are about equal), deaths from barbiturates and psychotherapeutic drugs, and deaths from strangulation, which show marked female excesses compared to males.

Although it was not the authors' intent to discuss injury theory, research, or prevention, their statistics are laced with incisive comments about the wide variations in incidence, explanations of many of the findings, and references to relevant work. In the process, they have also documented the substantial success of several injury control efforts.

An example is provided by childhood poisonings: "Since 1960, poisoning deaths among children younger than 5 years have decreased dramatically. The rate for poisoning by solids and liquids was 2.2 per 100,000 in 1960 and 0.5 in 1980 .... Between 1960 and 1980, the number of deaths from lead poisoning dropped from 78 to 2. Deaths from kerosene and other petroleum products dropped from 48 to 9, while those from aspirin dropped from 144 to 12 .... An especially steep decline in childhood poisoning death rates occurred after childproof packaging was required on all drugs and medications beginning in 1973. The 50 percent decrease in poisoning by all drugs and medications in the first three years (1973-1976) was substantially greater than the decrease in poisonings by other solids and liquids, most of which were not required to be packaged in childproof containers .... During 1968-1979, the period analyzed for most causes of death in this book, the 80 percent decline in poisoning death rates for children ages 1-4 exceeded that for any other major cause of childhood injury death."

In 1930, 348 people died in elevator failures. With improved elevator designs and government regulations and inspections, such deaths, despite huge increases in elevator use, have become so rare that they are no longer recorded separately in the nation's vital statistics.

The dramatic change in injury deaths, whether inadvertent or deliberate, that can result from correcting an environmental hazard is also illustrated by what happened when coal gas (which had a higher carbon monoxide content) was replaced by natural gas. In 1947, domestic piped gas caused about 1,000 unintentional deaths and was the agent in some 1,200 suicides. In 1980, after the change to natural gas, the corresponding totals were only 61 and 23 deaths, a decrease of more than 90 percent.

Despite such examples, the injury picture presented in this book is generally grim. It resembles the situation in the history of infectious diseases before the sanitary revolution and subsequent preventive and therapeutic measures. In contrast, the magnitude and characteristics of the injury problem documented in this book make it clear that the country and the relevant professions have a huge amount of catching up to do to bring injury control to the level of success already achieved with the infectious diseases and the level being approached with respect to malignancies and afflictions of the cardiovascular system. The data in the book are a baseline against which that objective will long be measured. Thorough familiarity with this book will long be necessary for professional literacy in the fields with which it deals and in those to which it relates. In addition, the data and commentary this book provides will long be invaluable resources for insurers, public health workers, and, in fact, for everyone concerned with the occurrence, reduction, and cost of injuries of all kinds.

William Haddon, Jr., M.D.
President
Insurance Institute for Highway Safety

Preface

This book would never have been written without the work of the pioneers who placed the study and control of injuries on a solid, scientific basis. They had the ability to ask the right questions, find ways to answer them, and disturb a lot of people with the results.

Hugh De Haven established the science of biomechanics of injury. His interest in human injury tolerance and the dynamics of injury causation began when he was almost killed in a World War I airplane crash. During months of recuperation, he contemplated the reasons for his survival, refusing to attribute it to chance. De Haven's subsequent analysis of survival of falls from great heights led to his discovery that, under favorable conditions, the body can tolerate 200 times the force of gravity. This meant that in high-speed crashes of automobiles and airplanes — as well as in falls from heights — "serious injury was not a sure, necessary, or acceptable result."

Subsequent workers such as Col. John Stapp and Dr. William Haddon, Jr., also refused to accept injuries as inevitable. John Stapp advanced our knowledge of human injury tolerance. William Haddon developed the conceptual frameworks that form the basis for understanding and controlling injuries.

The irresistible stimulus for beginning *The Injury Fact Book* came from my students, who are required to explore an injury problem that is of particular interest to them. With few exceptions, they tell me that their biggest surprise is the scarcity of data. How could a trip to the library yield so little information on carbon monoxide poisoning or farm machinery injuries or homicide in rural areas, when publications about problems of far less consequence take up entire shelves?

The pioneers and students set the stage. The Insurance Institute for Highway Safety provided the resources, both human and financial, that made it possible. The National Center for Health Statistics and the National Highway Traffic Safety Administration collected and made available the data for most of the analyses. I am grateful to them all and to each of the individuals cited on the following page.

Susan P. Baker

Acknowledgments

The team of co-workers who produced this book includes:

Research Support Alison M. Trinkoff, Jacqueline L. Rattiner, Judith S. Samkoff

Computing Support Deborah N. Sandroni

Editing Support Anne L. Fleming

Word Processing Stacey A. Church, Karen S. Whibley

Production Nina Minschwaner

Secretarial Support Diane M. Reintzell

Readers who generously contributed suggestions include James N. Eastham, Jr., Susan G. Gerberich, William Haddon, Jr., Janine Jagger, Trudy A. Karlson, Ben Kelley, Jess F. Kraus, John H. Read, Leon S. Robertson, Carol W. Runyan, George W. Rutherford, Stephen P. Teret, Allan F. Williams, and Garen J. Wintemute.

1 Introduction

Injuries are the most serious public health problem facing developed societies. In the United States, they account for the majority of deaths among children and young adults. Throughout the world, injuries are now the leading cause of death during half of the human lifespan.[14] Once overshadowed by more common causes of death and illness, injuries have grown in relative importance as many diseases have been controlled.

The absolute magnitude of the problem is equally sobering. About eight million people alive today in the United States can be expected to die from injuries.[13] The risk of injury while traveling, working, playing, or even sleeping is such that most people sustain a significant injury at some time during their lives. Few escape the tragedy of fatal or permanently disabling injury to a relative or friend. Nevertheless, this widespread human damage too often is taken for granted.

Comparatively little public attention is given to injuries and their prevention except during the aftermath of a disaster, even though on an average day the number of injury deaths in the United States is several times the toll of a major air disaster. The amount of scientific attention directed at the injury problem is miniscule compared to that for many other health problems.[10,11] Misunderstanding of this problem and its components has resulted in widespread failure to apply even available knowledge and technology to its solution.

The occurrence of injuries is largely determined by characteristics of the environment, particularly environmental modifications by human organizations. The incidence and severity of injury are greatly influenced by demographic factors such as age, sex, and race, as well as by economic, temporal, and geographic effects (figure 1-1). The influence of these is so great that death rates from many injuries differ a hundredfold or more among various groups of people. Specific injuries differ greatly in their distribution in space, time, and populations.

Injuries are caused by acute exposure to physical agents such as mechanical energy, heat, electricity, chemicals, and ionizing radiation, interacting with the body in amounts or at rates that exceed the threshold of human tolerance. In some cases (for example, drowning and frostbite) injuries result from the sudden lack of essential agents such as oxygen or heat.[3-7] However, about three-fourths of all injuries, in-

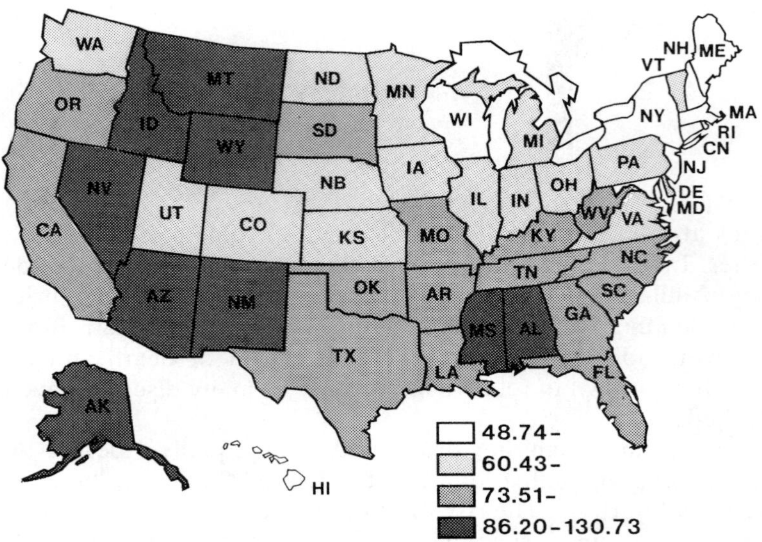

Figure 1-1. Death Rates from All Injuries by State, Per 100,000 Population, 1977-1979

cluding most from vehicle crashes, falls, sports, and shootings, are caused by mechanical energy (figure 1-2).

Although there are no sharp scientific distinctions between injury and disease, injuries usually are perceived almost immediately after contact with the causal agent.[5] Because injuries and the events leading to them are generally more obvious and close together in time than are diseases and the events that precede them, the role of human behavior is often erroneously assumed to be more important to injury causation than to disease causation. In fact, human behavior is important to both. For example, wearing shoes and cooking food are behaviors that can influence susceptibility to disease, even though symptoms of hookworm or amebic dysentery may not be apparent until months after a person walks barefoot in dirt infested with hookworm larvae or eats uncooked vegetables containing amebic cysts. There is no basis for the widespread assumption that modifying human behavior is any more important in preventing injuries than diseases.[6]

This book includes detailed information on many of the factors surrounding injuries — the man-made systems and products involved, the groups at greatest risk, and effective ways to protect people from injuries. The circumstances under which injuries occur, the etiologic

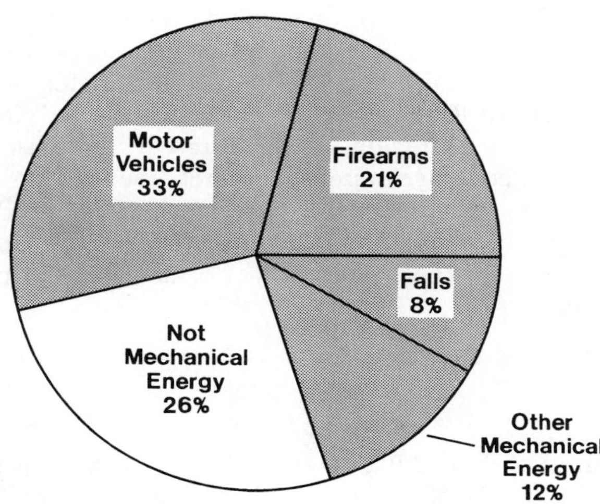

Figure 1-2. Percent of All Injury Deaths Caused by Mechanical Energy, 1980

agents, and the characteristics of the people involved are examined. Chapter 2 summarizes the importance of injuries in relation to other prominent health problems. Subsequent chapters describe injury mortality and, in cases where good population-based studies are available, nonfatal injuries.

The organization of the book is influenced by the International Classification of Diseases (ICD) E-codes, which determine the categories of most national mortality data on injuries. Since these codes are subdivided according to apparent "intent" of injury (i.e., unintentional, suicidal, or homicidal), Chapters 3-6 are organized on the basis of intent. Chapters 7-20 are organized on the basis of injury etiology; the chapter on poisoning, for example, includes details on suicidal as well as unintentional poisonings. To minimize repetition, the reader is sometimes referred to another chapter.

The analyses in Chapters 3-15 are primarily of injury deaths during 1977-1979, the most recent years for which detailed mortality data were available in mid-1983 for deaths other than those related to motor vehicles. Most of these data were collected by the U.S. Department of Health and Human Services, National Center for Health Statistics (NCHS). Chapters 16-20 summarize data on deaths from motor vehicle-related injuries. Most of these detailed data were obtained from the U.S. Department of Transportation, National Highway Traffic Safety Administration (NHTSA). Data from the 1980 census provided denominators for the rates throughout the book,* except for trendline calculations which were based on interpolations between census years.

The purpose of this book is to improve understanding of the nature and magnitude of the injury problem in the United States. Although it includes some discussion of ameliorative approaches, there is no comprehensive coverage of injury research, theory, or prevention, since these have been comprehensively discussed elsewhere.[1-9,12] This book is a thorough documentation of the injury problem. Most of the information presented is new, the product of analyses not previously published in any form.

Notes

1. Baker, S.P., and P.E. Dietz. "The Epidemiology and Prevention of Injuries." In *The Management of Trauma*, edited by G.D. Zuidema, R.B. Rutherford, and W.F. Ballinger, II. Philadelphia: W.B. Saunders Company, 1979.

2. Berger, L.R. "Childhood Injuries: Recognition and Prevention." *Current Problems in Pediatrics* (November 1981): 1-59.

3. Gibson, J.J. "The Contribution of Experimental Psychology to the Formulation of the Problem of Safety — A Brief for Basic Research." In *Behavioral Approaches to Accident Research*. New York: Association for the Aid of Crippled Children, 1961, pp. 77-89.

4. Haddon, W., Jr. "A Note Concerning Accident Theory and Research with Special Reference to Motor Vehicle Accidents." *Annals of the New York Academy of Sciences* 107 (May 22, 1963): 635-646.

5. Haddon, W., Jr. "Advances in the Epidemiology of Injuries as a Basis for Public Policy." *Public Health Reports* 95 (1980): 411-421.

6. Haddon, W., Jr., and S.P. Baker. "Injury Control." In *Preventive and Community Medicine*, edited by D. Clark and B. MacMahon. Boston: Little, Brown and Company, 1981, pp. 109-140.

7. Haddon, W., Jr., E.A. Suchman, and D. Klein. *Accident Research: Methods and Approaches*. New York: Harper and Row, 1964.

8. Robertson, L.S. *Injuries: Causes, Control Strategies, and Public Policy*. Lexington, MA: Lexington Books, 1983.

9. Teret, S.P., S.P. Baker, A.M. Trinkoff, and S. De Francesco. *Report of the National Conference on Injury Control*. The Johns Hop-

*Using estimates of the 1978 population as a denominator for calculating death rates during 1977-1979 would have made little difference in our findings, given the relatively small change in the population and the extremely large differences between the various demographic groups compared.

kins School of Hygiene and Public Health, May 18-19, 1981. Atlanta: The United States Public Health Service, Centers for Disease Control, 1981.

10. Terris, M. "The Paradox of the Missing Institute." *Journal of Public Health Policy* 4 (1983): 394-397.

11. Trunkey, D.D. "Trauma." *Scientific American* 249 (1983): 28-36.

12. Waller, J.A. *Injury Control: A Guide for Health and Safety Professionals to the Causes and Prevention of Trauma*. Lexington, MA: Lexington Books, in press.

13. Whitfield, R., P. Zador, and D. Fife. "Expected Mortality from Injuries." Washington, DC: Insurance Institute for Highway Safety, 1984.

14. Wintemute, G.J. "The Size of the Problem." *Injury Prevention in Developing Countries*, edited by G.J. Wintemute, S.P. Baker, D. Mohan, and S.P. Teret. Baltimore: The Johns Hopkins University, 1984.

2 Injuries in Relation to Other Health Problems

Health expenditures in the United States have been rising much faster than the gross national product in recent years. Policymakers and health professionals are increasingly aware that the resources needed for health care are limited and that available resources must be used more efficiently. Allocations of resources for research and for prevention and treatment of disease and injury should be made on the basis of the relative importance of various causes of morbidity and mortality in the population and the potential for effective intervention. This chapter documents the importance of injuries in relation to other health problems in the United States.

Injuries as a Cause of Death

The number of deaths in a population during a particular period is commonly used to describe and compare public health problems. Mortality data of this type are widely used, in part because deaths are well defined and usually tabulated in some detail. Most of the analyses presented in this book focus on mortality. In keeping with standard public health practice, results are generally summarized by death rates, defined as the number of deaths per 100,000 population each year.

One death in every 12 in the United States results from injury. Injuries are the fourth leading cause of death, claiming more than 160,000 lives each year. In 1980, the death rate for injuries (71 per 100,000 people) was surpassed only by the rates for heart disease (336), cancer (184), and cerebrovascular disease (stroke) (75).[6]

For more than four decades of life — specifically, ages 1-44 — injuries are the leading cause of death (figure 2-1).[6] As is true of cancer and other disease groups, injuries include a number of subgroups. One single subgroup of injuries, those related to motor vehicles, is the most common cause of death for ages 1-34.

The age-specific death rates for injuries far surpass those for cancer and heart disease for ages 1 through 44 (figure 2-2).[6] From age 1 through 4, injuries cause almost half of all deaths and result in 3 times the number of deaths from congenital anomalies, the second leading cause. From age 5 through 34, injury deaths exceed deaths from all other

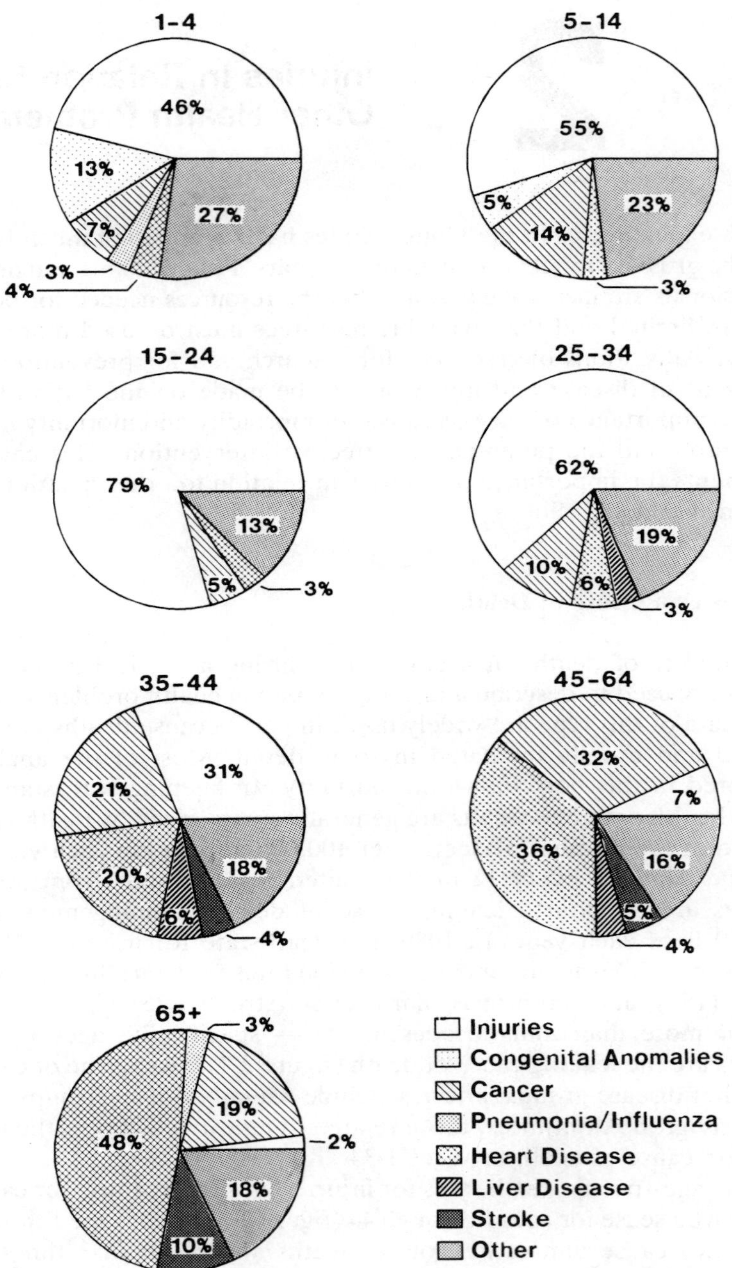

Figure 2-1. Percent of All Deaths by Cause and Age, 1980

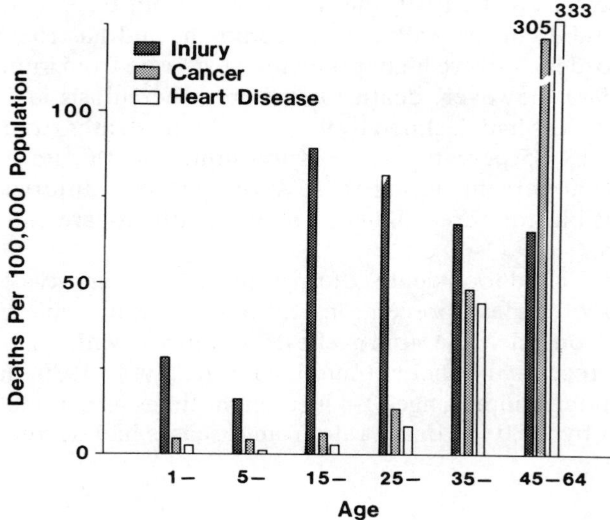

Figure 2-2. Death Rates by Cause and Age, 1980

causes combined. From age 35 through 44, they continue to outnumber deaths from any other single cause.[6]

After age 45, injuries account for fewer deaths than several other health problems, such as heart disease, cancer, and stroke. Despite the decrease in the proportion of deaths due to injury, the death rate from injuries is actually higher among the elderly than among younger people. In absolute numbers, injuries remain important throughout life. For example, each year some 30,000 people age 65 or older die from injuries.[6]

Children under one year old are often omitted from published injury statistics, even though injury deaths now surpass deaths from pneumonia during the first year of life and are outranked only by congenital anomalies and perinatal conditions. At this age, injury deaths outnumber by about 40 to 1 deaths from cystic fibrosis, although the latter are more common during the first year of life than at any other age and are the object of considerable public concern.

Trends in Mortality from Injuries and Other Causes

Injuries have always been a serious problem. Yet until a few decades ago, their importance was overshadowed by the prominence of many infectious diseases. In 1910, the death rates from three major disease groups — tuberculosis, influenza/pneumonia, and gastroenteritis and related disorders — were higher than the death rate from injuries (figure 2-3). By 1980, however, death rates from tuberculosis and gastro-intestinal disorders had declined by 99 percent, and deaths from influenza/pneumonia by 85 percent, whereas the injury death rate declined by only about 30 percent during these seven decades. Injuries presently are responsible for three times as many deaths as are influenza and pneumonia.

Trends in childhood deaths during the past 50 years vividly illustrate the success of disease prevention and amelioration, which have long been based on scientific approaches, in contrast with injury control, which only recently has been treated scientifically. In 1930, deaths from diseases among children ages 1-4 were eight times as common as injury deaths, but by 1980 the death rate from diseases had decreased almost

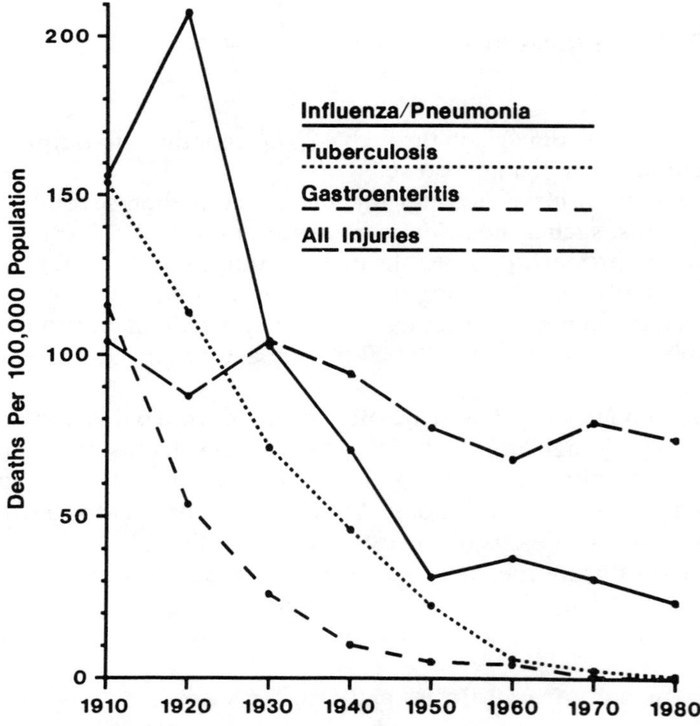

Figure 2-3. Death Rates from Injuries and Infectious Diseases by Year, 1910-1980

to the level of the injury rate, which had declined by only half (figure 2-4). Among children ages 5-14, the two death rates converged in the 1960s. For ages 15-24 the injury death rate by 1980 was almost three times that from diseases, whereas the opposite was true in 1930.

Societal Costs

Mortality comparisons, useful as they are for policymakers, illustrate only one part of the nation's health burden. Nonfatal health problems are also significant because of the demands they place on the health care system as well as the suffering and inconvenience of involved individuals and their families and associates. Comparing the relative impact of nonfatal health problems is a complex matter because of the substantially different outcomes of various health conditions. One com-

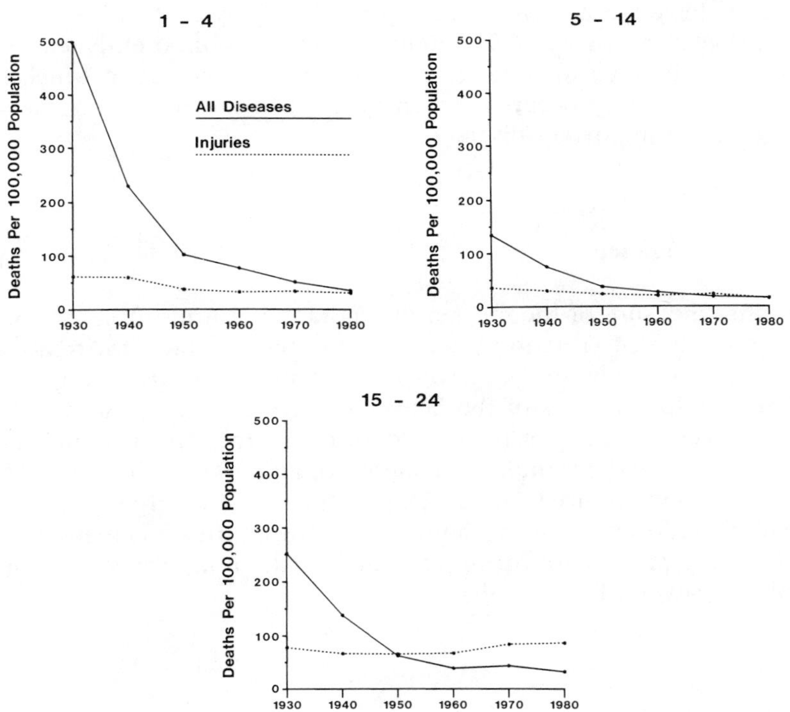

Figure 2-4. Death Rates from All Diseases and Injuries by Year and Age Group, 1930-1980

parative approach involves computing the societal costs associated with health problems and thus using dollars as a basis for comparison.

Such approaches are not universally accepted. Comparisons of the impact of health problems in economic terms must always be treated with caution because effects such as pain, grief, and family or social disruption cannot be measured in these terms. On the other hand, key effects such as loss of productivity (indirect costs to society) and the use of medical and other resources (direct costs) can be measured and compared in dollars for various health problems.

The total cost to society of all injuries is unknown. However, for motor vehicle crash injuries occurring in 1975, the total societal cost was estimated at almost $15 billion in 1975 dollars, over $20 billion in 1980 dollars.[3-4] A more recent estimate for motor vehicle injuries put the cost to society at over $25 billion in 1980 dollars.[8]

The societal cost of motor vehicle injuries, compared to other leading causes of death, is second only to the cost of cancer (figure 2-5).* The direct costs (expenditures for goods and services) resulting from motor vehicle crash injuries are approximately twice the direct costs of coronary heart disease.[3,4] The indirect costs (loss of potential earnings) are especially high for injuries because the average age at which fatal or disabling injury occurs is much lower than the corresponding ages for the most important diseases.

Physician Contacts

Another measure of the burden that nonfatal injuries place on society is the number of visits to physicians and other contacts for treatment. Injuries resulted in 99 million physician contacts in 1980, compared to 72 million for diseases of the heart, the second leading cause of such visits, and 64 million for respiratory diseases, the third leading cause.[7]

Emergency department visits also are an important element of the direct costs of injuries. Over 25 percent of *all* emergency room or hospital clinic visits are for the treatment of injuries.[7] The annual cost of this emergency care for more than 30 million injured Americans is probably several billion dollars.

---

*These results ranking motor vehicle injuries second to cancer are based on the incidence of new cases in one year. Other results based on the prevalence of specific health conditions in one year ranked all injuries combined second to heart disease.[2]

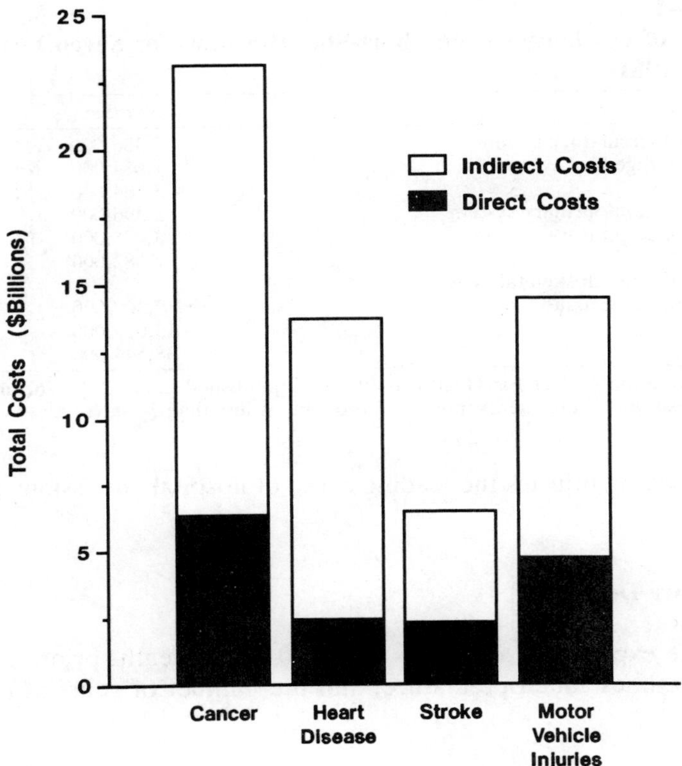

Source: Reprinted with permission of the publisher, from *The Incidence and Economic Costs of Major Health Impairments* by H.S. Hartunian, C.N. Smart, and M.S. Thompson (Lexington, Mass.: Lexington Books, 1981).

Figure 2-5. Societal Costs Associated with the Annual Incidence of Cancer, Coronary Heart Disease, Stroke, and Motor Vehicle Injuries, 1975

Hospital Admissions

The number of people who are admitted to hospitals for treatment provides another basis for comparing health problems in terms of the resources utilized. Injuries necessitate about 3.6 million hospital admissions each year, almost one of every ten admissions at short-stay hospitals. For all ages combined, injury admissions are outranked only by diseases of the circulatory and digestive systems (table 2-1). In 1979, there were 2.3 million injury admissions for people younger than 45

Table 2–1
Number of Discharges from Short-Stay Hospitals for Seven Leading Causes, 1981

Conditions	*Number*	*Percent*
Diseases of circulatory system	5,336,000	14
Diseases of digestive system	4,684,000	12
Injuries	3,584,000	9
Diseases of genitourinary system	3,496,000	9
Diseases of respiratory system	3,475,000	9
Neoplasms	2,582,000	7
Diseases of musculoskeletal system and connective tissue	2,308,000	6
Other	13,079,000	34
Total	38,544,000	100

Source: National Center for Health Statistics, unpublished data, 1981. Includes non-federal hospitals where the average length of stay is less than 30 days.

years, making injuries the leading cause of hospital admissions for this age group.[5]

Premature Deaths

Since life expectancy at birth is about 70 years, deaths prior to age 70 are sometimes called premature, and the number of years of life that

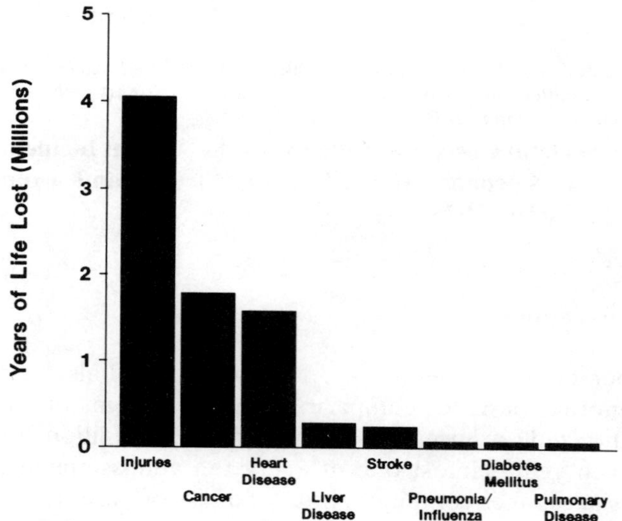

Figure 2-6. Potential Years of Life Lost Prior to Age 70 from Eight Leading Causes of Death, 1980

would have remained are considered years of life lost prematurely. For each cause, the difference between age 70 and the age at death is used to calculate the total number of years of life lost because of death prior to age 70.[1] There are more than 4 million potential years of life lost prematurely each year because of injuries, compared to less than 2 million each for cancer and heart disease and 0.3 million each for liver disease and cerebrovascular disease (stroke) (figure 2-6). Even when injury deaths from homicide and suicide are not included, the remaining unintentional injury deaths result in almost 3 million potential years of life lost prematurely, a greater loss than for any single disease.[1]

Notes

1. Centers for Disease Control. "Table V. Years of Potential Life Lost, Deaths, and Death Rates, by Cause of Death, and Estimated Number of Physician Contacts, by Principal Diagnosis, United States." *Morbidity and Mortality Weekly Report* 31 (1982): 599.

2. Cooper, B.S., and D.P. Rice. "The Economic Cost of Illness Revisited." *Social Security Bulletin* (1976): 21-36.

3. Hartunian, N.S., C.N. Smart, and M.S. Thompson. "The Incidence and Economic Costs of Cancer, Motor Vehicle Injuries, Coronary Heart Disease, and Stroke: A Comparative Analysis." *American Journal of Public Health* 70 (1980): 1249-1260.

4. Hartunian, N.S., C.N. Smart, and M.S. Thompson. *The Incidence and Economic Costs of Major Health Impairments: A Comparative Analysis of Cancer, Motor Vehicle Injuries, Coronary Heart Disease and Stroke*. Lexington, MA: Lexington Books, 1981.

5. Haupt, B.J., and E. Graves. *Detailed Diagnoses and Surgical Procedures for Patients Discharged from Short-Stay Hospitals: United States, 1979*. DHHS Publication No. (PHS) 82-1274-1. Washington, DC: U.S. Department of Health and Human Services, 1982.

6. National Center for Health Statistics. "Advance Report of Final Mortality Statistics, 1980." *Monthly Vital Statistics Report* 31 (September 1983): 22-26.

7. National Center for Health Statistics. "Physician Visits: Volume and Interval Since Last Visit, United States 1980." *Vital and Health Statistics* 10 (1983): 27, 58-59.

8. National Highway Traffic Safety Administration. "The Economic Cost to Society of Motor Vehicle Accidents." Technical Report DOT HS-806-342. Washington, DC: U.S. Department of Transportation, January 1983.

3 Overview of Injury Mortality

Unlike diseases, injuries are often classified on the basis of the behaviors and events that preceded them and the imputed intent of the people involved. The commonly used major subdivisions of injury deaths are homicide, suicide, and unintentional (or accidental*). Although the events leading to intentional and unintentional injuries may differ widely, the mechanisms of injury and the injuries themselves are typically identical or similar.For example, ingesting a toxic substance produces the same outcome even though the spectrum of behavior can range from completely unintentional, as when a person is not aware of the presence or nature of a drug or its potential effect, to suicidal self-poisoning. In addition, many of the basic preventive strategies are the same. Reductions in the carbon monoxide content of cooking and heating gas in England reduced both unintentional and suicidal deaths without corresponding increases in suicide by other means.[1,6] Similarly, the crashworthy fuel systems that have virtually eliminated postcrash fire deaths in Army helicopters are equally effective regardless of whether a crash occurs on training maneuvers or as a result of combat.[12]

More than 160,000 Americans died of injuries in 1980. Of these deaths, 66 percent were classed as unintentional and 32 percent as intentional; for the remainder the intent was unknown (figure 3-1). Unintentional injury deaths included approximately 53,000 resulting from motor vehicle crashes and 53,000 from other events. Of approximately 51,000 intentional injury deaths, 27,000 were classified as suicide and 24,000 as homicide and legal intervention. An additional 4,000 deaths (predominantly by poisoning, shooting, or drowning) were of undetermined intent.[11]

Age and Sex

The death rate from injuries varies greatly with age (figure 3-2). It is highest for ages 75 and older; for ages 75-84 it is more than double the

*The word *accident* erroneously implies that injuries occur by chance and cannot be foreseen or prevented. In much scientific work the descriptor *accident* is gradually being replaced by more appropriate terms, such as *unintentional injury*, descriptions of the injuries (e.g., fractured tibia), or specification of the injury-producing event, such as a motor vehicle crash.

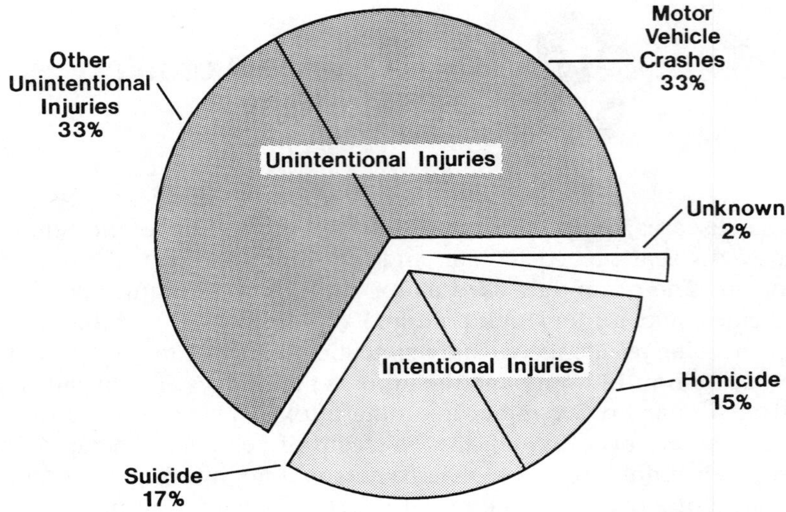

Figure 3-1. Percent of Injury Deaths by Manner of Death, 1980

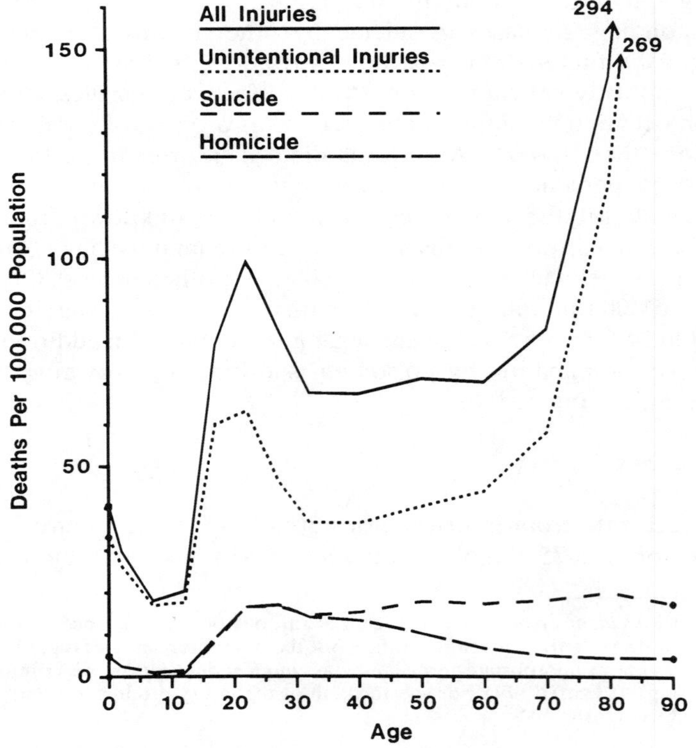

Figure 3-2. Injury Death Rates by Age, 1977-1979

overall rate for all ages combined. For ages 85 and older the death rate is almost 300 per 100,000 population. The *lowest* injury death rate is for ages 5-14. The next age group, 15-24, has a particularly *high* death rate. The shape of the curve for all fatal injuries combined is basically determined by the high death rates from unintentional injuries among young children, young adults, and the elderly.

The homicide rate is highest for ages 20-29, but among adults the suicide rate for both sexes combined shows little variation with age.

In addition to differences by age, injury death rates also vary by sex (figure 3-3; note that this figure has a different scale for unintentional injury in order to facilitate comparison of the pattern with those for suicide and homicide). Males have much higher rates in each category of injury death. For unintentional injury, male death rates have one peak in the 20-24 age group and another among the elderly. For suicide, there are also two peaks, one in the 20-24 age group and a

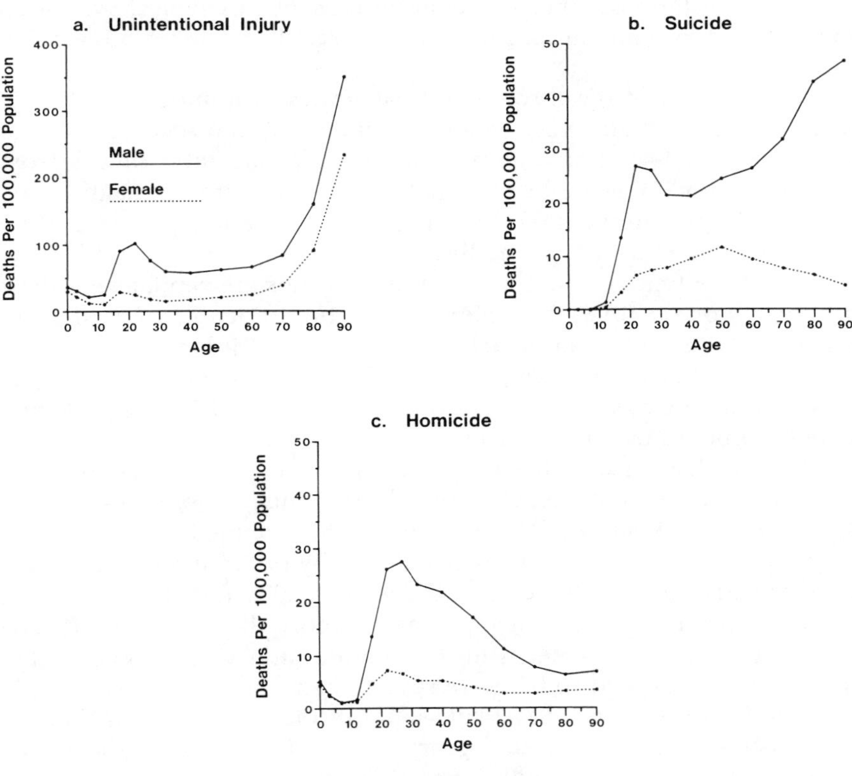

Figure 3-3. Death Rates from Unintentional Injury, Suicide, and Homicide by Age and Sex, 1977-1979

higher peak in the over-75 age group. For homicide, the single peak occurs in the 25-30 age group.

Among females, the highest suicide rates occur in the late forties. (That many women experience menopause at this age suggests the importance of research in this area.) For unintentional injury and homicide, peaks among females occur at ages 15-19 and 20-24, respectively. These peaks are at slightly younger ages than the corresponding peaks for young adult males, in part because in many social relationships females are generally somewhat younger than males.

The overall death rate for unintentional injuries is more than twice as high for males as for females (67 vs. 27 per 100,000 population). In the case of intentional injuries, male rates are more than three times as high as female rates (19 vs. 6 per 100,000 population for suicides and 14 vs. 4 for homicides). The higher rates for males in large part reflect differences in the likelihood of involvement in hazardous activities. These differences may be partly innate and partly a result of societal expectations; for example, hazardous jobs are typically assigned to men, and in many groups men are expected to drink more alcohol than women.

Within each of the three major categories of injury, the ratios of male to female deaths vary widely depending on the specific cause of injury (figure 3-4). For example, the male:female ratio ranges from 0.5:1 (1:2) for homicide by strangling to 52:1 for firearm deaths classified as "legal intervention," a category comprised of people shot by law-enforcement agents in the line of duty.

For some types of fatal injury, the sex ratios are similar regardless of intent. For example, the male:female ratio for deaths from firearms ranges between 4.9:1 and 6.3:1 for unintentional injury, suicide, and homicide. Other examples include deaths from sharp instruments (3.2:1 to 4.7:1) and deaths from barbiturates (0.7:1 and 1.0:1 for suicide and unintentional injury, respectively).

Unlike death rates, the nonfatal injury rates for males are only slightly higher than for females. Based on estimates from the National Health Interview Survey (NHIS), injuries that are medically treated or result in at least one day of restricted activity occur annually at a rate of about 364 per 1,000 males and 259 per 1,000 females, a ratio of 1.4:1.[10] Since male injury death rates are more than twice the female rates, the smaller differences in the nonfatal injury rates suggest that injuries to males tend to be more severe than those to females.

The best estimates of the per capita incidence of injuries that are serious enough to result in emergency room visits come from the Northeastern Ohio Trauma Study.[2] For these more serious injuries, the male:female ratio is slightly higher — 244 per 1,000 males compared

Ratio	*Unintentional Injury*	*Suicide*	*Homicide*
52:1			Firearm (legal intervention)
29:1	Electricity (non-home)		
22:1	Fall from ladder/scaffold		
19:1	Machinery		
17:1	Struck by falling object		
12:1	Drowning (boat)		
10:1	Motorcyclist		
7:1			
	Fall from structure		
	Explosion		
	Lightning		
	Firearm		
6:1			
	Pedestrian (train)	Domestic gas	
		Firearm	
5:1			
	Drowning (non-boat)		Firearm
	Airplane crash		Beating
	Cutting/piercing		
	Electricity (home)		
	Bicyclist		
4:1			
	Opiate poisoning	Hanging	Cutting/stabbing
	Suffocation		
	Motor vehicle exhaust	Cutting/piercing	
3:1			
	Alcohol poisoning		
	Excessive cold		
	Motor vehicle occupant		
	Pedestrian		
	Fall from other level		
	Excessive heat	Motor vehicle exhaust	
2:1			
	Pedestrian (non-traffic)	Jumping	
	Exposure		
	Housefire		
	Aspiration (food)		
	Natural disaster		
	Aspiration (non-food)		
	Fall on stairs		
	Hot substance	Drowning	
1:1	Fall on level — — — — — — — —	— — — — — — — —	— — — — — —
	Barbiturate poisoning	Barbiturate poisoning	
		Psychotherapeutic drugs	
1:2			
			Strangulation

Figure 3-4. Male: Female Ratios of Death Rates by Cause, 1977–1979

to 148 per 1,000 females, a 1.6:1 ratio. For these injuries, male rates exceed female rates until about age 55 (figure 3-5). Among older people, the rate is slightly higher among females than males, largely because of falls.[7] For both sexes, injury rates are highest at ages 15-24. In contrast to the age-related pattern for fatal injuries and hospital admissions, for which the rates are highest among the elderly, the rates for injuries treated in hospital emergency rooms are lowest after age 65.

The number of deaths occurring for every 1,000 injuries treated in hospital emergency rooms shows a very different pattern with age than the population-based injury and death rates (figure 3-5). The ratios of deaths per 1,000 injuries are higher among young adults than children, suggesting that the injuries sustained are, on the average, more severe after age 15. The increase in deaths at these ages (16 and older) in large part reflects increasing involvement in serious motor vehicle crashes. Large increases in the number of deaths per 1,000 injuries among the elderly reflect their greater likelihood of serious complications and poorer prognosis after injury.

The elderly also have the highest rates of hospitalization for injuries

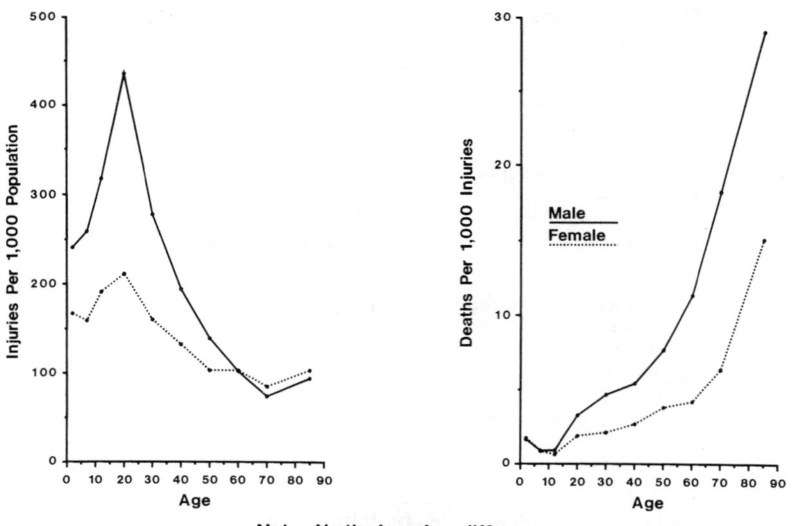

Source: Reprinted with permission from: D. Fife, J.I. Barancik, and B.F. Chatterjee, "Northeastern Ohio Trauma Study II: Injury Rates by Age, Sex, and Cause," *American Journal of Public Health,* 1984. Copyright, American Public Health Association.

Figure 3-5. Rates of Injuries Requiring Emergency Room Visits by Age and Sex, and Ratios of Deaths to Injuries, Northeastern Ohio, 1977

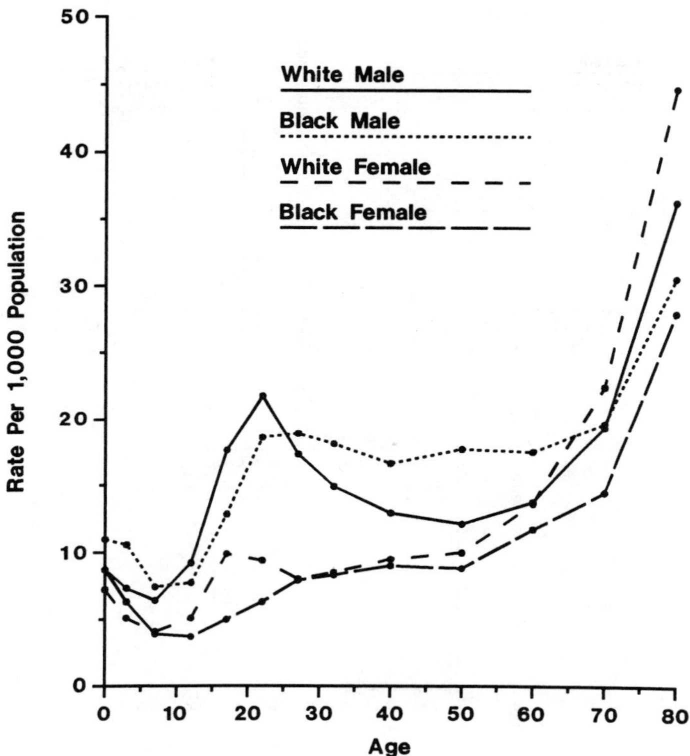

Figure 3-6. Short-Stay Hospital Discharge Rates for Injuries by Age, Race, and Sex, Maryland 1981

at acute-care hospitals (figure 3-6).* These rates are due to higher rates of admissions for fractures of the extremities, especially fractures of the hip, which are primarily fractures of the neck of the femur and intertrochanteral fractures (figure 3-7)** (see also Chapter 10). Hospitalization rates for intracranial and other internal injuries, lacerations, and dislocations are highest at ages 15-24, and sprains of the back and neck are most prominent at ages 35-44. Fractures of the arm resulting in hospital admission have high rates at ages 5-14 as well as among the elderly. These rates are determined not only by the incidence of the respective injuries but also by factors (such as age and injury severity) that influence the likelihood of admission after injury. Nevertheless,

*Rates shown were calculated using unpublished hospital discharge data for Maryland and corresponding census data.
**Rates shown in figure 3-7 are based on unpublished data from NCHS for 1981.

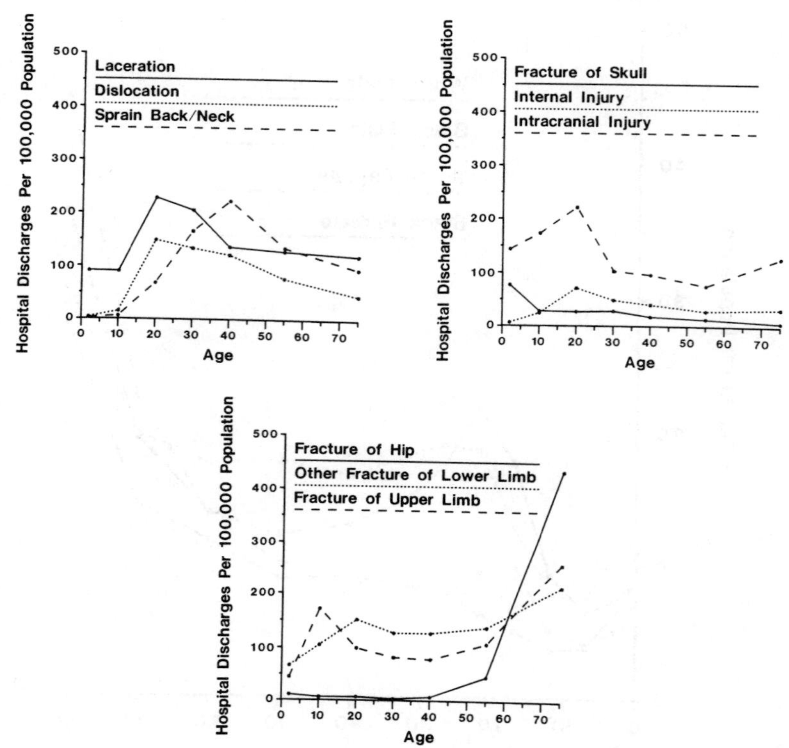

Figure 3-7. Short-Stay Hospital Discharge Rates for Injuries by Age and Type of Injury, NCHS Hospital Discharge Survey, 1981

the shapes of the curves shown here for various fracture groups are roughly similar to the curves for incidence rates based on x-rays rather than hospitalization.[5]

Race and Per Capita Income

Injury death rates vary substantially among racial and economic groups. Native Americans (Indians, Eskimos, and Aleuts) have the highest death rates from unintentional injury, blacks have the highest homicide rates, and whites and Native Americans have the highest suicide rates (figure 3-8). Asian Americans (Chinese, Japanese, Koreans, Hawaiians, Filipinos, and Guamanians) have the lowest rates of death from unintentional injury, suicide, and homicide.

Rates of hospital admission for injuries were calculated for whites

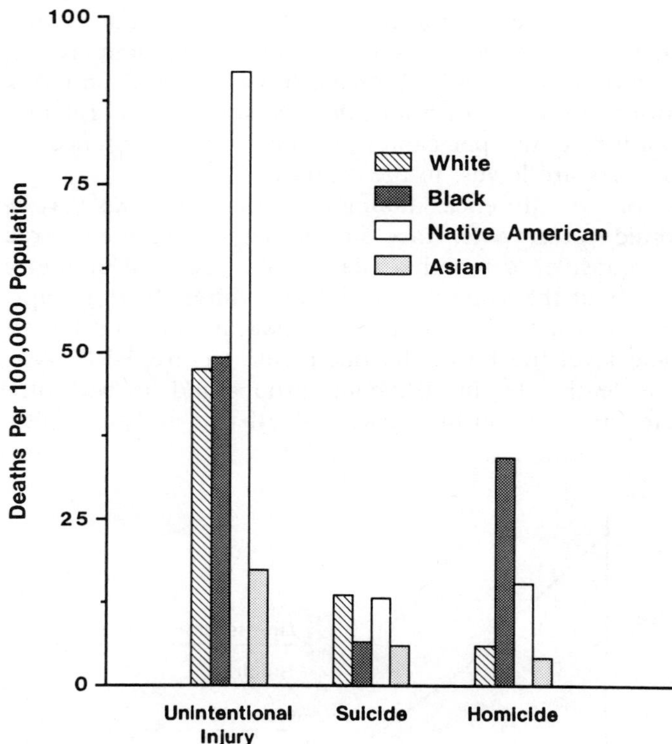

Figure 3-8. Death Rates from Unintentional Injury, Suicide, and Homicide by Race, 1977-1979

and blacks in Maryland (figure 3-6). The peaks seen among whites of both sexes at ages 15-24 are not as pronounced for black males and are not present for black females. Among children and middle-aged adults, admission rates are highest for black males.

National mortality data do not include information on individual economic status, but considerable evidence indicates that injury rates vary substantially among different economic groups.[3,9,13] In this book analyses of injury rates by economic group have been made on the basis of the per capita income of the area of residence of each fatally injured individual.* For unintentional injuries, the death rate varies

*For counties that include cities of 250,000 or more, the per capita income was calculated separately for city and noncity residents. For other counties, "area of residence" is synonymous with county. These analyses probably reduce the differences that would be seen if injured people could be categorized on the basis of their personal or family incomes, because within any area there can be large differences in income.

substantially with per capita income, decreasing from 71 per 100,000 in the lowest-income areas to 34 in the highest-income areas (figure 3-9). This relationship holds for both motor vehicle and non-motor vehicle unintentional injuries. For homicides and suicides, the relationship between death rate and per capita income is not pronounced, although homicide rates are lowest in the wealthiest areas.

Some of the differences among races in injury rates may be related to economic status. When race and per capita income of area of residence are considered together, death rates from all unintentional injuries are about the same for blacks and whites. Both groups have an inverse relationship between income levels and death rates: the higher the income level the lower the death rate (figure 3-10). Asians have the lowest death rates in all income groups and, as with other races, show an inverse relationship between death rate and per capita income.

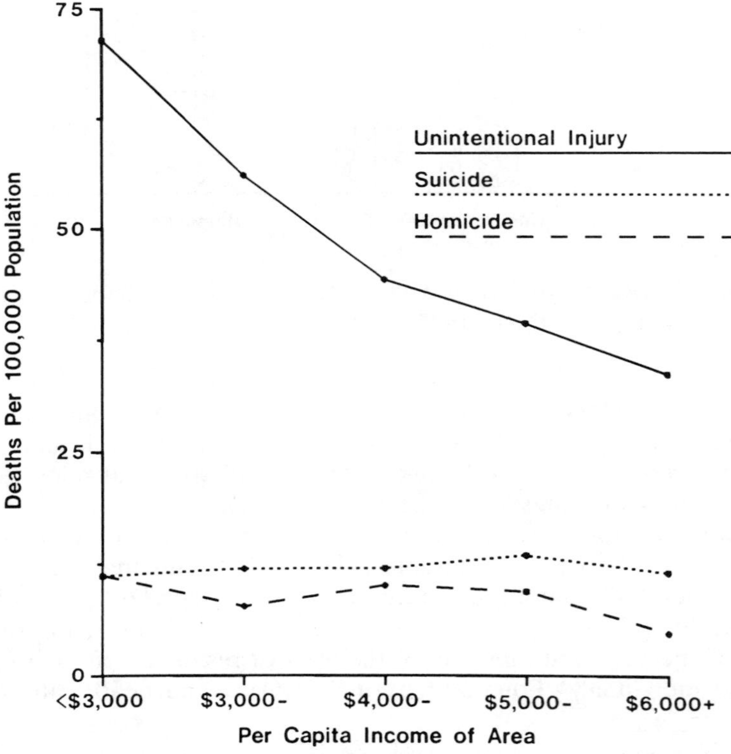

Figure 3-9. Death Rates from Unintentional Injury, Suicide, and Homicide by Per Capita Income of Area of Residence, 1977-1979

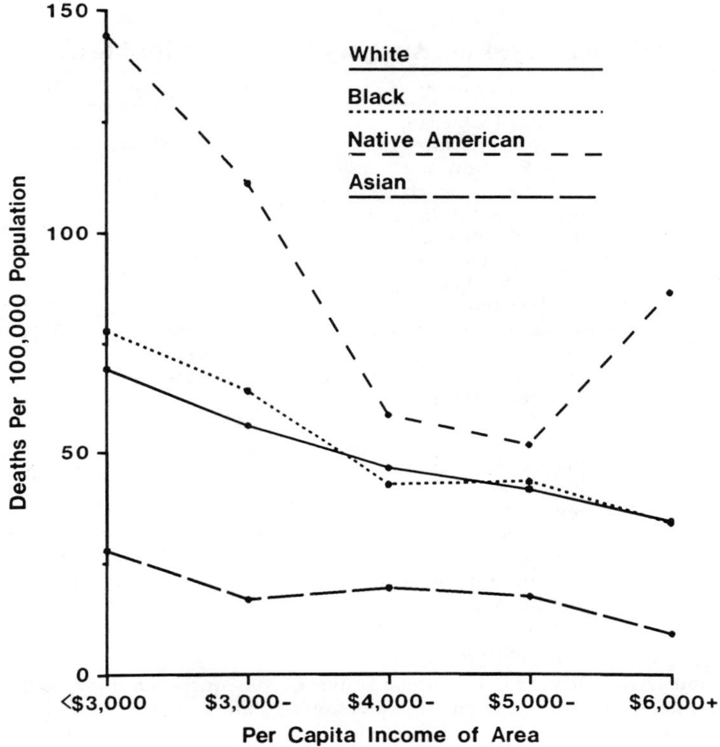

Figure 3-10. Death Rates from Unintentional Injury by Per Capita Income of Area of Residence and Race, 1977-1979

Native Americans have the highest death rates, with especially high rates in low-income areas. Unlike the other racial groups, the trend of lower death rates in high-income areas is reversed for Native Americans, in part because many Native Americans live in Alaska, where cost of living, per capita income, and injury death rates are extremely high.

Urban/Rural and Geographic Differences

The U.S. population was subdivided into five groups for the purpose of comparisons on the basis of place of residence (table 3-1). Counties that are part of the U.S. Census Bureau's Standard Metropolitan Sta-

Table 3–1
Population Subdivisions Used for Analyses by Place of Residence

Designation	*Description*	*Number of Areas*	*1980 Population*
Six largest cities	Residents of Chicago, Detroit, Houston, Los Angeles, New York, and Philadelphia, each of which has 1 million or more population	6 cities	17,531,000
Other large cities	Residents of cities with population between 250,000 and 1 million	52 cities	23,497,000
Other SMSAs	Residents of metropolitan (SMSA) counties, excluding residents of cities of 250,000 or more	724 counties or parts of counties	129,170,000
Rural nonremote	Residents of nonmetropolitan counties that do not meet the definition of "rural remote"	1,846 counties	51,665,000
Rural remote	Residents of nonmetropolitan counties that are not adjacent to an SMSA and have no settlement as large as 2,500 persons[a]	556 counties	4,543,000 4,428,000

[a]Larry Long and Diana DeAre, U.S. Bureau of the Census, provided a list of these counties, which they identified for their research on population migration.[8]

tistical Areas (SMSAs)* were divided into three groups: the six largest cities of 1,000,000 or more population, other large cities (populations 250,000 to 1,000,000), and other SMSAs. Counties not part of SMSAs were divided into two groups: "rural remote" counties not adjacent to an SMSA and with no town as large as 2,500, and other counties, termed "rural nonremote."[8] This categorization permitted the calculation of death rates for the most rural and the most urban areas, as well as for three intermediate groups. As with rates calculated by per capita income, death rates calculated by place of residence are based on the residence of the decedent, not the place of injury.

Unintentional injury death rates are highest in rural areas (figure 3-11). This is true for both motor vehicle and non-motor vehicle injury.

*An SMSA is a large population nucleus together with adjacent communities which have a high degree of economic and social integration. Areas qualify for establishment as a new SMSA by containing either a central city of 50,000 population, or a Census Bureau-defined urban area of 50,000 with a total metropolitan population of at least 100,000 (75,000 in New England).

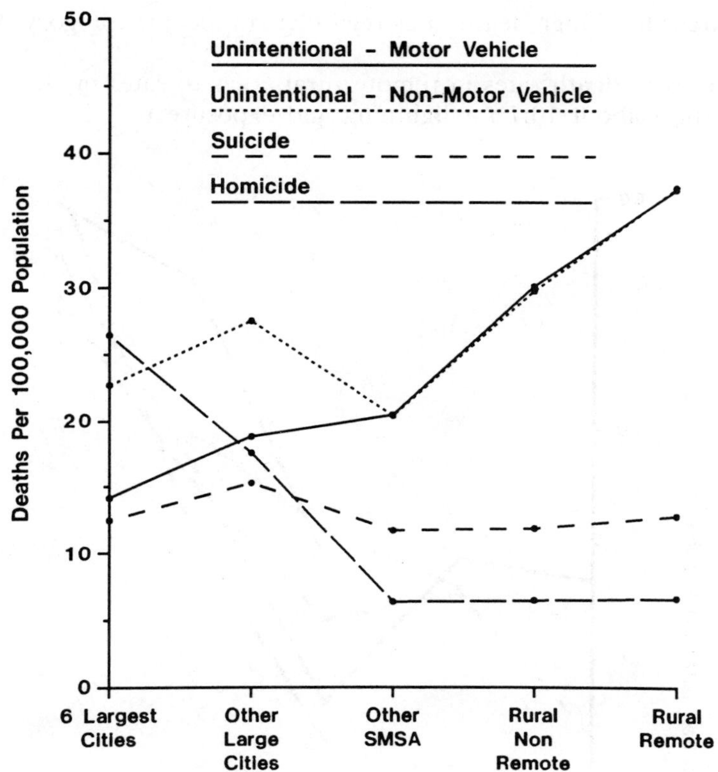

Figure 3-11. Death Rates from Unintentional Injury, Suicide, and Homicide by Place of Residence, 1977-1979

For these categories combined, the rate for the most rural areas (75 per 100,000 population) is twice the rate (37) for the largest cities. Homicide rates, on the other hand, are highest in large cities and show a fourfold difference by place of residence, ranging from a high of 26 in the largest cities and 18 in other large cities to a low of about 6 in less urban areas. Suicide shows the least variation by place of residence; the highest rates, in cities of 250,000-1,000,000 population, are only one-fourth greater than the rates for other areas.

In general, income is lowest in rural areas; 96 percent of all counties with a per capita income below $3,000 are rural counties that are not part of an SMSA. When income and place of residence are considered jointly, it is clear that economic differences do not account for the higher death rates for unintentional injuries in rural counties. The most rural areas have high death rates regardless of income category (figure 3-12).

Ratios of death rates in remote rural areas to rates in large cities range from about 10:1 for lightning and exposure to 1:29 for opiate

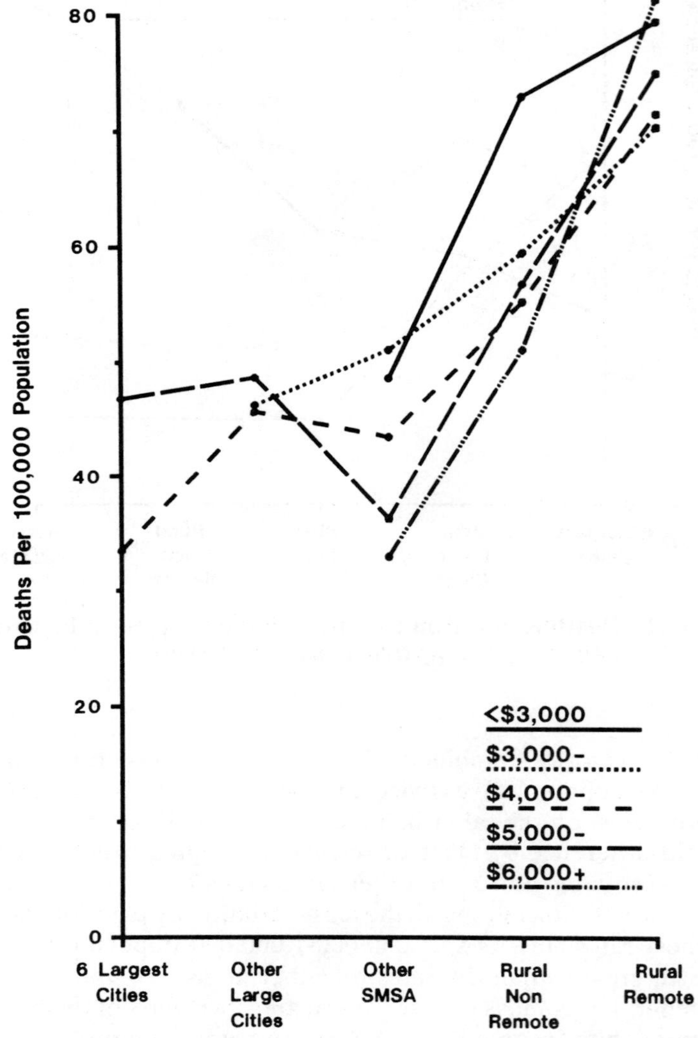

Figure 3-12. Death Rates from Unintentional Injury by Place of Residence and Per Capita Income of Area of Residence, 1977-1979

Ratio	*Unintentional Injury*	*Suicide*	*Homicide*
10:1	Lightning; exposure		
9.1	Machinery; natural disaster		
7:1	Firearm		
	Struck by falling object		
6:1	Pedestrian (non-traffic)		
	Excessive cold		
	Drowning (boat)		
5:1	Suffocation		
	Motor vehicle occupant		
4:1	Electricity (non-home)		
	Explosion		
3:1	Fall on level		
	Clothing ignition		
	Airplane crash		
	Aspiration (non-food)	Firearm	
2:1	Alcohol poisoning		
	Electricity (home)		
	Motor vehicle exhaust		Beating
	Drowning (non-boat)		
	Cutting/piercing		
	Motorcyclist		
	Aspiration (food)		
	Fall from ladder/scaffold		
	Housefire		
	Bicyclist	Motor vehicle exhaust	
1:1	----------	----------	----------
	Hot substance		
	Excessive heat		
	Pedestrian		
	Pedestrian (train)	Drowning	
	Fall on stairs	Hanging	
1:2	Fall from structure	Psychotherapeutic drugs	Firearm (legal intervention)
		Cutting/piercing	
		Domestic gas	
1:3			Firearm
1:4	Barbiturate poisoning		
1:5		Barbiturate poisoning	
1:6			
1:7			Cutting/stabbing
1:10			Strangulation
1:20		Jumping	
1:29	Opiate poisoning		

Figure 3-13. Rural:Urban Ratios of Injury Death Rates by Cause, 1977-1979

poisoning (figure 3-13). These differences underscore the importance of the physical environment in determining injury death rates. High buildings and heroin, for example, are especially present in large cities, whereas farm machinery and firearms are especially prevalent in rural areas.

In addition to urban/rural variations, pronounced geographic patterns characterize injury death rates (figure 3-14). Rates from unintentional injuries and suicides tend to be highest in the western states, while homicide rates are generally highest in southern states. The death rates for unintentional injury range among all states from a low of 33 in New York and Hawaii to a high of 97 in Alaska; for suicide, from a low of 8 in New Jersey to 22 in Nevada; and for homicide, from less than 2 in North Dakota and New Hampshire to 16 in Louisiana.* The magnitude of these differences reflects the great diversity among the states in population characteristics and exposure to hazards. Many of these relationships will be discussed in later chapters in connection with specific causes of death.

State-specific death rates, like other death rates presented in this book, have not been adjusted for age or other population characteristics that may differ from state to state, as is often done with health statistics. Except for falls, the age-adjusted death rates for most injuries differ very little from the actual (unadjusted) death rates.[7] In contrast, for most causes of injury there are fourfold to twentyfold differences in death rates among the various states. Age-adjustment would not change the patterns illustrated and would only slightly accentuate or reduce the differences in the actual rates. The use of unadjusted rates permits others to replicate the analyses in this book and portrays the actual rates of death in various population subgroups.

Temporal Variation

With the exception of suicides, injury deaths occur most frequently on weekends, peaking on Saturdays (figure 3-15). Suicides show less variation by day of week than the other two injury groups. The greatest numbers occur on Mondays; the fewest occur on Fridays, Saturdays, and Sundays.

---

*The highest rate (27) in figure 3-14c is for Washington, D.C. Although not a state, its rate was taken into consideration when the maps were subdivided to show the 10 highest areas, the 15 next-to-highest, the 16 next-to-lowest, and the 10 lowest.

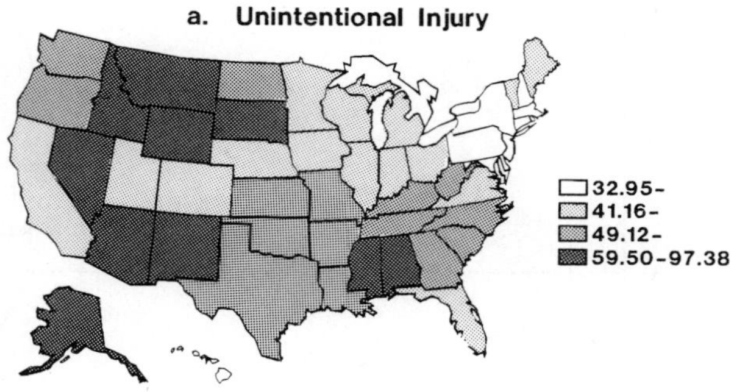

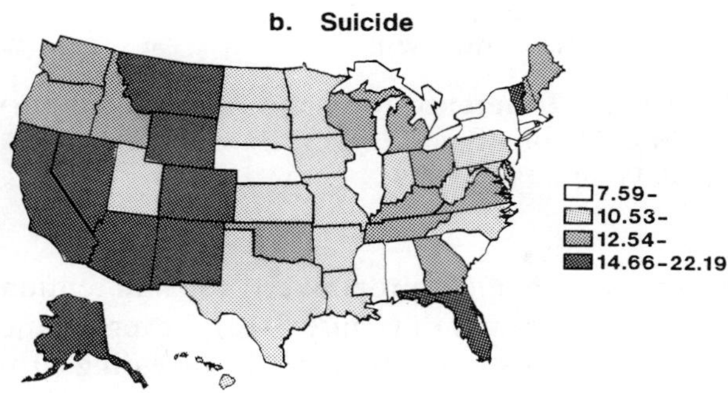

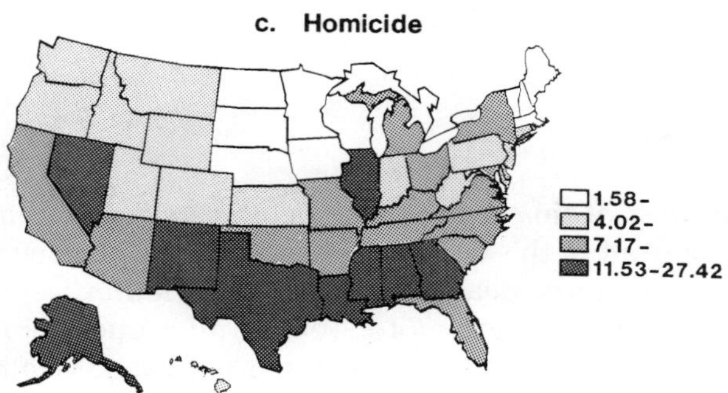

Figure 3-14. Death Rates from Unintentional Injury, Suicide, and Homicide by State, Per 100,000 Population, 1977-1979

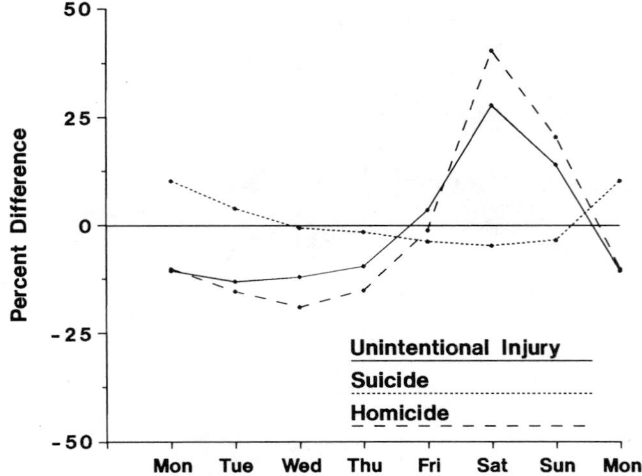

Figure 3-15. Percent Difference from the Average Number of Deaths from Unintentional Injury, Suicide, and Homicide by Day of Week, 1977-1979

Seasonal variation is most pronounced for unintentional injuries, with July being the peak month (figure 3-16). Several major causes of death contribute to this summertime peak, including drowning, motorcycle crashes, and electric current injuries. (As with later figures showing month of death, figure 3-16 does not adjust for the number of days in each month or the number of weekends in each month during the years studied. Such adjustment would tend to reduce some of the monthly variation shown in this graph.)

Historical Trends

Throughout most of this century, the death rate from injuries has declined. Virtually all of this decline has occurred in the general category of unintentional injury deaths not related to motor vehicle crashes (figure 3-17). While the non-motor vehicle injury death rate declined by 71 percent between 1910 and 1980, the per capita death rate from motor vehicle crashes increased approximately tenfold between 1910 and 1930, and there has been relatively little change since that time. The homicide rate varied from a low of less than 5 in 1910 to a high of more than 11 in 1980, with an earlier peak during the 1930s. In contrast, the suicide rate has shown less fluctuation.

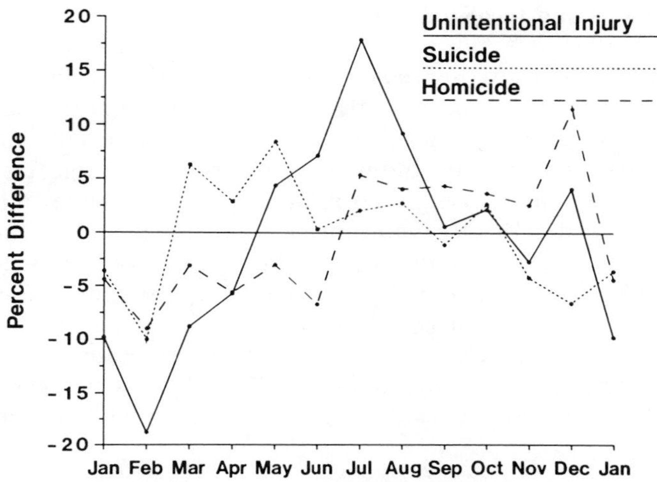

Figure 3-16. Percent Difference from the Average Number of Deaths from Unintentional Injury, Suicide, and Homicide by Month, 1977-1979

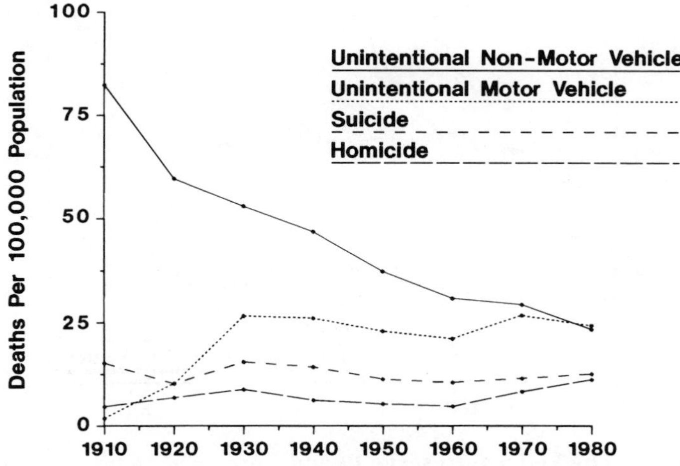

Figure 3-17. Death Rates from Unintentional Injury, Suicide, and Homicide by Year, 1910-1980

Injury Deaths and the Economy

When the economy is depressed, suicides and homicides reportedly increase and motor vehicle deaths decrease.[4] The national economic indicator most commonly used to quantify these associations has been the Federal Reserve Board Industrial Index of Production (IIP), which since 1950 has been strongly correlated with the annual number of motor vehicle deaths. Virtually every drop in the index during this period has been accompanied by a reduction in motor vehicle deaths (figure 3-18). It is important to note that this correlation is not due to increases or decreases in vehicle mileage. During the 1981-1982 economic slowdown, vehicle mileage increased while motor vehicle deaths declined in parallel with the economy. Correlations between the IIP and suicides and homicides are not as strong as with motor vehicle

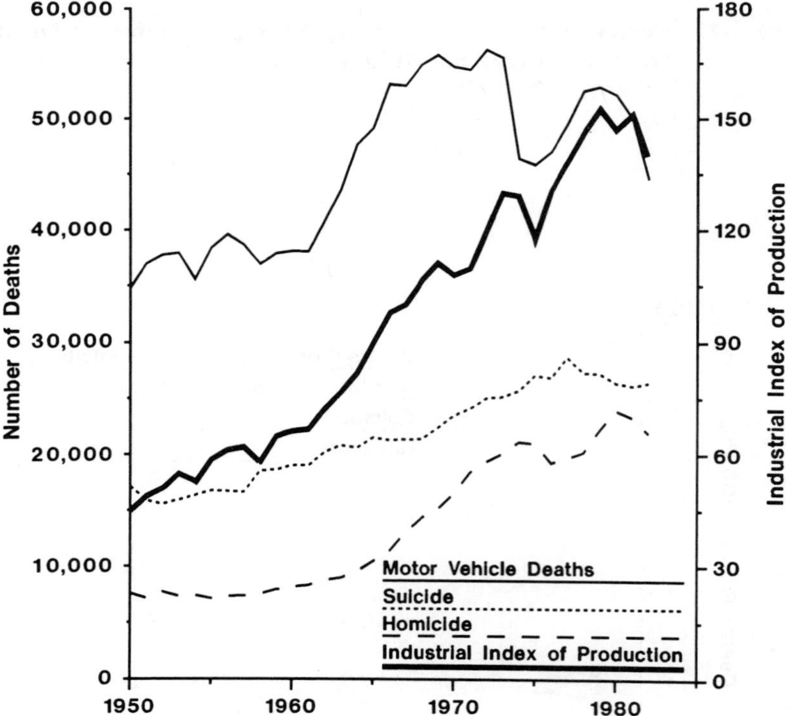

Figure 3-18. The Federal Reserve Board Industrial Index of Production and Deaths from Motor Vehicle Crashes, Suicide, and Homicide by Year, 1950-1982

deaths. To date, no empirical research has adequately explained the correlations between injury death rates and economic indicators.

Notes

1. Alphey, R.S., and S.J. Leach. "Accidental Death in the Home." *Royal Society of Health Journal* 3 (1974): 97-102, 144.

2. Barancik, J.I., B.F. Chatterjee, Y.C. Greene, E.M. Michenzi, and D. Fife. "Northeastern Ohio Trauma Study: I. Magnitude of the Problem." *American Journal of Public Health* 73 (1983): 746-751.

3. Barancik, J.I., and M.A. Shapiro. "Pittsburgh Burn Study. Pittsburgh and Allegheny County, Pennsylvania, 1 June 1970-15 April 1971." Washington, DC: U.S. Consumer Product Safety Commission, May 1976.

4. Brenner, M.H. "Estimating the Social Costs of National Economic Policy: Implications for Mental and Physical Health, and Criminal Aggression." In *Achieving the Goals of the Employment Act of 1946, Thirtieth Anniversary Review. Volume 1: Employment. A Study Prepared for the Joint Economic Committee, Congress of the United States*. Washington, DC: U.S. Government Printing Office, October 26, 1976.

5. Buhr, A.J., and A.M. Cooke. "Fracture Patterns." *The Lancet* 1 (1959): 531-536.

6. Hassall, C., and W.H. Trethowan. "Suicide in Birmingham." *British Medical Journal* 1 (1972): 717-718.

7. Iskrant, A.P., and P.V. Joliet. *Accidents and Homicide*. Cambridge, MA: Harvard University Press, 1968.

8. Long, L., and D. DeAre. "Repopulating the Countryside: A 1980 Census Trend." *Science* 217 (1982): 1111-1116.

9. Mierley, M.C., and S.P. Baker. "Fatal House Fires in an Urban Population." *Journal of the American Medical Association* 249 (1983): 1466-1468.

10. National Center for Health Statistics. "Persons Injured by Class of Accident and Whether Activity Restricting, 1981." Unpublished data from the National Health Interview Survey, 1982.

11. National Center for Health Statistics. "Advance Report of Final Mortality Statistics, 1980." *Monthly Vital Statistics Report* 31 (September 1983): 22-26.

12. Singley, G.T., III. "Army Aircraft Occupant Crash-Impact Protection." *Army Research, Development and Acquisition Magazine* (July-August 1981): 10-12.

13. Wise, P.H. "Differential Childhood Mortality in Boston." *American Journal of Diseases of Children* 137 (1983): 538.

4 Unintentional Injury

Unintentional injuries cause more than 100,000 deaths annually and are the fourth leading cause of death in the United States. Table 4-1 shows the numbers of deaths from the 20 leading causes of unintentional injury death. Motor vehicle crashes, falls, drownings, housefires, and poisonings cause three-fourths of all deaths from unintentional injuries.

Age and Sex

The relative importance of various causes of fatal injury varies substantially with age (figure 4-1). Motor vehicle crashes are the most

Table 4–1
Twenty Leading Causes of Unintentional Injury Death, 1980

Cause	*Number of Deaths*
1. Motor vehicle crashes (traffic)	51,930
2. Falls	13,294
3. Drowning	7,257
4. Fires and burns	6,016
5. Poisoning by solids and liquids	3,089
6. Firearms	1,955
7. Aspiration of food	1,943
8. Airplane crashes	1,494
9. Machinery	1,471
10. Aspiration of non-food material	1,306
11. Motor vehicle crashes (non-traffic)	1,242
12. Electric current	1,095
13. Struck by falling object	1,037
14. Mechanical suffocation	872
15. Excessive cold	707
16. Poisoning by motor vehicle exhaust	611
17. Pedestrians hit by trains	450
18. Exposure or neglect	415
19. Explosions	339
20. Collision with object or person	318

Source: National Center for Health Statistics, unpublished data, 1980.

Note: Deaths from adverse effects of drugs, surgery, or medical care are included in most statistics for unintentional injury. These deaths, numbering 2,437 in 1980, are excluded from the table and are not discussed in this book, but they are included in any total figures or analyses for all unintentional injuries, in order to keep totals consistent with those published elsewhere. Also excluded from the table are deaths attributed to excessive heat; they numbered 1,700 in 1980, about seven times the average annual number in 1977–1979.

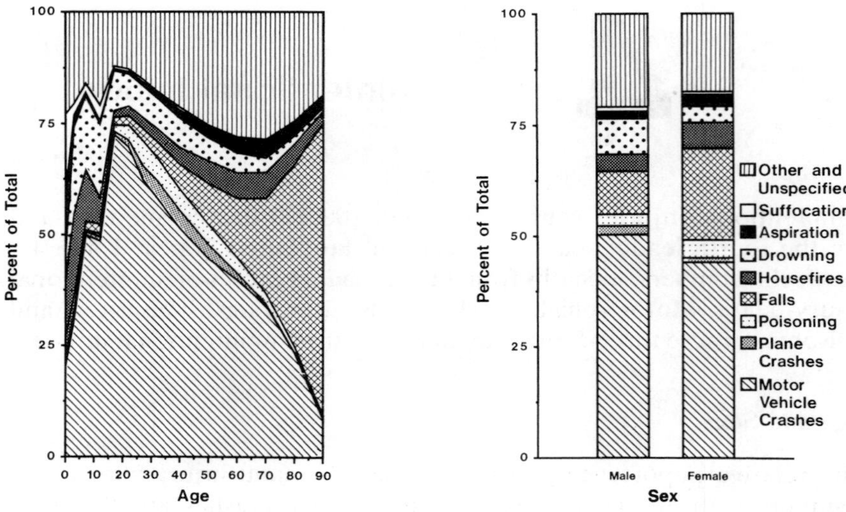

Figure 4-1. Percent of Unintentional Injury Deaths by Age and Cause, and by Sex and Cause, 1977-1979

frequent cause of fatal injury for ages 1-74, and falls are the most frequent cause for ages 75 and older. Drowning is the second leading cause of unintentional injury death for ages 1-44 and the third leading cause for all ages combined. Falls account for one-fifth of all unintentional injury deaths among females, compared to one-tenth among males (figure 4-1).

Looking at the proportions of injury deaths by cause indicates which causes are most important among specific groups of people, but it does not tell which groups have the highest mortality *rates* per 100,000 population. For example, firearms cause 8 percent of all unintentional injury deaths at ages 10-14 compared to 3 percent at ages 15-19, but the death *rate* from this cause is highest at ages 15-19. In an analysis of various causes of death for ages 15-19, the high injury death rates from many other causes eclipse deaths from firearms, despite the high death rate from this cause relative to other ages.

The death rates by age for all unintentional injuries combined form a J-shaped curve with an intermediate peak at ages 15-24 (figure 3-2). The shape of this curve, however, does not hold for individual causes of fatal injury. Mortality patterns for 12 categories of unintentional injury by age and sex exhibit widely differing patterns (figure 4-2).*

*To emphasize the variety of patterns, the vertical axes in this figure have different scales for various causes of death. As with many other figures in this book, the causes of death are arranged in a manner intended to call attention to similarities as well as differences in the patterns.

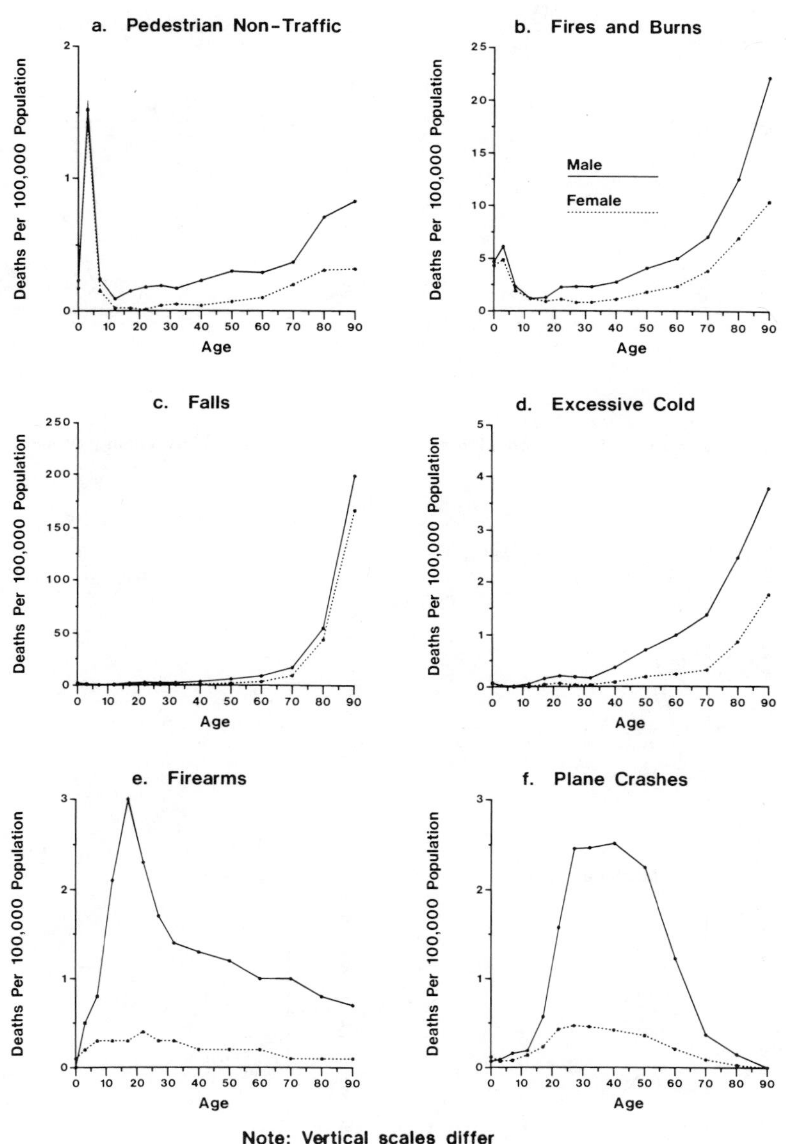

Figure 4-2. Death Rates from Unintentional Injury by Age, Sex, and Cause, 1977-1979

Some causes of death — for example, deaths from firearms — have one especially high-risk age group (figure 4-2e). The more complex patterns — for example, deaths from poisoning by solids and liquids — usually reflect the composite nature of a group of injury deaths

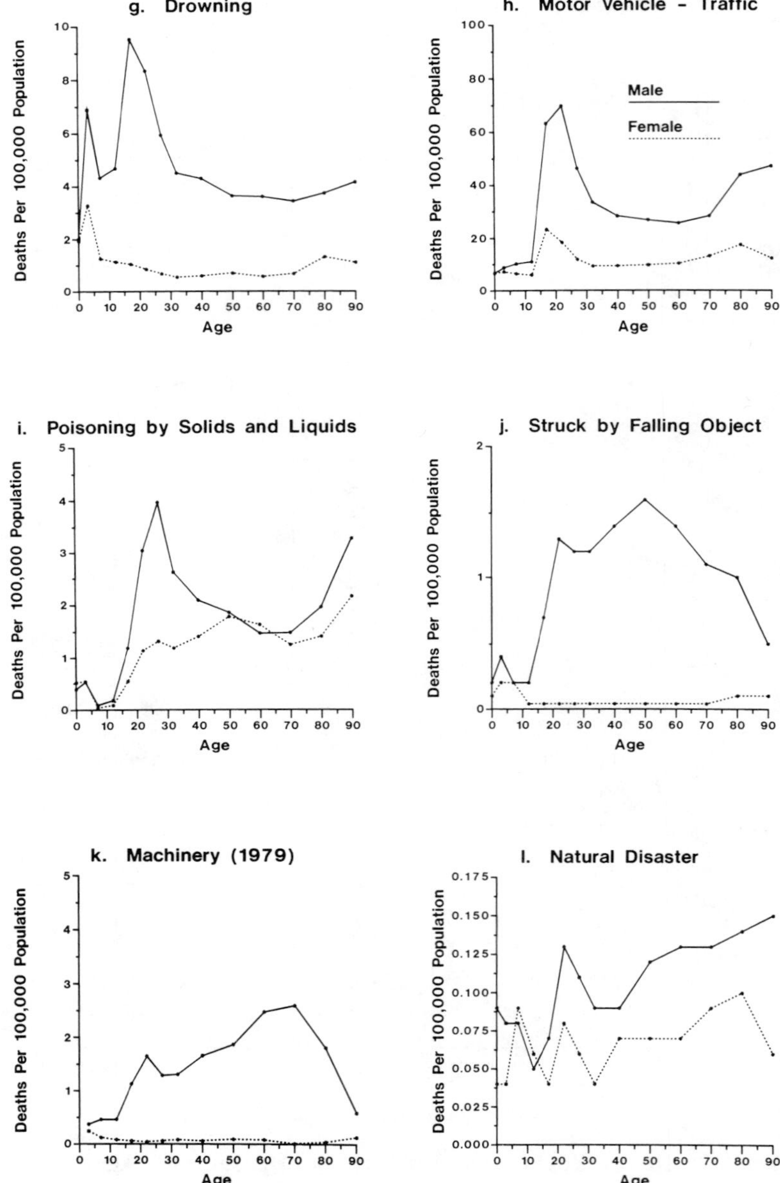
g. Drowning
h. Motor Vehicle - Traffic
i. Poisoning by Solids and Liquids
j. Struck by Falling Object
k. Machinery (1979)
l. Natural Disaster
Deaths Per 100,000 Population
Age
Male
Female
Note: Vertical scales differ

Figure 4–2 *(continued)*

(figure 4-2i). In this case, poisoning deaths from several groups of toxic substances with distinctive age and sex patterns are included. (Chapter 15 includes more detailed information on poisoning.)

Unlike other types of unintentional injury, deaths from natural disasters (e.g., floods, earthquakes, and tornados) do not have dramatic age-and sex-related patterns (figure 4-2l), presumably because people of both sexes and all ages are comparably exposed. The somewhat higher death rate among the elderly from disasters probably reflects their reduced ability to escape such situations, greater susceptibility to injury per se, and higher case-fatality rates when they are injured.

Elderly people have the highest death rates from many causes, including pedestrian injuries, excessive cold, falls, fires and burns, and farm machinery (figure 4-2). Among people age 70 or older, the extremely steep rise in fatal falls is substantially greater than the increase in deaths from any other cause (figure 4-3).

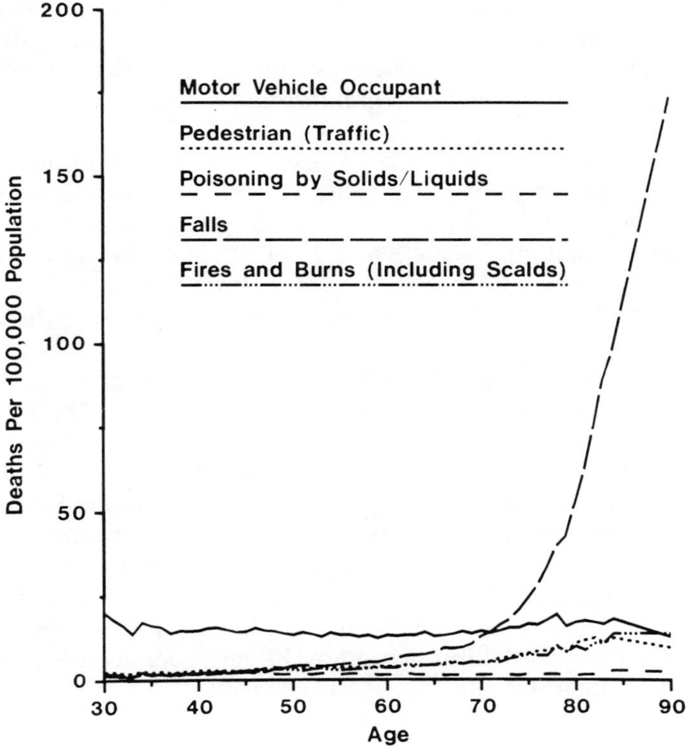

Figure 4-3. Death Rates from Unintentional Injury by Age and Cause, for Ages 30 and Older, 1977-1979

The higher injury death rates among the elderly result from a combination of factors, including decreasing ability to perceive and avoid hazards such as moving automobiles; musculoskeletal, proprioceptive, and other changes increasing their likelihood of falling; greater likelihood of injury when subjected to a given force, and poorer outcome following injury.[1,4,5]

The importance of exposure (the opportunity of being injured) as a factor in death rates is suggested by the decline after age 70 or 80 in death rates from some causes including firearms (figure 4-2e). Machinery-related deaths — which occur predominantly on farms, about half involving tractors — decline sharply after age 75 (figure 4-2k).

For most causes of death that are typically work-related, such as deaths from falling objects, the death rate is relatively constant throughout the working ages (figure 4-2j). The rates shown are based on the entire population and include deaths that are not work-related. Some occupational injury rates adjusted for the numbers of workers and days of work have revealed high rates of nonfatal injury among workers in their thirties and forties.[7] A study of work-related injury deaths in Maryland has indicated that when the number of workers is taken into account, males ages 25-44 are at greatest risk of fatal, on-the-job injury. The male:female ratio for such deaths was 75:1.[2]

High death rates in the 15-24 age group — for example, from firearms, drownings, and motor vehicles — partly reflect increasing use by males, beginning in their early teens, of potentially lethal products such as guns and motorcycles. The role of cultural patterns of expected behavior in relation to injuries — for example, what is regarded as appropriate behavior by young adult males compared to females — needs further research.

An increase in death rates from many causes begins at about age 10. Motor vehicle occupant death rates increase steeply between ages 15 and 18, then decline for people in their twenties (figures 4-4a and 4-4c). Other causes of death in this age group are dwarfed by motor vehicle occupant death rates and therefore are graphed separately, using different vertical scales (figures 4-4b and 4-4d). Among males, motor vehicle death rates and drownings peak at age 18, while the highest death rates for motorcyclists* and pedestrians are at age 20. Death rates from falls are high at ages 18-22 but, unlike many injuries, do not decrease markedly thereafter. Firearm deaths are unusual in having their highest death rates at ages 14-17.

---

*The death rates shown here for motorcyclists are based on National Center for Health Statistics data and are somewhat lower than the rates from the Fatal Accident Reporting System used as the basis for analyses in Chapters 16-20 (see Appendix). The same age pattern is illustrated using both data sets.

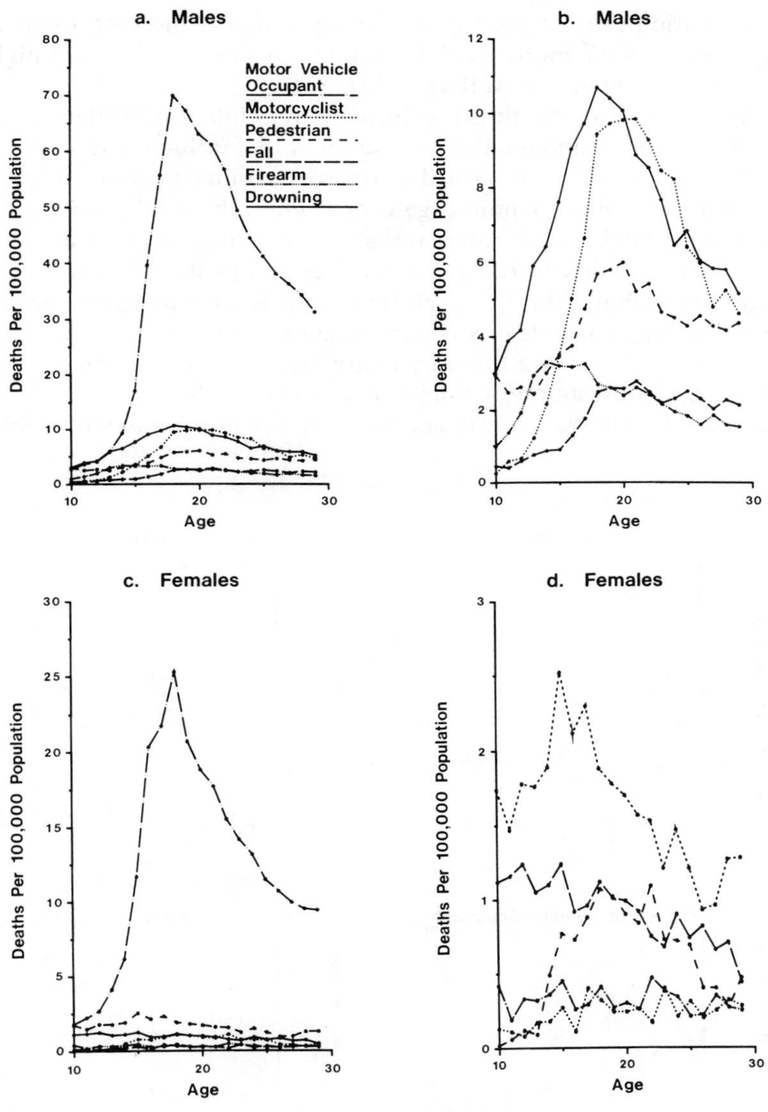

Figure 4-4. Death Rates from Unintentional Injury by Age, Sex, and Cause, for Ages 10-29, 1977-1979

Death rates for females are graphed using different scales from those used for males, in order to make age-related patterns discernible (figures 4-4c and 4-4d). Rates for females are much lower and show less dramatic peaks at slightly earlier ages than is the case for males. An exception is the motor vehicle occupant death rate, which is highest at age 18 for females as well as males.

The patterns of death rates during early childhood reflect various aspects of physical and mental development that influence susceptibility to injury: recognition of hazards, curiosity, ability to perform certain tasks (for example, opening a gate or riding a bicycle), and need for supervision. High death rates among very young children are partly due to their inability to recognize hazards and protect themselves. An example is a child who is struck by a vehicle in a driveway or other off-road place. Such deaths occur predominantly in the first year or two of life, and they are the only major type of injury death for which the rate is highest among young children (figure 4-2a).

Figure 4-5 shows specific age patterns for nine causes of uninten-

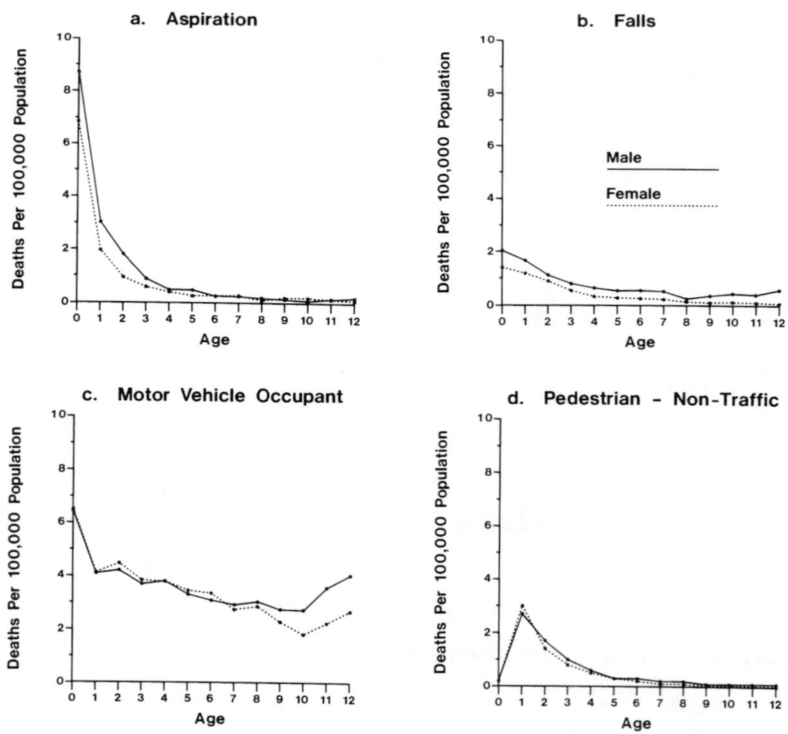

Figure 4-5. Death Rates from Unintentional Injury by Age, Sex, and Cause, for Ages 0-12, 1977-1979

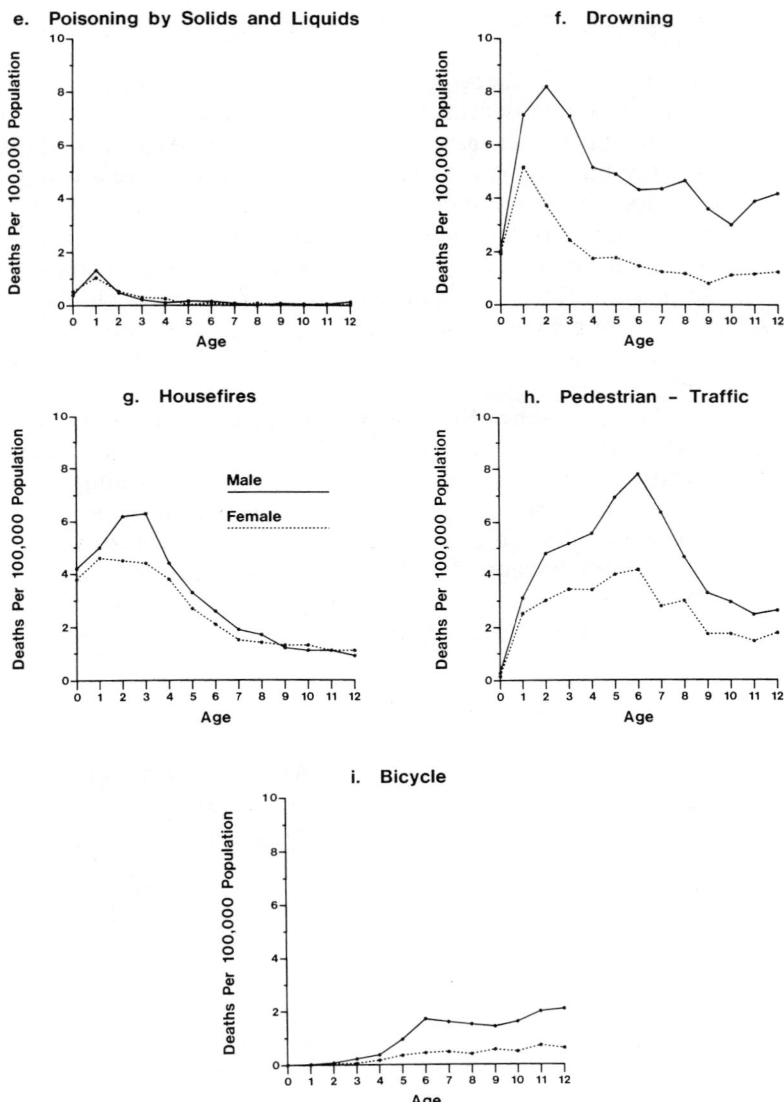

Figure 4–5 *(continued)*

tional injury deaths during the preteen years. Aspiration, fall, and motor vehicle occupant deaths decrease after the first year of life, as do nontraffic pedestrian and suffocation deaths (not shown here). Pedestrian and bicyclist deaths in traffic peak at age 6 and then decline.

Deaths from many of these causes increase again during the teenage years.

During childhood, there is little difference between the sexes in motor vehicle occupant deaths, which generally involve no initiative on the part of the child. The ratio of male to female deaths is highest for drowning, bicycling, and pedestrian deaths in traffic; these are activities the child is more likely to have initiated. For nonfatal injuries treated in emergency departments, higher rates among male children are evident beginning in the first year of life.[6] As in the case of teenagers and young adults, sex differences in injury rates among young children raise questions regarding societal norms and parental expectations in influencing their activities and behaviors, as well as the role of innate biological differences.

During the first year of life, the major causes of injury death differ in their distribution by month of age (figure 4-6). Motor vehicle occupant deaths are most common at 1-2 months. Drowning rates are high in the perinatal period, possibly reflecting the inclusion of some unidentified homicides. Housefire death rates are lowest for the youngest babies, perhaps because families with infants are less likely to be sound asleep during the early morning hours when most housefires occur (see Chapter 12). Deaths coded as aspiration and suffocation,

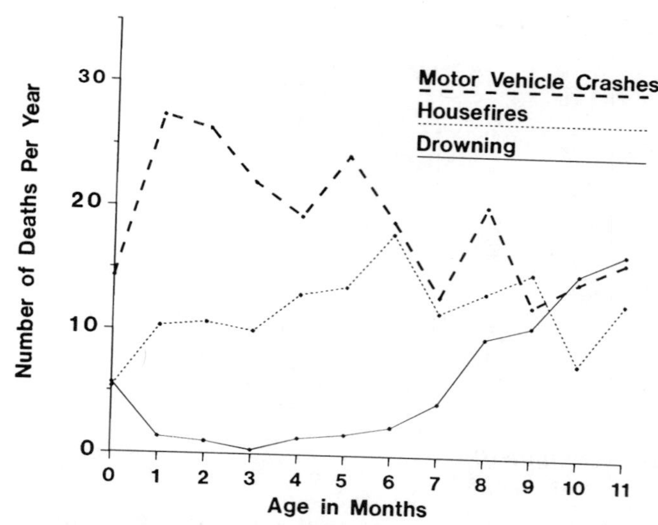

Figure 4-6. Average Number of Deaths Per Year from Housefires, Drowning, and Motor Vehicle Crashes by Month of Age, for Ages 0-11 Months, 1977-1979

the other major categories of fatal unintentional injury during infancy, occur primarily during the first 5 months (see Chapter 14). (Homicide rates are also high in the first few months of life.)

Race and Per Capita Income

There are differences by race not only in overall death rates from unintentional injuries (figure 3-8) but also in age-specific patterns (figure 4-7). Native Americans have the highest rates at all ages. Whites have the second highest rates among teenagers and the elderly. Unlike rates for other races, those for blacks do not peak between ages 15 and 24, and they increase after age 25.

Motor vehicles are the major cause of fatal unintentional injury for

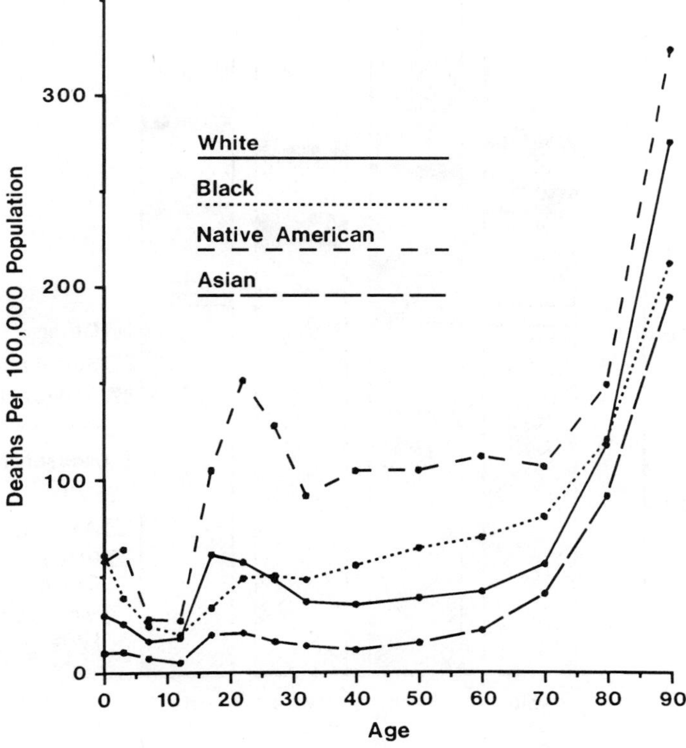

Figure 4-7. Death Rates from Unintentional Injury by Age and Race, 1977-1979

each racial group, but the relative importance of other causes differs (figure 4-8). Falls are the second leading cause of unintentional deaths among whites. Drownings are second or third among each racial group. Among blacks, the death rate from housefires almost equals their high drowning rate.

Of the causes of death that have substantial proportions occurring in industrial sites or mines (figure 4-9), three — explosions, collisions with objects or persons, and being "caught or crushed" — have death rates that are 24-29 percent higher for blacks than for whites. Death rates from electric current and machinery, on the other hand, are 79 and 61 percent higher, respectively, for whites.

Death rates are high in low-income areas for most categories of unintentional injury (figure 4-10). Causes of death showing this pattern

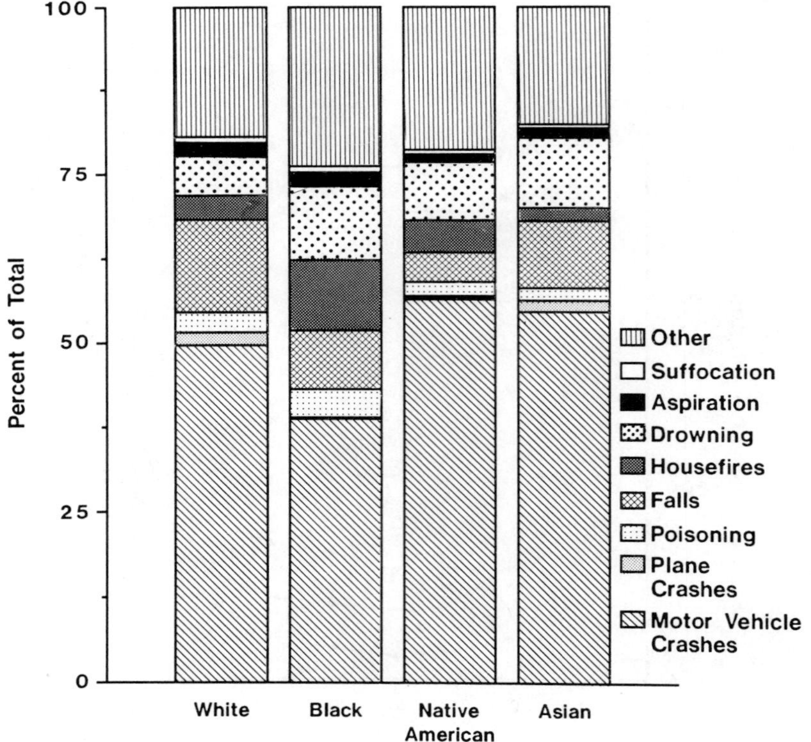

Figure 4-8. Percent of Unintentional Injury Deaths by Race and Cause, 1977-1979

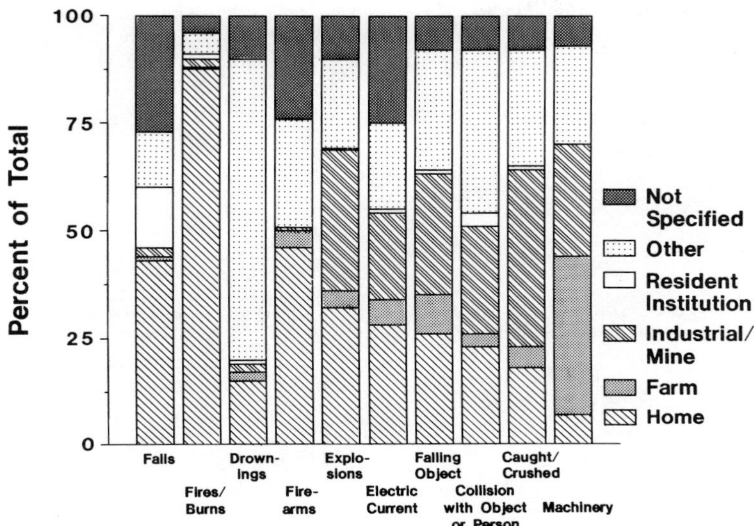

Figure 4-9. Percent of Unintentional Injury Deaths by Place and Cause, 1979

include those related to excessive cold, fires, firearms, aspiration of nonfood objects, and machinery or falling objects. The pattern of death rates from natural disasters may be due in part to the greater protection against tornados that is generally offered by housing in high-income areas, and the fact that floodplains are often low-income areas. Deaths from airplane crashes increase with per capita income (see also Chapter 8). Deaths from falls do not show a strong relationship with income.

Urban/Rural and Geographic Differences

For most unintentional injuries, death rates are highest in the more rural areas (figure 4-11). These high rates are in part related to certain causes of injury (for example, machinery and electricity) among people living or working on farms. Although farm workers constitute only 4 percent of U.S. workers,[3] 38 percent of all deaths identified as machinery-related occur on farms, as do 7 percent of all deaths from electricity and 10 percent from falling objects (figure 4-9).

There is pronounced geographic variation among unintentional injury deaths (figure 4-12). The high death rates in southern and mountain states for many causes reflect the fact that much of the population lives in rural areas, where injury death rates tend to be high. For falls, the

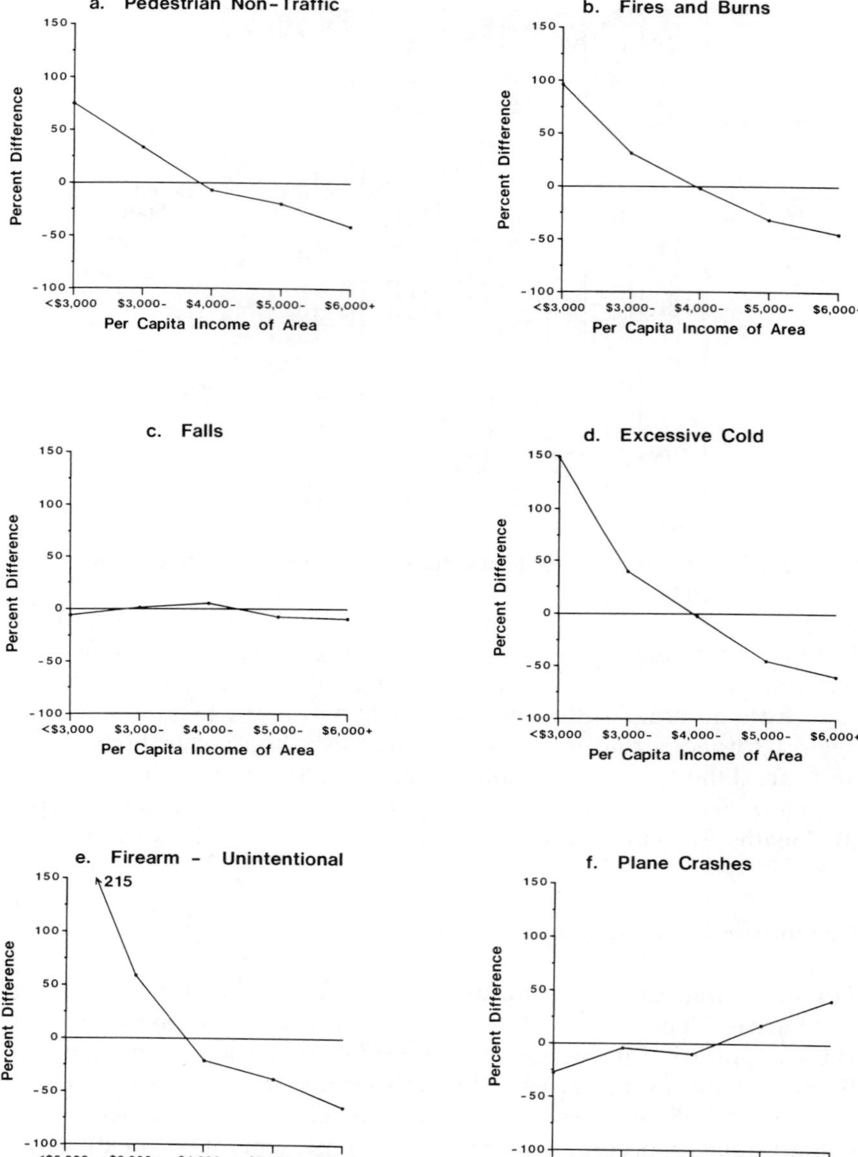

Figure 4-10. Percent Difference from the Average Death Rates from Unintentional Injury by Per Capita Income of Area of Residence and Cause, 1977-1979

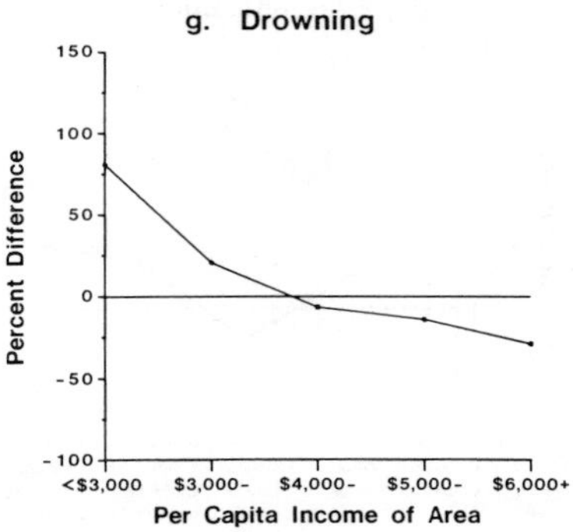

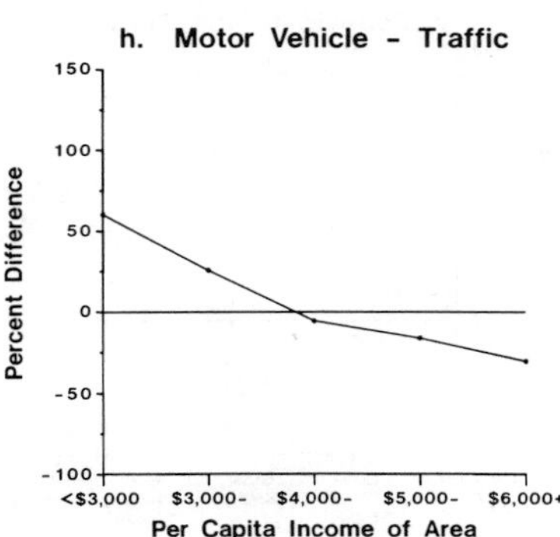

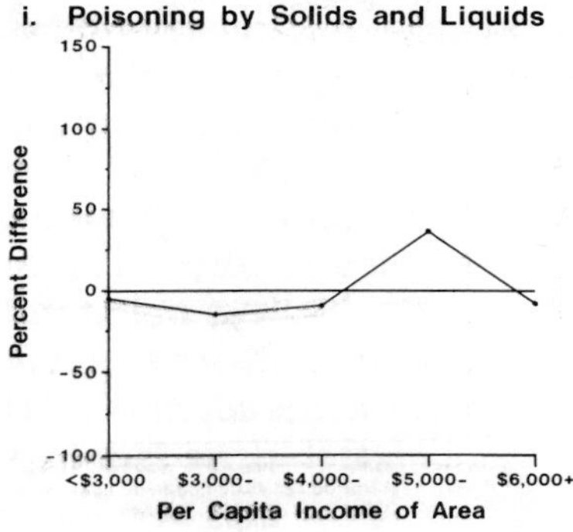

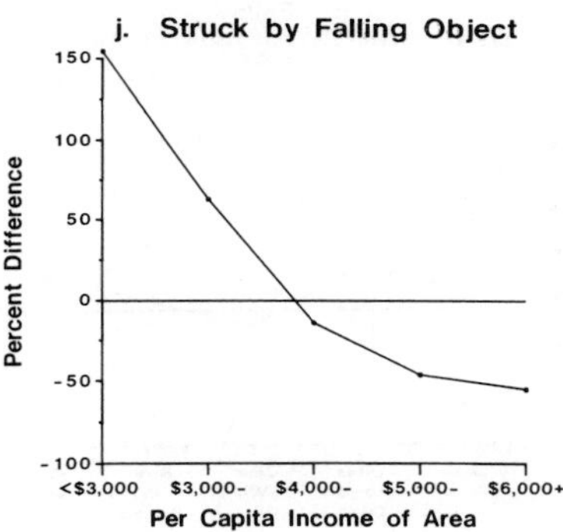

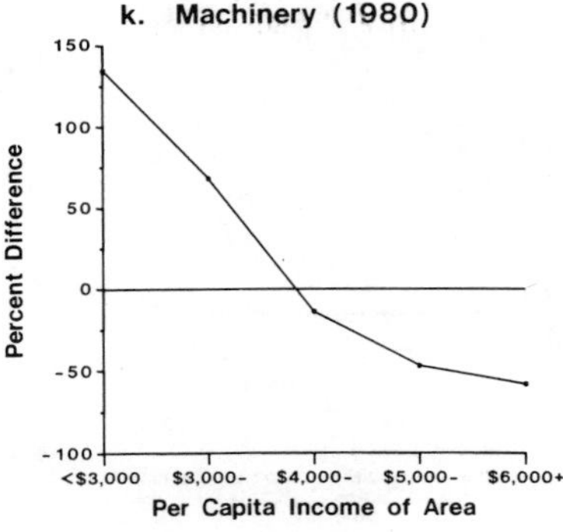

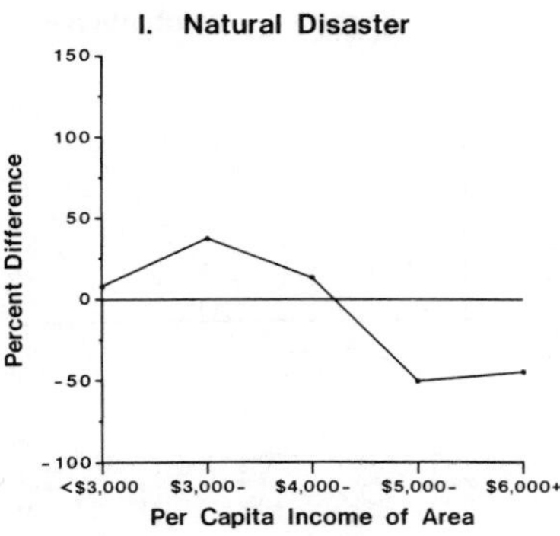

Figure 4-10 *(continued)*

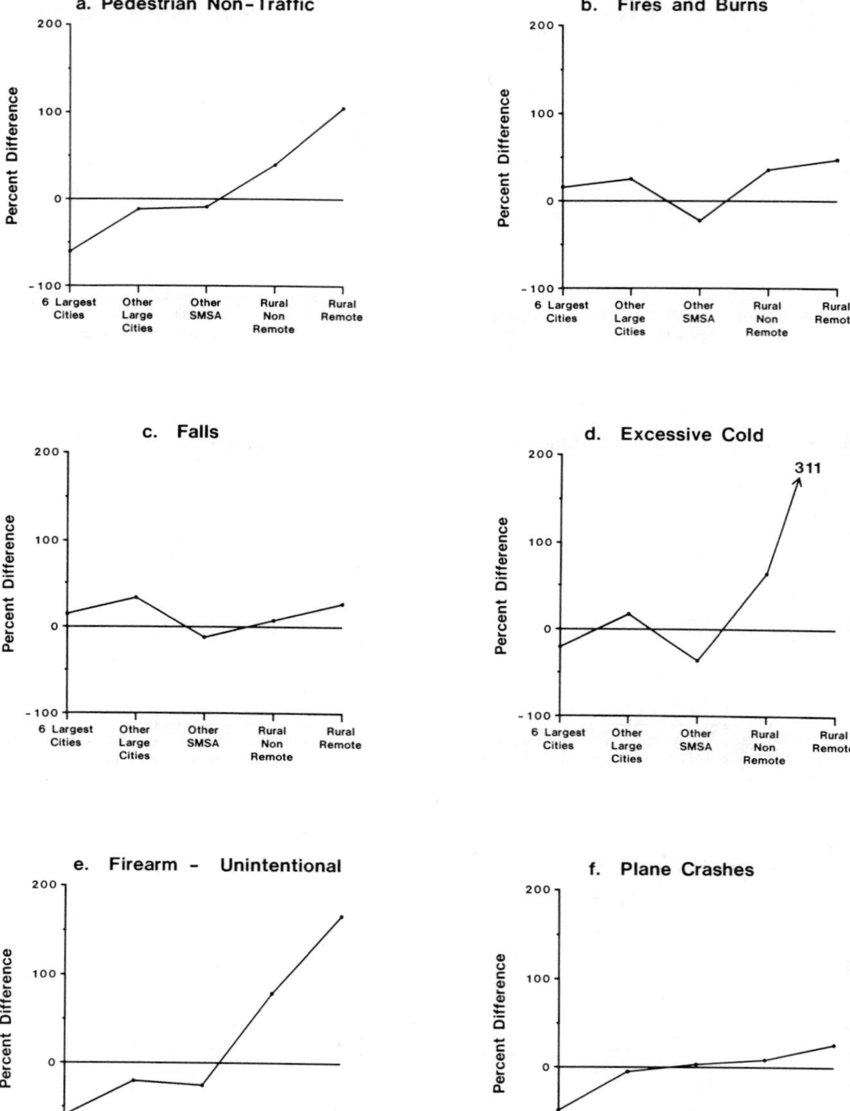

Figure 4-11. Percent Difference from the Average Death Rates from Unintentional Injury by Place of Residence and Cause, 1977-1979

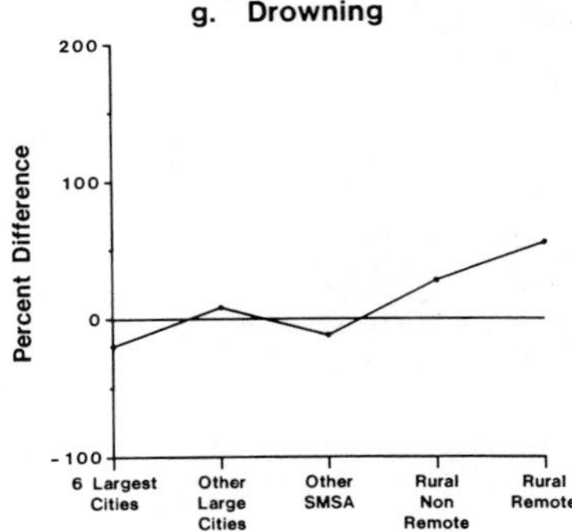

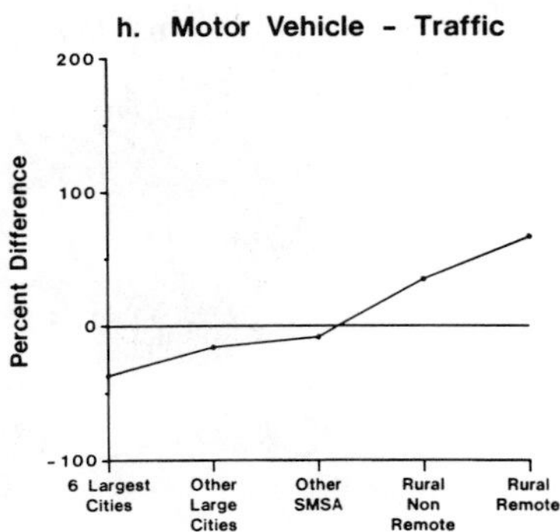

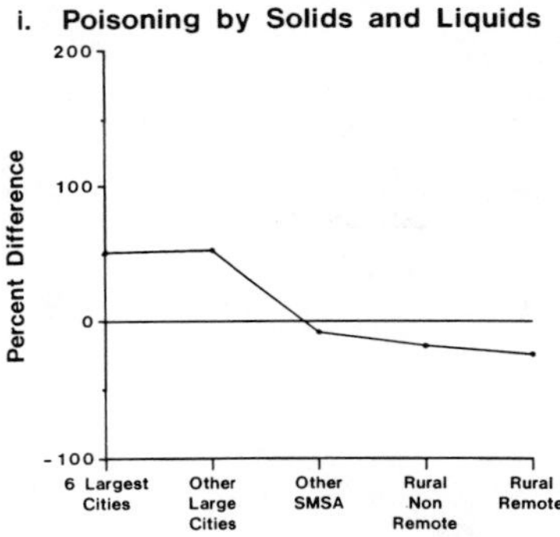

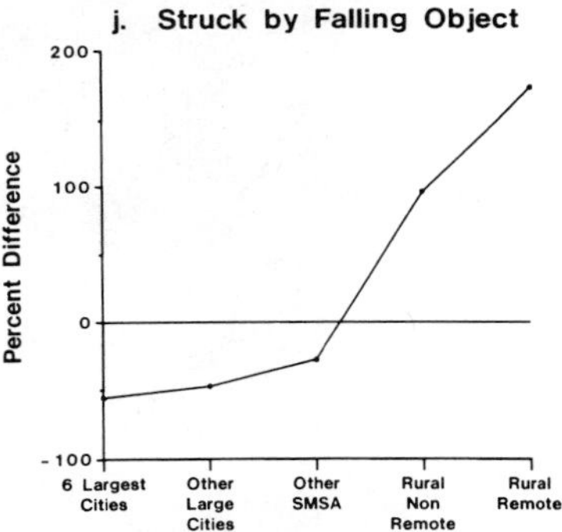

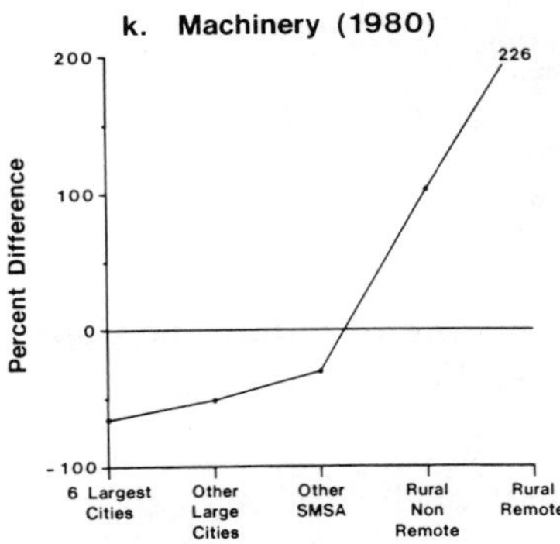

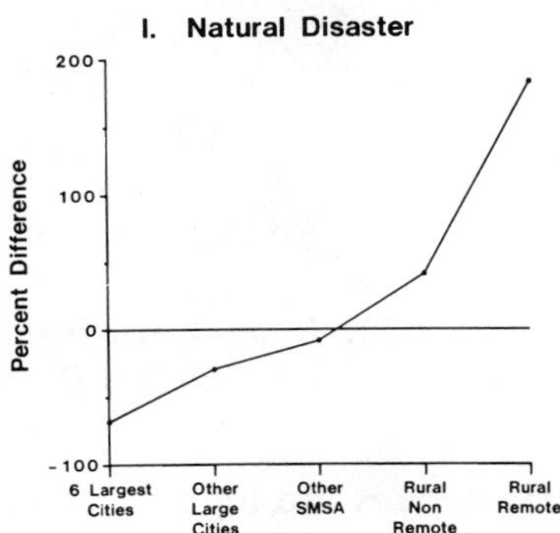

Figure 4-11 *(continued)*

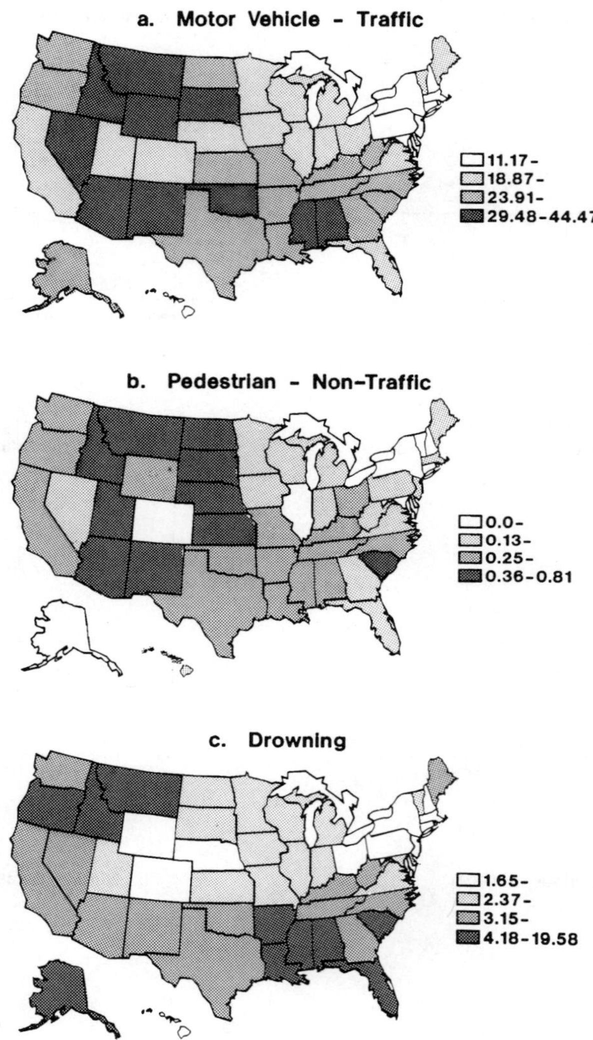

Figure 4-12. Death Rates from Unintentional Injury by State and Cause, Per 100,000 Population, 1977-1979

death rates are highest in the northern half of the country, an unexplained pattern that persists when death rates are age-adjusted. As in the case of urban/rural differences, these dramatic regional variations illustrate the importance of the environment as a determinant of injury death rates.

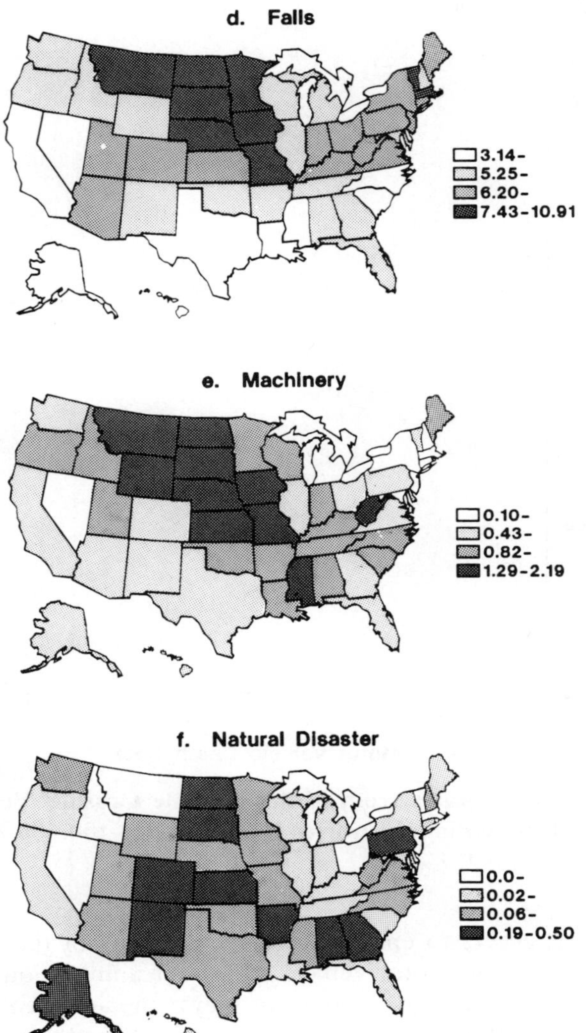

Figure 4–12 *(continued)*

There is a generally unrecognized correlation between state death rates from motor vehicle injuries and those from other unintentional injuries (figure 4-13). This close correlation suggests common factors in initiating circumstances (for example, high alcoholism rates would influence the incidence of most categories of injuries) and in other

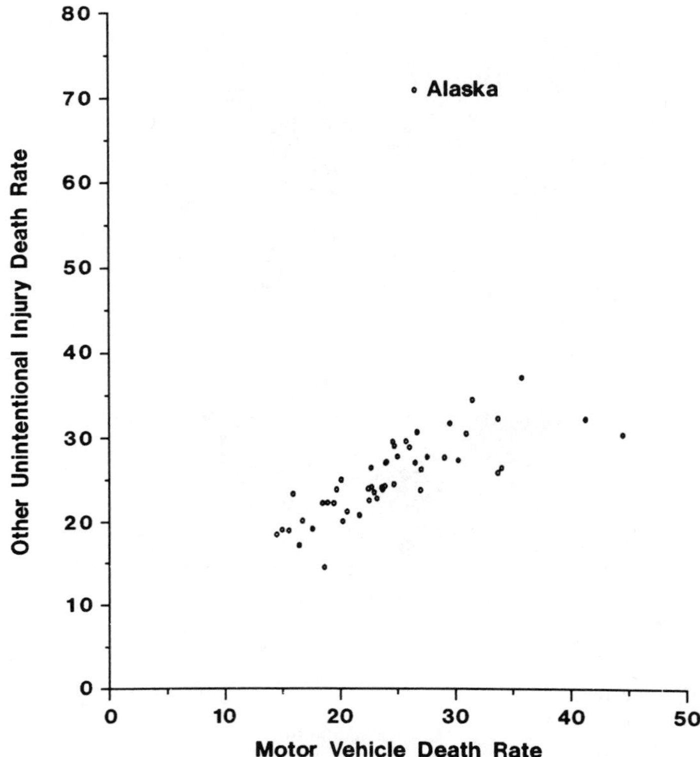

Figure 4-13. Death Rates from Motor Vehicle Crashes Versus Other Unintentional Injuries by State, Per 100,000 Population, 1977-1979

factors such as access to emergency care. In many of the states with high death rates from motor vehicle and other unintentional injuries, much of the population lives far from major medical centers; this is especially true in Alaska, which has the highest death rate from unintentional injuries. If the rates shown in figure 4-13 were for travel and nontravel injury deaths, Alaska would fall much closer to the line for other states, since a substantial portion of the injury deaths in that state result from airplane crashes and water transport.

Temporal Variation

Almost all causes of death from unintentional injury have weekend peaks, generally coinciding with increased social and recreational ac-

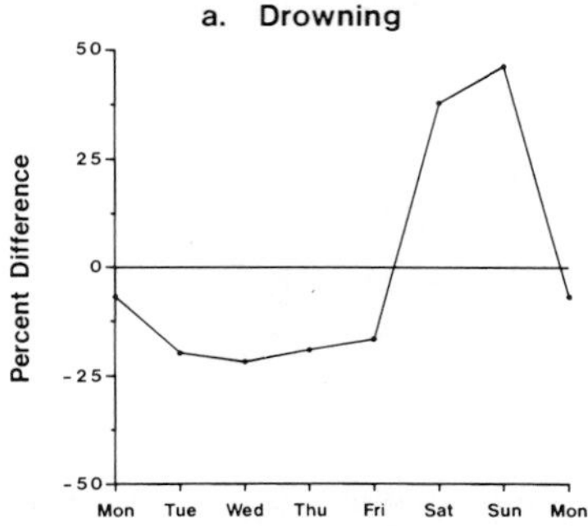

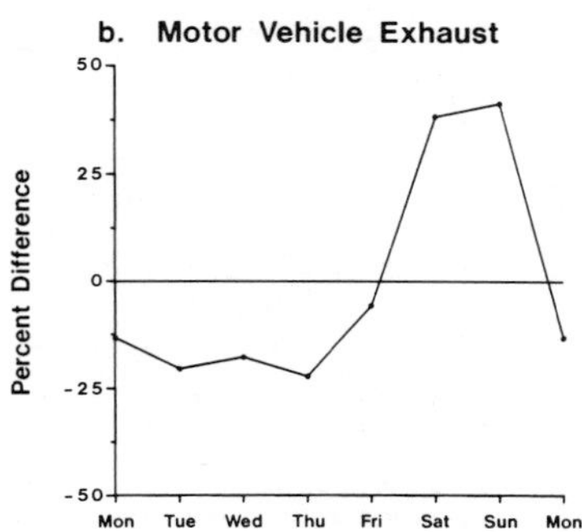

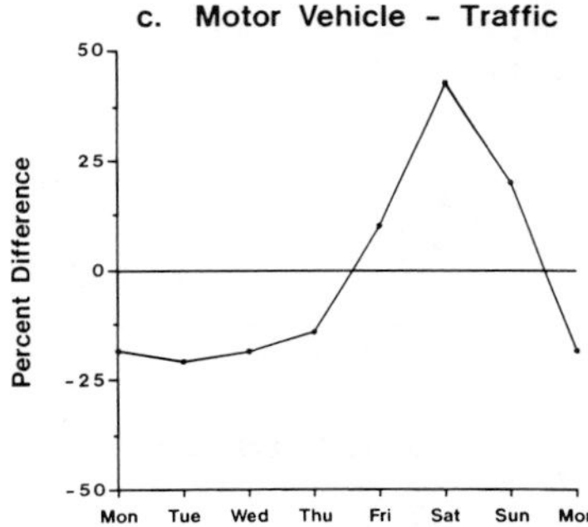

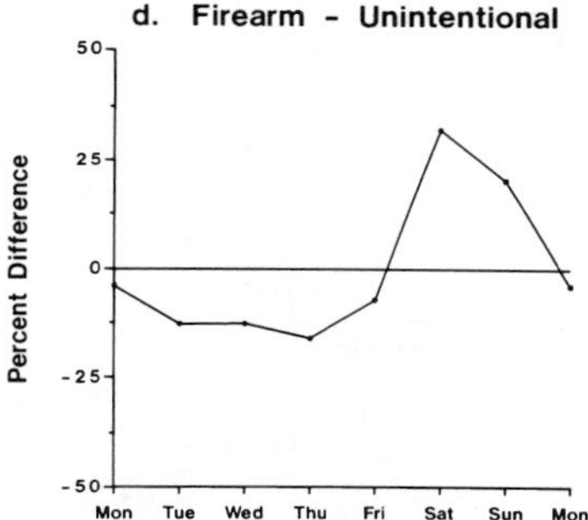

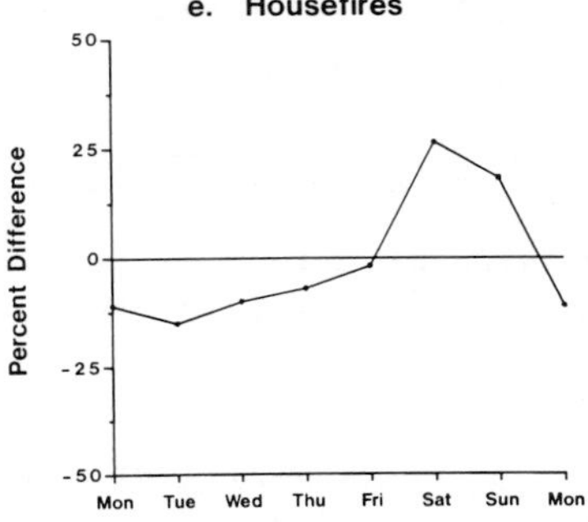

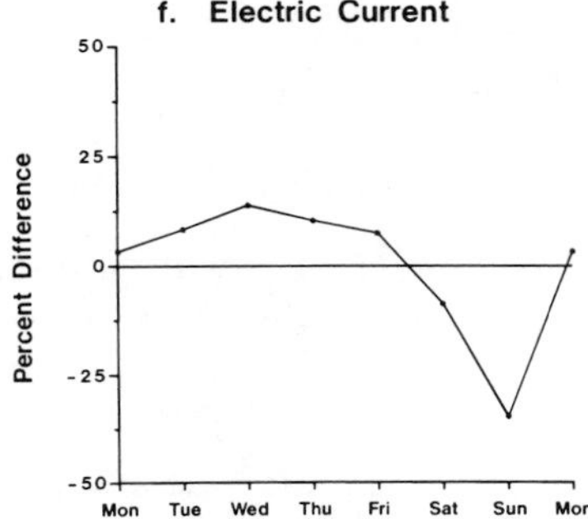

Figure 4-14. Percent Difference from the Average Number of Unintentional Injury Deaths by Day of Week and Cause, 1977-1979

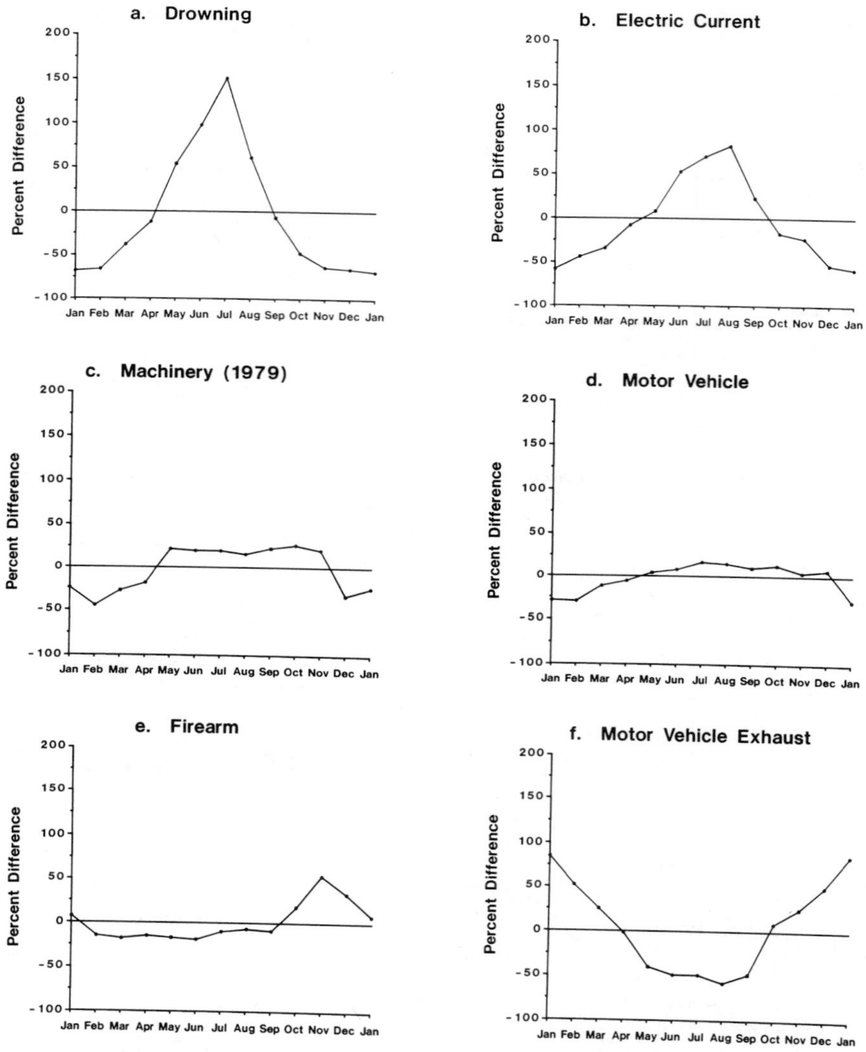
a. Drowning
b. Electric Current
c. Machinery (1979)
d. Motor Vehicle
e. Firearm
f. Motor Vehicle Exhaust
Percent Difference
200
150
100
50
0
-50
-100
Jan Feb Mar Apr May Jun Jul Aug Sep Oct Nov Dec Jan

Figure 4-15. Percent Difference from the Average Number of Unintentional Injury Deaths by Month and Cause, 1977-1979

tivity and greater alcohol use (figure 4-14). An exception is death from electric current, which occurs least commonly on Sundays, presumably because of the occupational nature of many electrocutions. The data analyzed are based on date of death rather than date of injury; con-

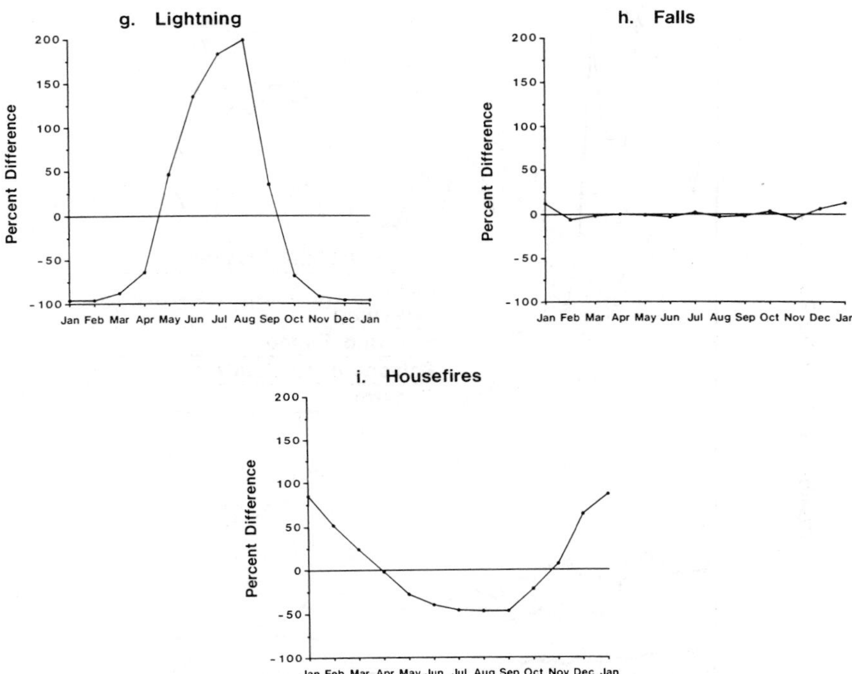

Figure 4-15 ***(continued)***

sequently, they may obscure temporal differences in the occurrence of injuries that usually are not rapidly fatal (e.g., falls and clothing ignition (not shown)).

The death rate from all unintentional injuries is slightly higher in the summer (figure 3-16). Ten percent of the deaths occur in July, compared to 7 percent in February. The summer excess is especially prominent in drownings and deaths from lightning or electric current (figure 4-15). In addition, motorcyclist and bicyclist deaths, discussed in Chapters 19 and 20, have very pronounced summer peaks. Deaths from housefires and unintentional poisoning by motor vehicle exhaust peak in wintertime. Most other types of unintentional poisonings show little monthly variation. Deaths from fatal falls are slightly more common in December and January; the slight wintertime excess, which may be due partly to icy conditions, might be more marked except for the long periods that often elapse between fall injury and death.

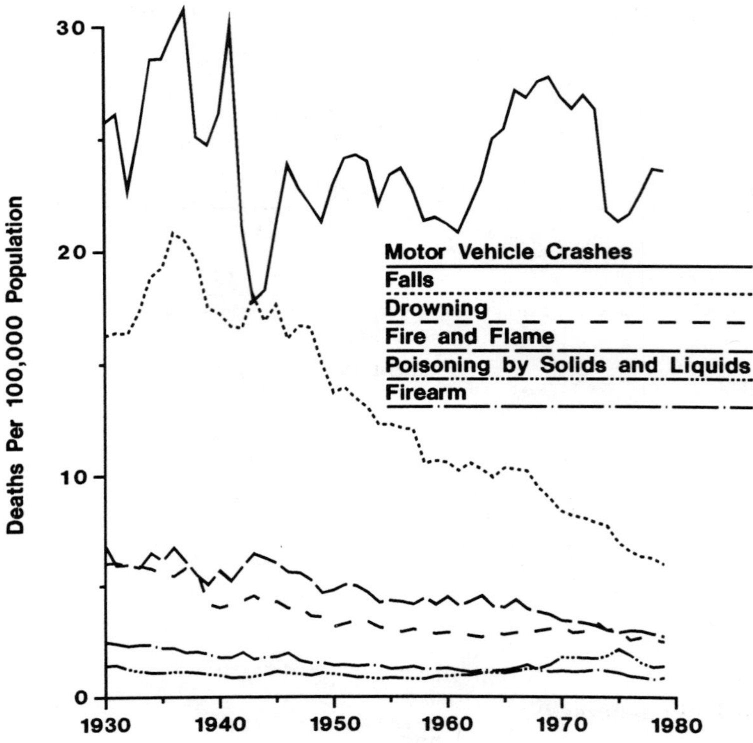

Figure 4-16. Death Rates from Unintentional Injury by Year and Cause, 1930-1979

Historical Trends

From 1930 to 1980, the overall death rate from unintentional injuries declined by almost 60 percent, from 113 to 47 per 100,000 population. This decline, however, has been far from uniform (figure 4-16, table 4-2). The rates for deaths related to motor vehicles and poisoning have changed relatively little. The housefire death rate has increased somewhat despite the fact that exposure, in terms of time spent in houses, is not likely to have increased.

The greatest *absolute* drop occurred in the death rate from falls. The greatest *proportional* decreases have occurred in deaths related to nonfarm machinery, lightning, and burns other than housefires (table 4-2). For all of these, the rates in 1980 were one-fifth or less of the 1930 rates. Deaths attributed to suffocation and aspiration have also decreased dramatically, but this is largely an artifact caused by changes

Table 4–2
Percent Change in Unintentional Injury Death Rates from 1930 to 1980, by Cause

Cause	Death Rate per 100,000 Population 1930	1980	Percent Change
Farm machinery	0.25	0.36	+44%
Aircraft	0.48	0.66	+38%
Housefires and other conflagrations	1.62	2.14	+32%
Motor vehicle occupants	15.44	16.39	+6%
Poisoning by solids and liquids	1.44	1.36	−6%
Electric current	0.80	0.48	−40%
Drowning, excluding water transport	6.05	2.66	−56%
Pedestrians	9.99	4.23	−58%
Falls	16.27	5.85	−64%
Firearms	2.53	0.86	−66%
Poisoning by gases and vapors*	1.98	0.55	−72%
Non-farm machinery	1.40	0.29	−79%
Lightning	0.29	0.04	−86%
Other burns	5.30	0.51	−86%
All unintentional injuries	112.89	46.53	−59%

Sources: National Center for Health Statistics, unpublished data for 1980, and Bureau of the Census, Mortality Statistics for 1930.

*Poisoning by gases and vapors decreased mainly because of a 96% decrease in the death rate between 1947 and 1980 from utility gas piped to homes; data prior to 1947 not available for utility gas.

in classification of deaths from sudden infant death syndrome (SIDS or "crib death"), many of which were formerly attributed to suffocation or aspiration of food (see Chapter 14).

In recent decades, reductions in the unintentional injury death rate have been largely due to reductions in death rates among the middle-aged and elderly (figure 4-17). Unlike figure 4-17, which shows age-specific death rates during two years, figure 4-18 shows percent changes in age-specific death rates calculated from trendlines fitted to the data for the 12 years, 1968-1979. For all ages combined, the general trend was downward, with a 23 percent decline in the death rate for all unintentional injuries. There was about a 40 percent decrease in the unintentional injury death rate for ages 65 and older, compared to a decrease of only 8 percent in the death rate for ages 15-19. Figure 4-18 shows that the decline in rates among the elderly was greatest for females; much of this decrease was associated with reduced deaths from falls. For ages 15-24, rates declined much less for females than for males; therefore, the sex difference for these ages has decreased.

Since injury deaths from late complications occur more often among older people, the greater decrease in death rates for the oldest groups may reflect improvement in the ability of the medical care system to prevent complications or reduce their effects.

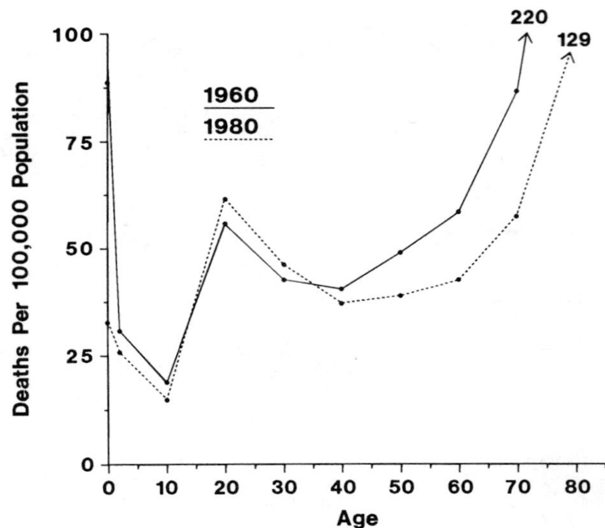

Figure 4-17. Death Rates from Unintentional Injury by Age, 1960 and 1980

Notes

1. Baker, S.P. "Determinants of Injury and Opportunities for Intervention." *American Journal of Epidemiology* 101 (1975): 98-102.

2. Baker, S.P., J.S. Samkoff, R.S. Fisher, and C.B. Van Buren. "Fatal Occupational Injuries." *Journal of the American Medical Association* 248 (1982): 692-697.

3. Bureau of the Census. "Farm Population of the United States: 1979." *Current Population Reports — Farm Population* 53 (1980): 8.

4. Haddon, W., Jr., P. Valien, J.R. McCarroll, and C.J. Umberger. "A Controlled Investigation of the Characteristics of Adult Pedestrians Fatally Injured by Motor Vehicles in Manhattan." *Journal of Chronic Diseases* 14 (1961): 655-678.

5. Hogue, C.C. "Injury in Late Life: Part I. Epidemiology." *Journal of the American Geriatrics Society* 30 (1982): 183-90.

6. Rivara, F.P. "Epidemiology of Childhood Injuries." In *Preventing Childhood Injuries, Report of the Twelfth Ross Roundtable on Critical Approaches to Common Pediatric Problems*, edited by A.B. Bergman. Columbus, OH: Ross Laboratories, 1982.

7. Robertson, L.S., and J.P. Keeve. "Worker Injuries: The Effects of Workers' Compensation and OSHA Inspections." *Journal of Health Politics, Policy and Law* 8 (Fall 1983): 581-597.

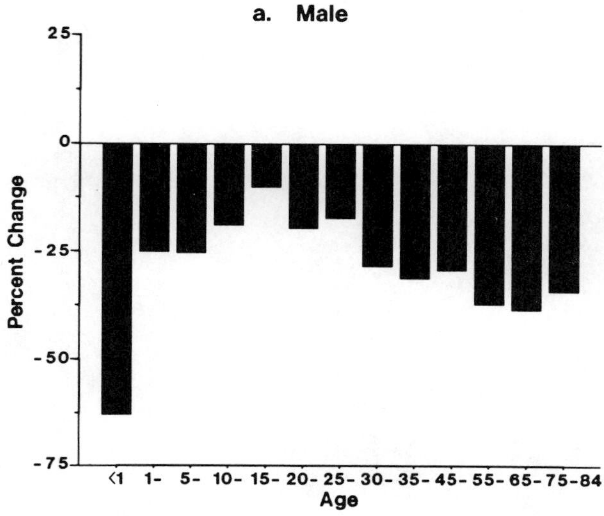

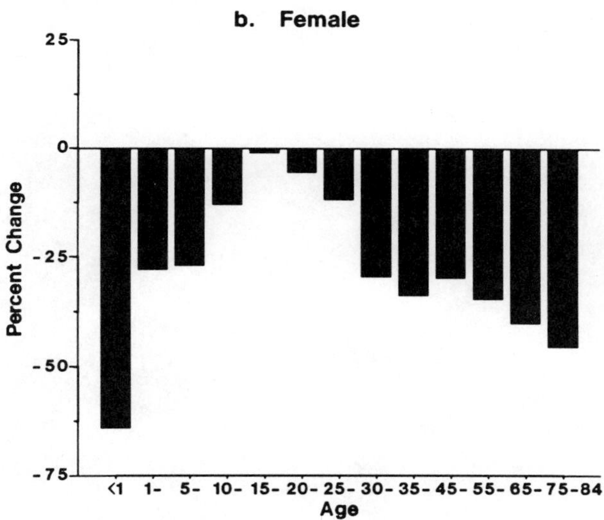

Figure 4-18. Percent Change in Death Rates from Unintentional Injury by Age and Sex, Based on 1968-1979 Trend

5 Suicide

Approximately 27,000 deaths in 1980 were classified as suicide, making this the tenth leading cause of death in the United States. For ages 15-34, suicide is the third leading cause, surpassed only by unintentional injury and homicide. Among white males, suicide is the seventh leading cause of death.

More than half of all suicidal deaths (57 percent) are caused by firearms. The next most frequent causes are hanging (14 percent), poisoning by ingestion of solids or liquids (11 percent), and carbon monoxide poisoning with motor vehicle exhaust (7 percent). Other means include jumping from high places (3 percent), drowning (2 percent), and cutting with a sharp instrument (1 percent).

Studies of nonfatal injuries that are deliberately self-inflicted (parasuicide) indicate that drug ingestion is the most common method, accounting for at least 70 percent of such cases. Although cutting with a sharp instrument accounts for only 1 percent of all suicides, wrist cutting is the second most common method of attempting suicide, accounting for about 15 percent of parasuicides.[5,6] Firearm injuries are relatively uncommon among parasuicides because of the high case-fatality rate from such injuries.

Age and Sex

Suicide is rare prior to age 15. Fewer than 1 percent of all suicides involve people under 15 years old. For males, the suicide rate increases steadily from age 10 to 24, declines until about age 34, and then begins to increase again (figure 3-3). The highest suicide rates are among elderly males. The rate for females increases until age 45-54 and then declines. Overall, the female suicide rate is one-third of the male rate. For both sexes combined, the highest incidence of parasuicide is at ages 20-24.[5]

Males and females differ substantially in their methods of committing suicide at various ages (figure 5-1). Firearms are used in 64 percent of male suicides but only 37 percent of female suicides. Firearms are the most common method of committing suicide for most age and sex groups. Among females ages 65 and older, poisoning is the predominant

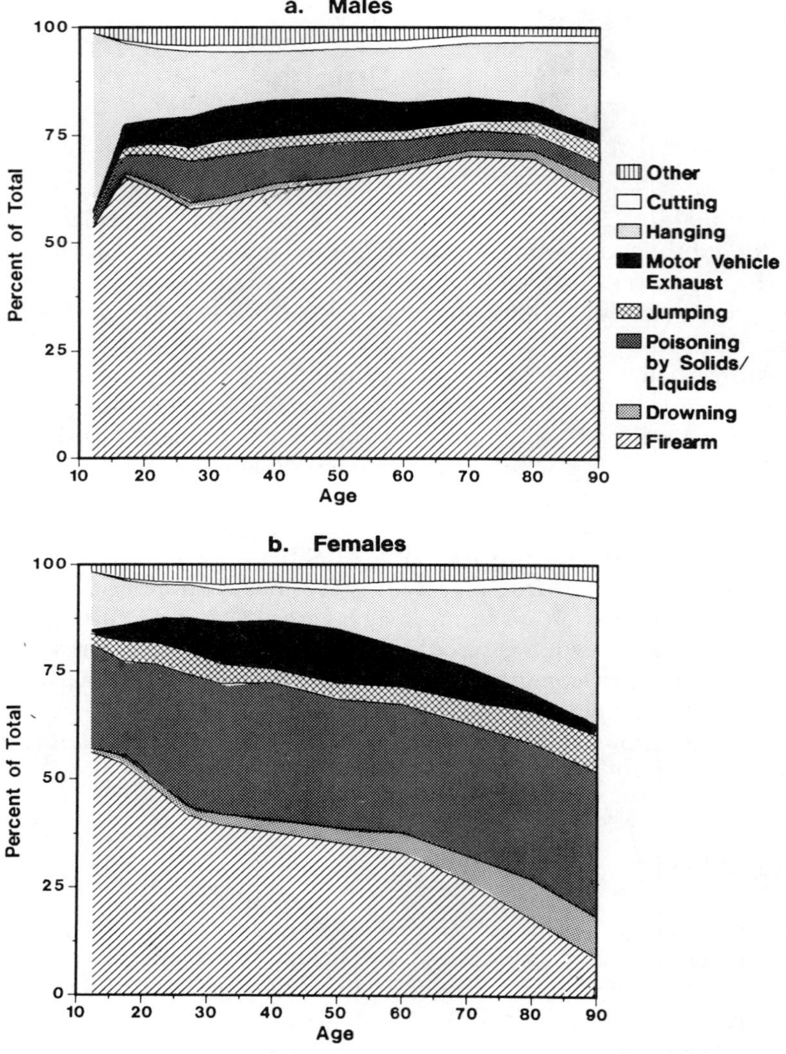

Figure 5-1. Percent of Suicides by Age, Sex, and Method, 1977-1979

means. Hanging is especially common in the youngest and oldest age groups. Among males age 10-14, 48 percent of all suicides are by hanging.

The age- and sex-specific mortality pattern for all methods of suicide combined reflects the pattern for firearms (figure 5-2a), because those are used in the majority of suicides. The patterns for hanging, jumping,

a. Firearm

Deaths Per 100,000 Population

Age

b. Hanging

Deaths Per 100,000 Population

Male

Female

Age

c. Jumping

Deaths Per 100,000 Population

Age

d. Cutting

Deaths Per 100,000 Population

Age

e. Poisoning, Solids and Liquids

Deaths Per 100,000 Population

Age

f. Drowning

Deaths Per 100,000 Population

Age

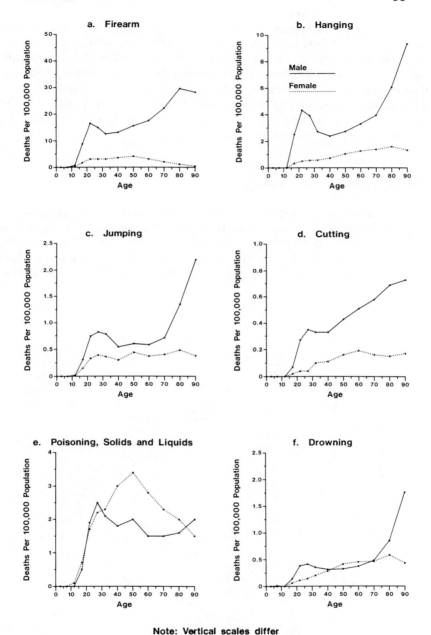

Note: Vertical scales differ

Figure 5-2. Death Rates from Suicide by Age, Sex, and Method, 1977-1979

and drowning are roughly similar (figures 5-2b, 5-2c, and 5-2f). Suicide by drowning exhibits the smallest difference by sex. Males and females have similar death rates for suicidal poisoning by solids and liquids until age 30, after which the death rate is substantially higher among females. Distinctive peaks in female death rates occur among women in their early forties for poisoning by solids and liquids, late forties for virtually all other categories of suicide, and again at ages 75-84 for suicide by firearms, hanging, drowning, and barbiturates.

Race and Per Capita Income

Suicide rates are highest among whites and Native Americans (14 and 13 per 100,000 population, respectively) and relatively low among Asians and blacks (6 for both groups). The age-specific patterns for these four racial groups show major differences (figure 5-3). Native Americans exhibit the sharpest peak at age 20-24 and have the highest suicide

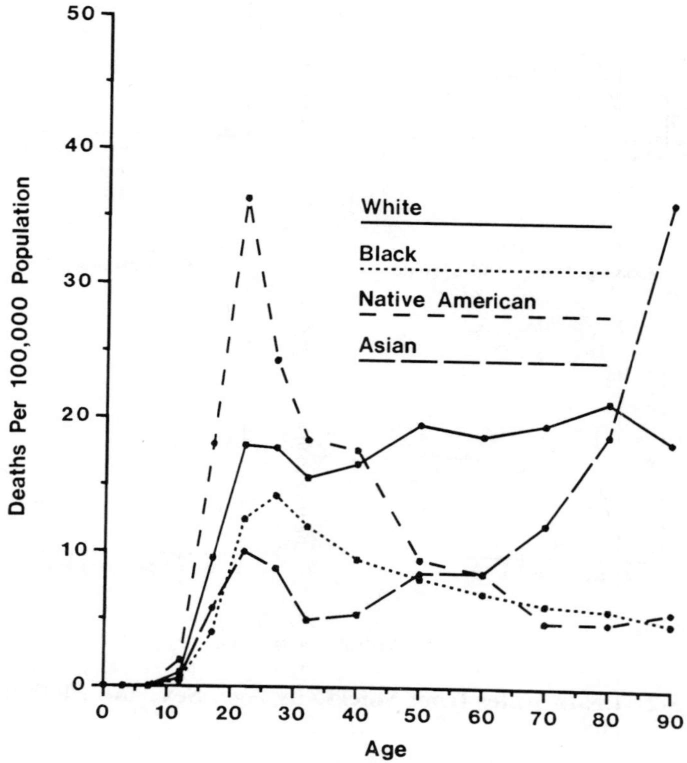

Figure 5-3. Death Rates from Suicide by Age and Race, 1977-1979

death rates up to age 44. Except for elderly Asians, whites have the highest rates after age 44.

The racial groups also differ in the methods employed to commit suicide (figure 5-4).[4] Firearms are used in only about one-fourth of suicides by Asians, compared to more than half of suicides by the other three groups. Hanging is the most common means among Asians, accounting for 35 percent of their suicides. It is the second most common means among blacks and Native Americans, accounting for about one-fifth of the suicides among the latter.[3]

After age 30, age- and sex-specific suicide rates show markedly different patterns for blacks and whites (figure 5-5). Among black males, the suicide rate declines after age 30. While the downward trend reverses at age 60, it does not show the dramatic rise that is apparent for white males. The rate for black females declines after age 30, while for white females it is highest at ages 45-54.

Overall suicide rates show little variation with per capita income of the area of residence (figure 3-9), but specific types of suicide show strong relationships with per capita income. Except for firearm suicides,

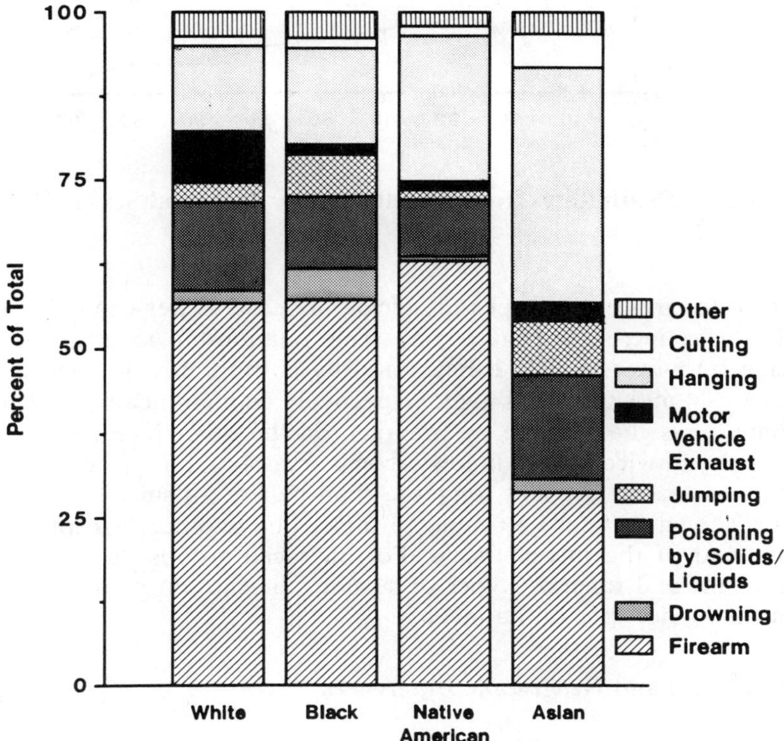

Figure 5-4. Percent of Suicides by Race and Method, 1977-1979

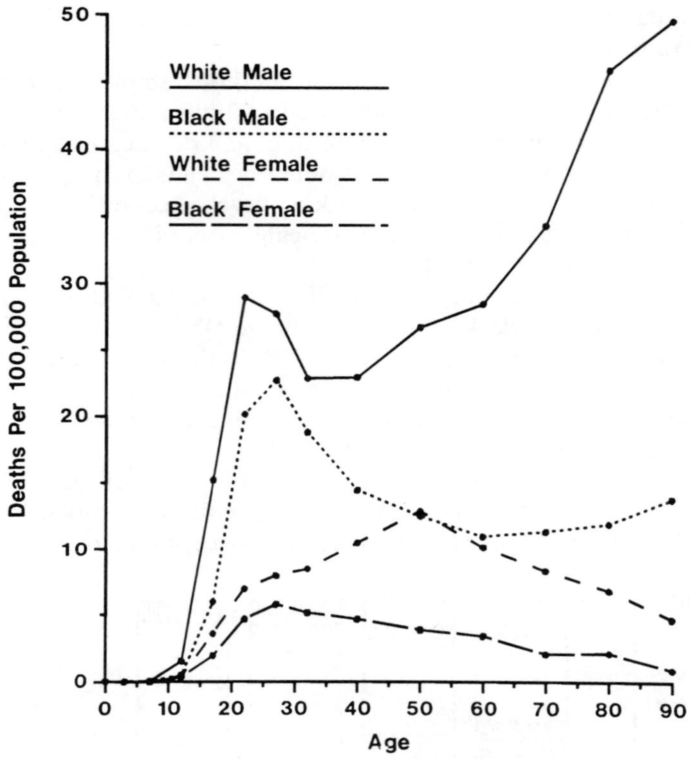

Figure 5-5. Death Rates from Suicide by Age, Race, and Sex, 1977-1979

death rates from most types of suicide increase as per capita income of the area increases (figure 5-6). This relationship is strongest for suicide by motor vehicle exhaust and by barbiturates, for which the rates are 11 and 8 times as high, respectively, in high-income as in low-income areas. For suicide by firearms, on the other hand, the death rate is about twice as high in low-income areas as in high-income areas. Because firearms account for more than half of all suicides, the two trends shown in figure 5-6 tend to offset one another, except at the upper end of the income scale. For all racial groups except Native Americans and for most types of suicide, the rate drops in the areas with the highest per capita income.

Urban/Rural and Geographic Differences

The suicide rate is highest in large cities for both blacks and whites (figure 5-7). Urban-rural patterns differ by type of suicide and to a

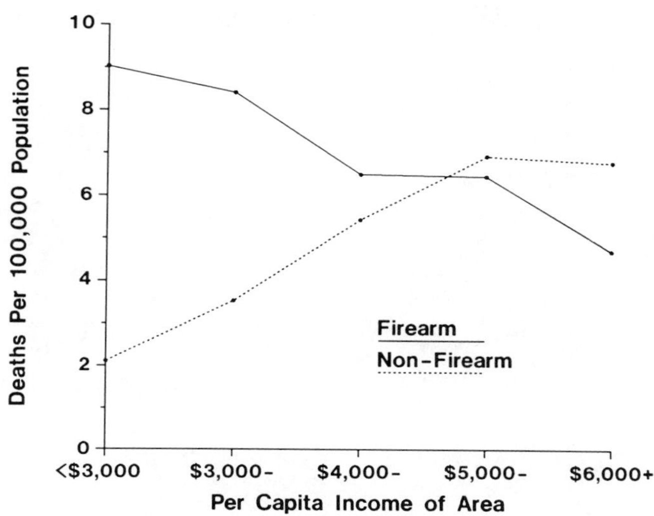

Figure 5-6. Death Rates from Firearm and Non-Firearm Suicide by Per Capita Income of Area of Residence, 1977-1979

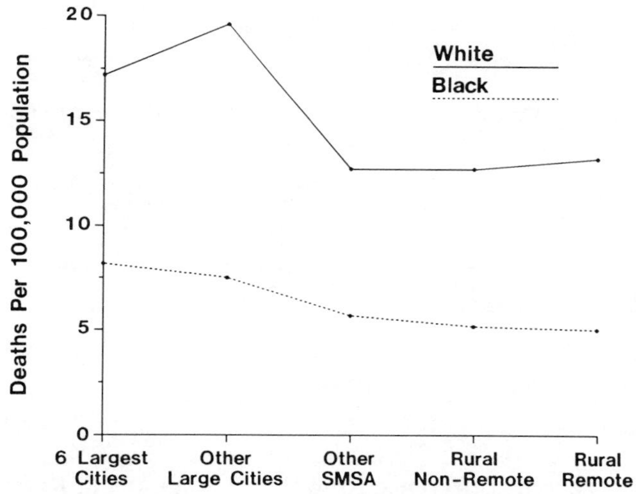

Figure 5-7. Death Rates from Suicide by Place of Residence and Race, 1977-1979

large extent reflect the availability of various methods (figure 5-8). Large cities, where tall buildings offer a ready means of committing suicide, have especially high rates of fatal jumps. Rates of suicidal poisoning by solids and liquids are also high in large cities, whereas

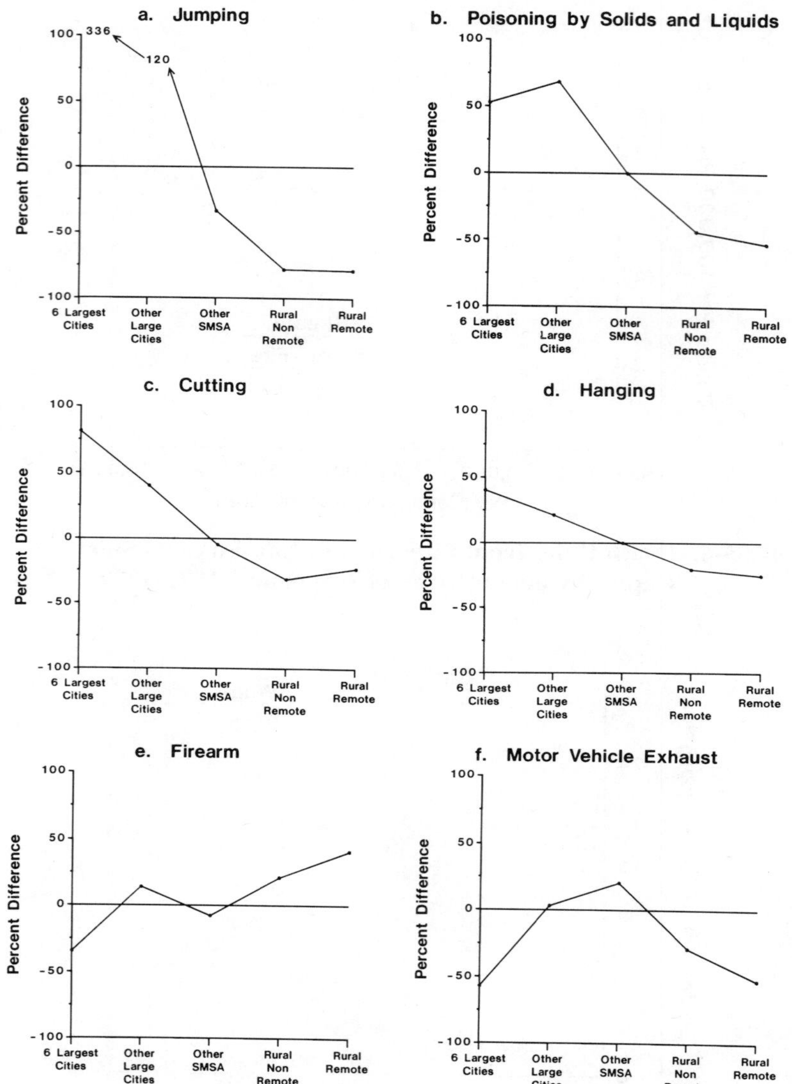

Figure 5-8. Percent Difference from the Average Death Rates from Suicide by Place of Residence and Method, 1977-1979

rates for firearm suicide are highest in rural areas, where gun ownership is most prevalent.[2] High rates of suicide by motor vehicle exhaust in areas of intermediate urbanization may reflect a greater prevalence of garages.

Suicide death rates range from a low of 8 per 100,000 population in New Jersey to a high of 22 in Nevada. Although rates for all types of suicide combined are generally highest in the western states, the geographic patterns differ depending on the method (figure 5-9). Rates

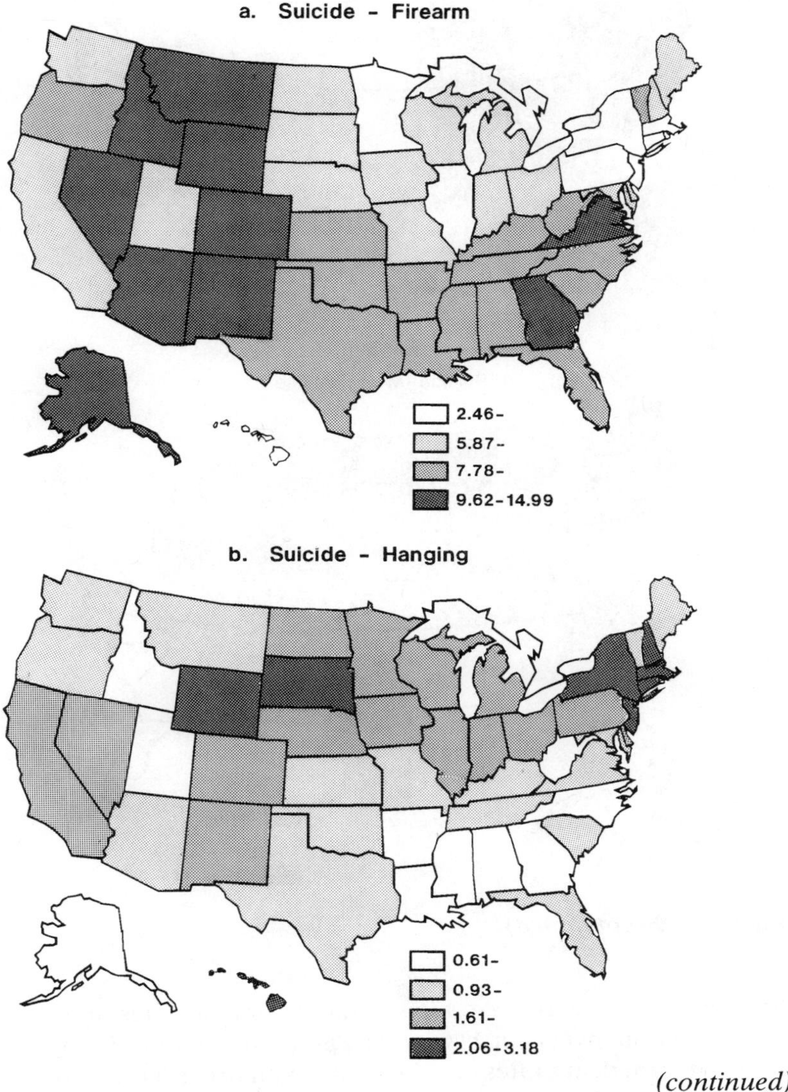

(continued)

Figure 5-9. Death Rates from Suicide by State and Method, Per 100,000 Population, 1977-1979

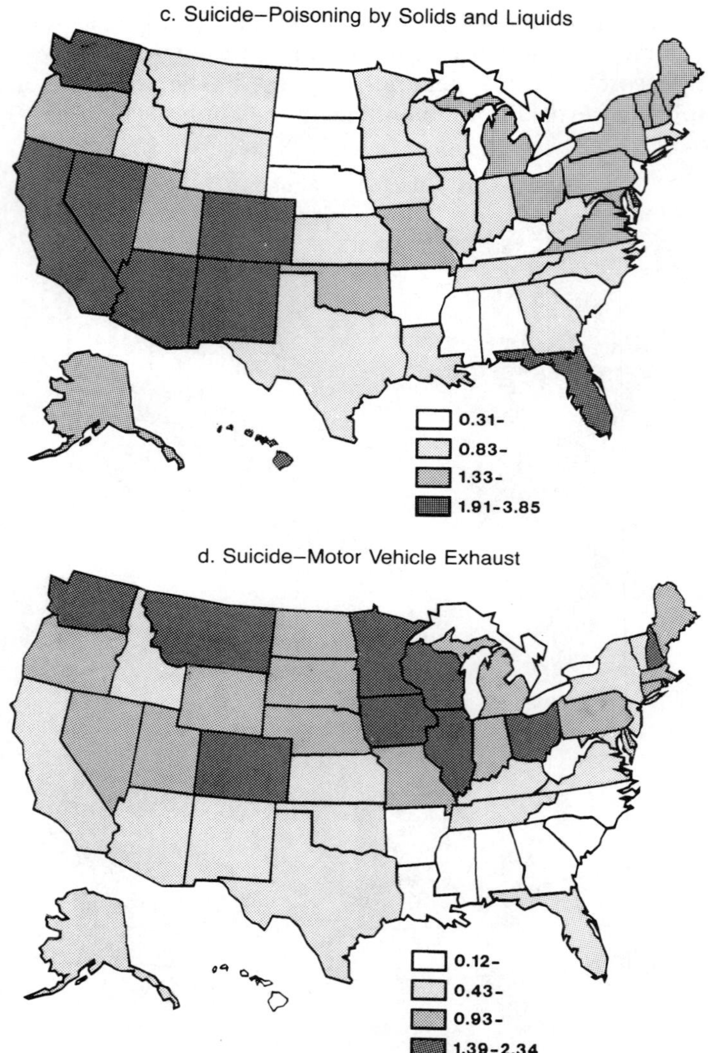

Figure 5–9 *(continued)*

for suicide by firearms are high in the mountain states and the South, where firearm ownership is generally greatest.[2] (Even within a southern state, firearm death rates are correlated with firearm ownership rates.[1]) The rate for suicide by hanging, the method most commonly used by the Asian group, is highest in Hawaii and the Northeast. Suicidal poisoning by solids and liquids is especially common in Florida and the West and Southwest, while the highest rates for poisoning by motor vehicle exhaust are in northern states, where garages may be more common. The geographic patterns for both of these categories of poisoning are roughly similar to the patterns for unintentional injury deaths from the same causes.

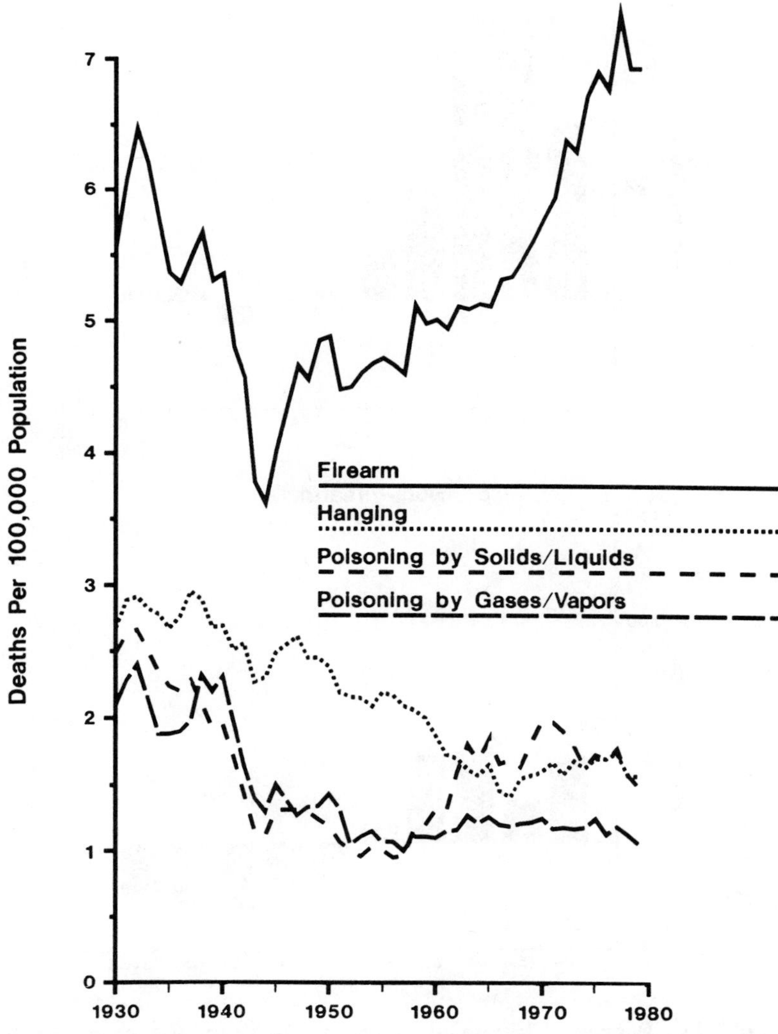

Figure 5-10. Death Rates from Suicide by Year and Method, 1930-1979

Temporal Variation

Suicides do not vary greatly by day of week, although more are recorded on Mondays than on any other day (figure 3-15). There is a slight peak

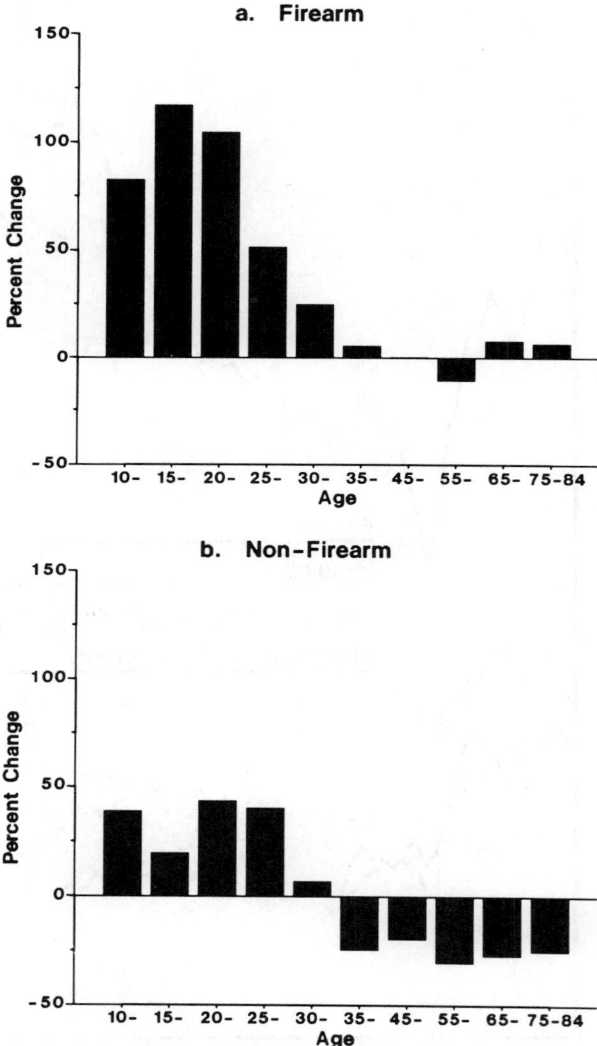

Figure 5-11. Percent Change in Death Rates from Firearm and Non-Firearm Suicide by Age, Based on 1968-1979 Trend

in the springtime and a December low in most years, but the seasonal fluctuations in suicides are much less marked than in unintentional injuries (figure 3-16).

Historical Trends

The overall suicide rate decreased from a high of 17 per 100,000 population in 1932 to about 10 in 1943-1944, then increased to 12 in 1980. Virtually all of the increase since 1963 has been in suicides by firearms (figure 5-10).

The general trend in the suicide death rate between 1968 and 1979 was upward, with an overall increase of about 14 percent. The rate for suicide by firearms increased by 30 percent, while suicide by all other means decreased by 2 percent. The largest increase was for ages 15-24, whose firearm suicide rate more than doubled (figure 5-11). For all ages and types of suicide combined, the trend in this period reflects a 20 percent increase in male rates and no change among females.

Notes

1. Alexander, G.R., R.M. Massey, T. Gibbs, and J. Altekruse. "Firearm-Related Fatalities: An Epidemiologic Assessment of Violent Death." *American Journal of Public Health*, in press.

2. Gallup, G.H. "Gun Registration." In *The Gallup Poll, Public Opinion 1972-1977, Volume One, 1972-1975*. Wilmington, DE: Scholarly Resources, Inc., March 28-31, 1975: 506-508.

3. Simpson, S.G., R. Reid, S.P. Baker, and S.P. Teret. "Injuries Among the Hopi Indians, A Population-Based Survey." *Journal of the American Medical Association* 249 (1983): 1873-1876.

4. Warshauer, M.E., and M. Monk. "Problems in Suicide Statistics for Whites and Blacks." *American Journal of Public Health* 68 (1978): 383-388.

5. Weissman, M.M. "The Epidemiology of Suicide Attempts, 1960 to 1971." *Archives of General Psychiatry* 30 (1974): 737-746.

6. Wexler, L., M.M. Weissman, and S.V. Kasl. "Suicide Attempts 1970-75: Updating a United States Study and Comparisons with International Trends." *British Journal of Psychiatry* 132 (1978): 180-185.

6 Homicide

The 24,000 homicide and legal intervention deaths in 1980 made this the eleventh leading cause of death for all ages combined. For ages 15-34, only unintentional injury surpassed homicide as a cause of death. Among blacks ages 20-34, homicide is the leading cause of death.

Firearms are used in two-thirds of all homicides. Other leading methods are cutting and stabbing with knives and other sharp instruments (18 percent) and strangulation (4 percent). The majority of homicides take place in the home and involve family members or other people who are known to the victim.[5]

Age and Sex

Homicide rates are highest for males ages 25-29 (figure 3-3). Among females, the death rates peak slightly earlier, at ages 20-24. Except when young children are killed, firearms are the most common means of homicide (figure 6-1). For young children, other assaults including

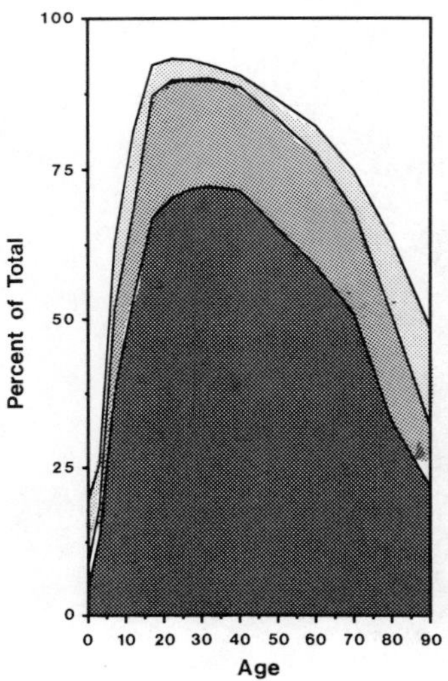

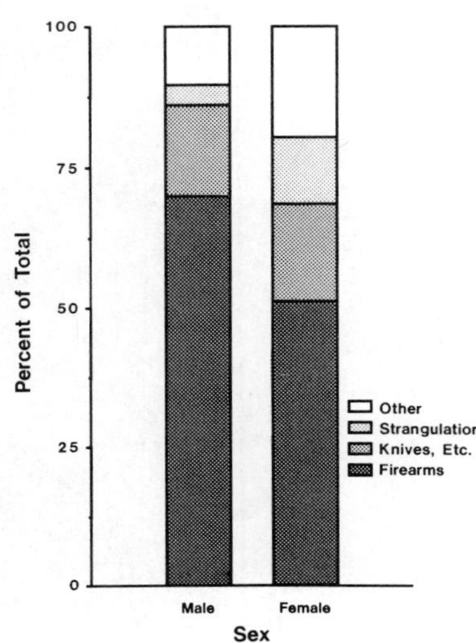

Figure 6-1. Percent of Homicides by Age and Method, and by Sex and Method, 1977-1979

beatings (with or without weapons) are the most common means of homicide.

Fatal assaults on children are usually inflicted by family members (figure 6-2).[4,7] Beginning at about age 15, deaths are more often the result of assault by nonfamily acquaintances. Assaults by strangers are most important among teenagers and the elderly, but they never comprise more than about one-fourth of all homicides. The higher proportion of stranger-committed homicides among people in their sixties or older is consistent with the larger proportion of homicides of older people committed in connection with robberies and other felonies.[4] For ages 15-59, homicides occur primarily in connection with arguments. Since this is the age group with the highest homicide rate, arguments are a precipitating factor in almost half of all homicides.[2]

Firearms are the most commonly used weapon in fatal assaults on both males and females. Cutting and stabbing account for almost one-fifth of homicides among both sexes (figure 6-1). Death by strangulation

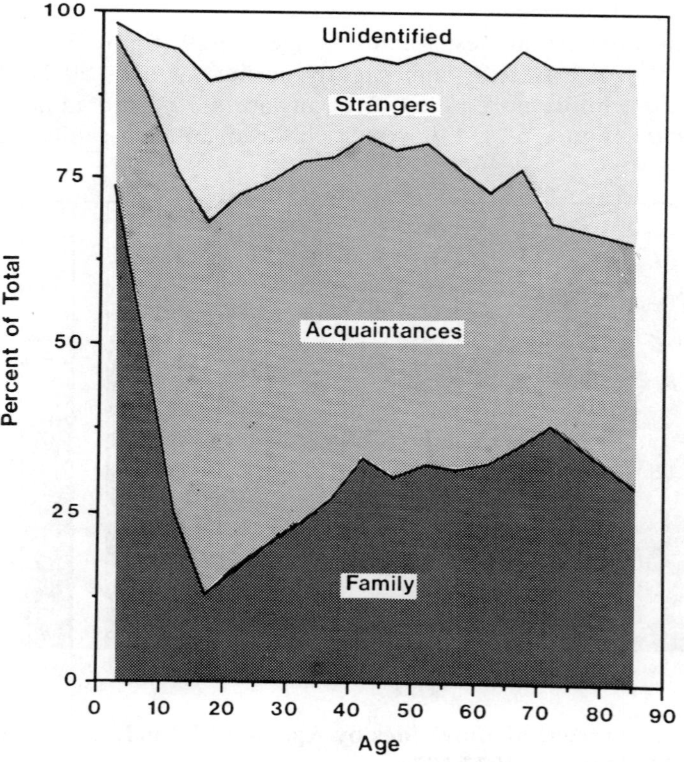

Figure 6-2. Percent of Homicides by Victim Age and Victim-Offender Relationship, FBI, 1981

causes 12 percent of homicides among females, but only 2 percent among males. Not only does strangulation account for a larger proportion of homicides in females, but the death *rate* is much higher than for males (figure 6-3). This particular sex difference is especially pronounced at ages 15-29 when strangulation often accompanies rape.[3]

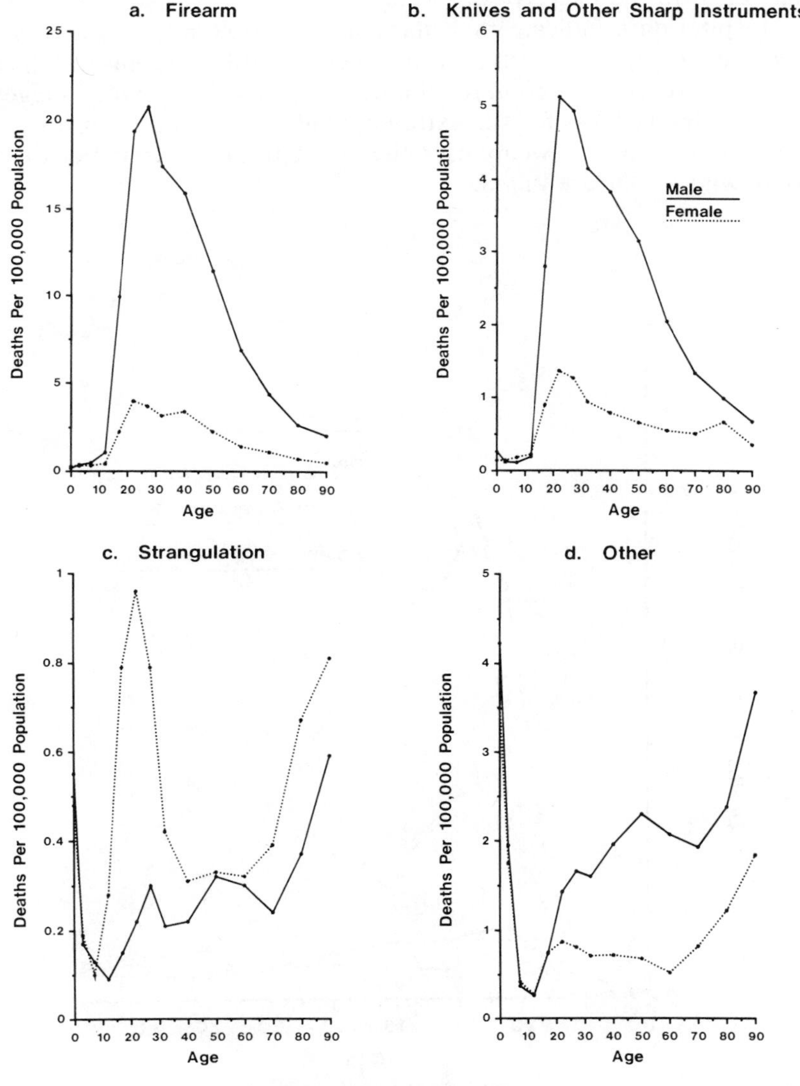

Figure 6-3. Death Rates from Homicide by Age, Sex, and Method, 1977-1979

The shape of the age- and sex-specific death rate curves for firearm homicides is virtually the same as for cutting and stabbing with knives and other sharp instruments, although the firearm rate is about four times as high. The resemblance in the shapes of these curves is closer than for other causes of injury death, suggesting important similarities between the circumstances involved and the populations at risk of being assaulted with the two types of weapons.

Hospital data indicate that many more people are assaulted with sharp instruments than with firearms. Yet the ratio of deaths to injuries is roughly five times as great for shootings.[8] The evidence thus suggests that the primary basis for the extremely high death rate from firearms is the lethality of the weapons rather than the characteristics of the people who kill or are killed.

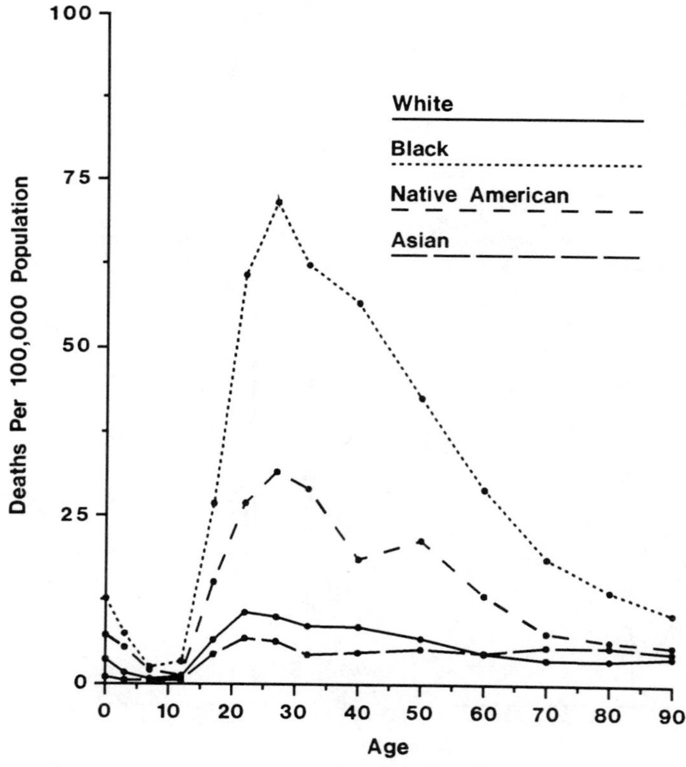

Figure 6-4. Death Rates from Homicide by Age and Race, 1977-1979

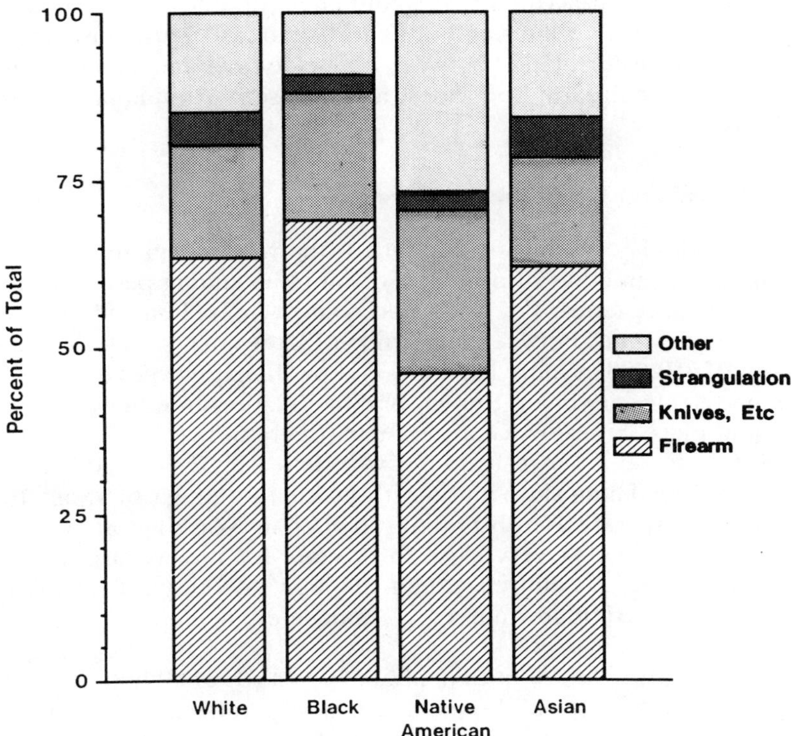

Figure 6-5. Percent of Homicides by Method and Race, 1977-1979

Race and Per Capita Income

Homicide rates are highest for blacks (34 per 100,000 population) and lowest for whites and Asians (6 and 4, respectively), with Native Americans in between (15). The age-specific rates for blacks and Native Americans have pronounced peaks at ages 25-29 (figure 6-4). The highest death rates among whites and Asians are at ages 20-24, but these peaks are less pronounced.

The method of injury is roughly similar among the four racial groups, except that for Native Americans cutting and stabbing cause a larger proportion of deaths, and firearms cause a smaller proportion, than for the other racial groups (figure 6-5). The preponderance of firearms among weapons used to kill Asians contrasts with the pattern seen for suicide by Asians, in which firearms are less commonly employed.

Homicide rates are more than twice as high in low-income areas as in high-income areas for all races combined (figure 3-9). This relationship is strongest for whites and in nonurban areas (figure 6-6). In general, the inverse correlation between homicide rates and income is most pronounced for firearm homicides, and is absent or minimal for other methods.

Urban/Rural and Geographic Differences

For all methods of homicide combined, the rate is four times as high among people in cities of a million or more as among people who do not live in large cities. For both blacks and whites, homicide rates do not differ very much between rural and SMSA residents excluding those in cities of 250,000 or more (figure 6-7). For all major types of homicide the highest rates are in large cities, and the relationships between death rates and place of residence are similar (figure 6-8).

Homicide rates range from a low of less than 2 per 100,000 population in New Hampshire and North Dakota to a high of about 16 in Louisiana. The rate is substantially higher in Washington, D.C. — about 27 per 100,000, very close to the rate for the six largest cities. Washington, D.C. is entirely urban. Its high rate may reflect the fact that a disproportionate number of homicides in metropolitan areas occur in inner cities.

Because firearms are used in about two-thirds of all homicides, the geographic pattern for all homicides generally reflects the geographic pattern for firearm homicides, with low rates in north central, northwest, and New England states and high rates in the South (figures 3-14c and 6-9a).

The geographic pattern for homicides not due to firearms differs from the pattern for firearm homicides in several important respects (figure 6-9b). In particular, New York and California have high rates of nonfirearm homicides — ranking second and third among all states, respectively — but their firearm homicide rates are not exceptionally high (seventeenth and twenty-first, respectively).

Another way of looking at the relationship of firearm to nonfirearm homicides is by mapping their ratios (figure 6-9c). Nationally, the ratio is almost 2:1. It is 3:1 or more in most southern states. In New England, on the other hand, the ratio is less than 1:1; that is, there are fewer homicides by firearms than by other means. These ratios reflect patterns of gun ownership, which is most common in the South and least common in the Northeast.[6]

Temporal Variation

Half of all homicides occur on Fridays, Saturdays, or Sundays, with the largest number (20 percent) occurring on Saturdays (figure 3-15).

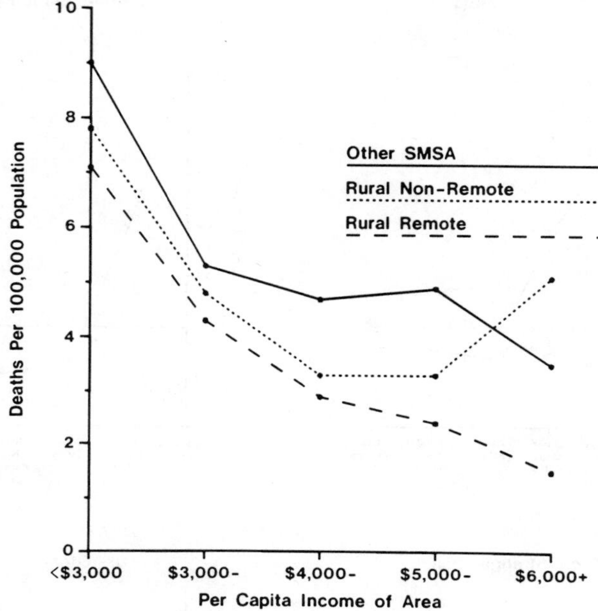

Figure 6-6. Death Rates from Homicide by Per Capita Income and Place of Residence for Whites, 1977-1979

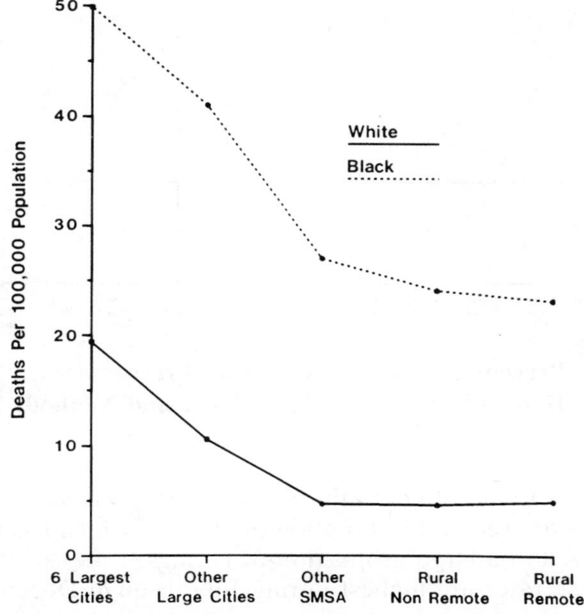

Figure 6-7. Death Rates from Homicide by Place of Residence and Race, 1977-1979

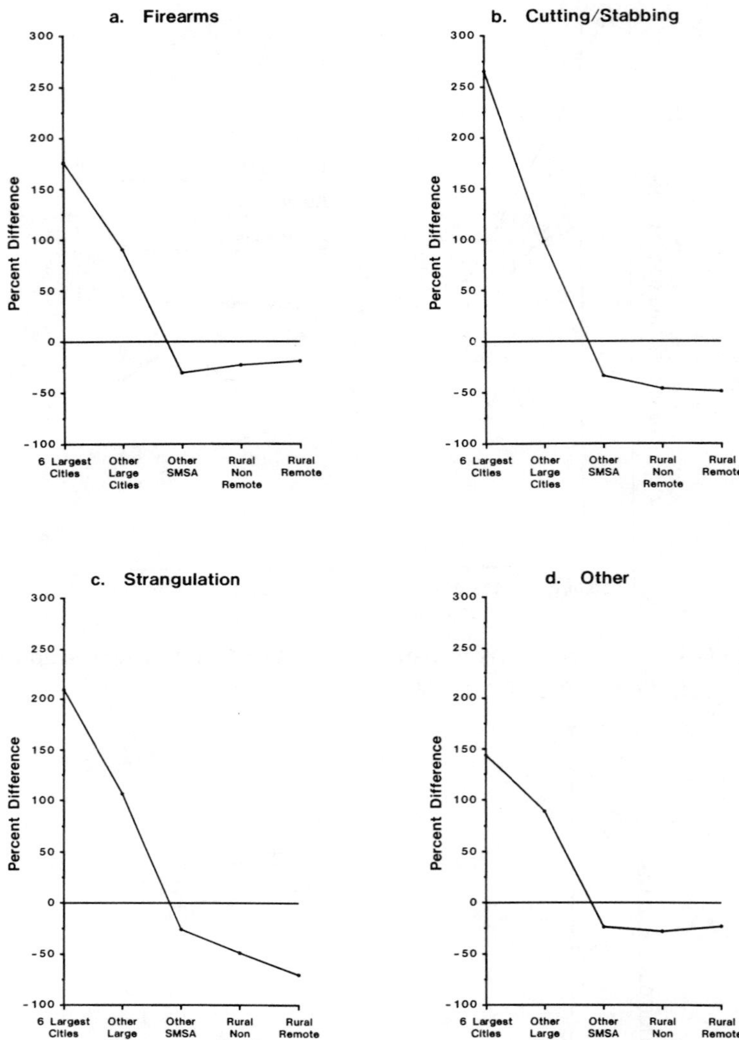

Figure 6-8. Percent Difference from the Average Death Rates from Homicide by Place of Residence and Method, 1977-1979

As with many unintentional injuries, the higher weekend incidence is partly owing to greater consumption of alcohol, which has been shown to be involved in a large proportion of killings.[1]

Homicide rates are highest during July through December (figure

a. Firearm Homicide

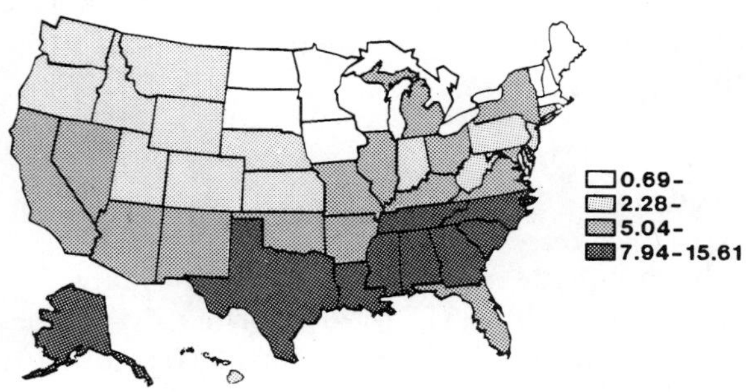

b. Non-Firearm Homicide

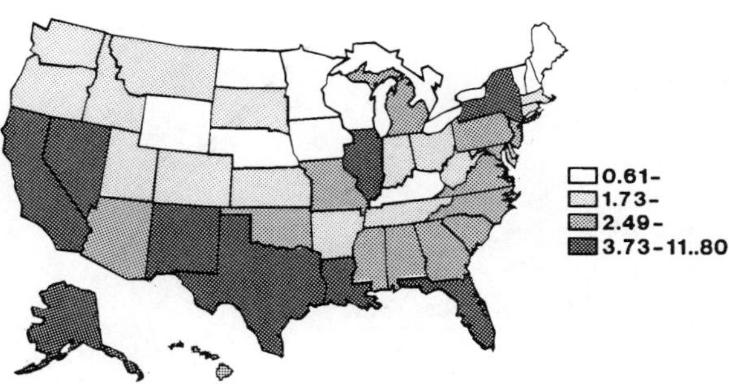

c. Ratio of Firearm to Non-Firearm Homicides

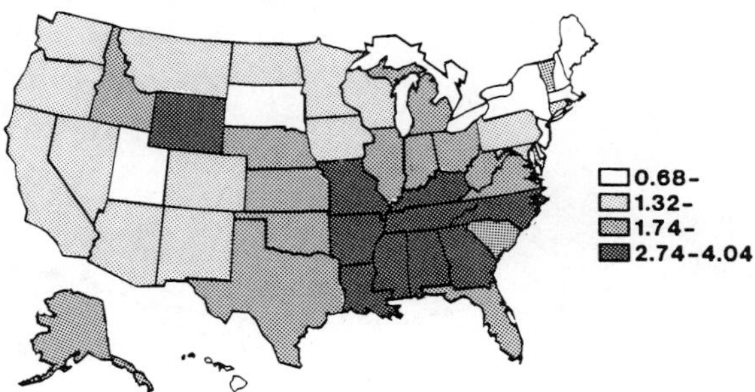

Figure 6-9. Death Rates from Homicide by State and Method, Per 100,000 Population, 1977-1979

3-16). Compared to unintentional injury deaths, this monthly variation in homicides is small, with the number of deaths in December, the peak month, only one-fifth greater than the number in February, the lowest month.

Historical Trends

Since 1930, the homicide rate has fluctuated widely (9 per 100,000 population in 1930, 4 in 1957, 11 in 1980), primarily because of changes in the death rate from homicide by firearms (figure 6-10). For other types of homicide, the trends have usually been in the same direction as for firearms, but in general the fluctuations have been much less, both proportionally and in absolute numbers. For example, between 1960 and 1980 the death rate from firearm homicide increased by 160

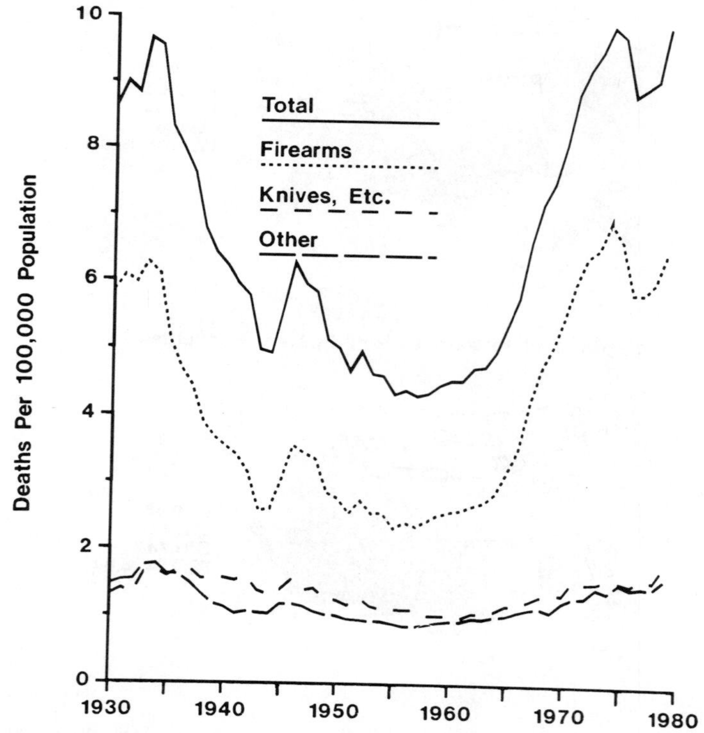

Figure 6-10. Death Rates from Homicide by Year and Method, 1930-1979

percent (from 2.6 to 6.8), while all other homicides increased by only 85 percent (from 2.0 to 3.7).

The greatest increases in homicide rates since 1968 have occurred among ages 1-19 and 75 or older; the death rate has increased by about 40 percent or more in these age groups (figure 6-11). Rates among children ages 5-9 showed the most marked increase, almost doubling between 1968 and 1979. The smallest changes occurred among children under 1 year old and at ages 25-64.

The trend in the homicide rates during 1968-1979 has been upward with a greater increase among females than males — 32 percent compared to 23 percent. Increases have been especially great for strangulation, for which the death rate doubled among both males and females. Rates for most other methods of homicide increased by about one-fourth.

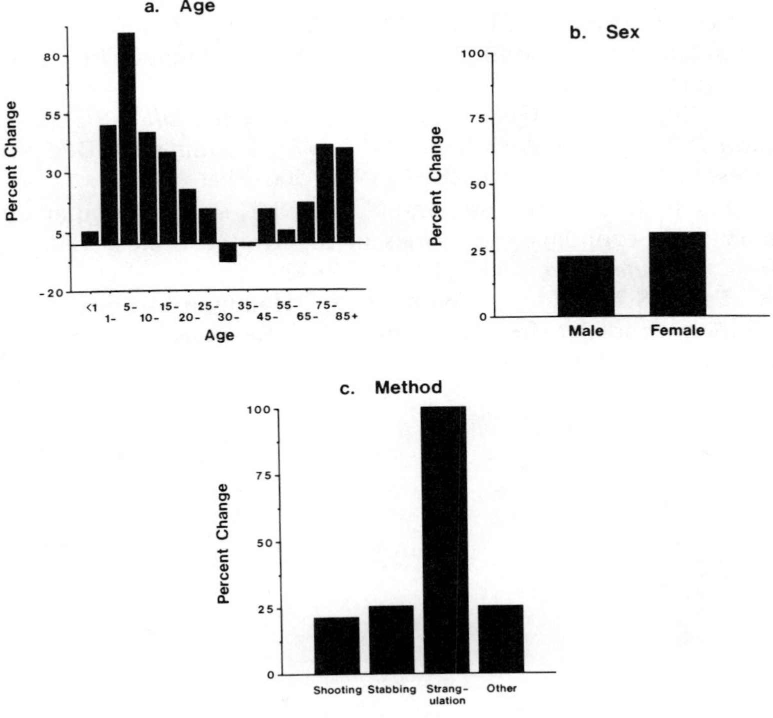

Figure 6-11. Percent Change in Death Rates from Homicide by Age, Sex, and Method, Based on 1968-1979 Trend

Notes

1. Baker, S.P., L.S. Robertson, and W.U. Spitz. "Tattoos, Alcohol, and Violent Death." *Journal of Forensic Sciences* 16 (1971): 219-225.

2. Centers for Disease Control. "Homicide — United States." *Morbidity and Mortality Weekly Report* 31 (1982): 594-602.

3. Dietz, P.E. *Social Factors in Rapist Behavior*. Philadelphia: University of Pennsylvania School of Medicine, Center for Studies in Social-Legal Psychiatry. Unpublished manuscript, 1977. Portions appear as a chapter in: Dietz, P.E. "SocialFactors in Rapist Behavior." In *Clinical Aspects of the Rapist*, edited by R. Rada. New York: Grune and Stratton, 1978.

4. Federal Bureau of Investigation. "Supplementary Homicide Report, 1981, By Age, Sex, Race, Within Relationship." Unpublished data, May 1983.

5. Federal Bureau of Investigation. *Uniform Crime Reports in the United States: 1981*. Washington, DC: U.S. Government Printing Office, August 26, 1982.

6. Gallup, G.H. "Gun Registration." In *The Gallup Poll, Public Opinion 1972-1977, Volume One, 1972-1975*. Wilmington, DE: Scholarly Resources, Inc., March 28-31, 1975: 506-508.

7. Jason, J., L.T. Strauss, and C.W. Tyler, Jr. "A Comparison of Primary and Secondary Homicides in the United States." *American Journal of Epidemiology* 117 (1983): 309-319.

8. Teret, S.P., and G.J. Wintemute. "Handgun Injuries: The Epidemiologic Evidence for Assessing Legal Responsibility." *Hamline Law Review* 6 (1983): 341-350.

7 Major Causes of Injury Death and Alternatives for Prevention

The leading cause of injury death is motor vehicle crashes, discussed in detail in Chapters 16-20. Chapters 7-15 present analyses of other major causes of injury death. Where population-based data were available, information on nonfatal injuries is also presented.

Mortality data from the National Center for Health Statistics, the major source of data in this section, are based on death certificate information which is subject to some limitations, the greatest being a lack of detail on the circumstances of injury. Since our knowledge of the circumstances of many fatal injuries is limited, analyses and discussions in Chapters 7-15 are less detailed than in Chapters 16-20, where many aspects of motor vehicle injuries are described in more detail because the data sources for such injuries typically contain more information.

The ninth edition of the International Classification of Diseases (ICD), used since 1979 to code National Center for Health Statistics data, adds some detail not previously available concerning the causes of injury.[18] It still does not specifically identify work- or recreation-related deaths.

Work-related deaths comprise a substantial component of the deaths from machinery and electric current (see Chapters 9 and 12). The largest number of deaths from occupational injuries involve road vehicles (see Chapters 16-20). Other major causes of job-related deaths are airplane crashes, falls, shootings, and burns (see Chapters 8, 10, 11, and 12). Information in these chapters is relevant to the causes and prevention of occupational injury. Since there are no national sources of detailed data on work-related deaths, no chapter is devoted to the subject.

Similarly, because of the dearth of systematically collected national data on sports fatalities, this book does not have a chapter on sports and recreational injuries. However, they are an important source of serious injuries and deaths including the majority of drownings, many firearm fatalities, 10 percent of all brain injuries,[11] 7 percent of spinal cord injuries,[12] and 13 percent of facial injuries treated in hospitals.[10] The best national estimates of injuries from specified sports come from the Consumer Product Safety Commission's sample of patients treated in emergency rooms and a review of sports-related deaths (table 7-1).[15]

Although the focus of this book is not injury prevention, Chapters

Table 7–1
Sports-Related Injuries (1980) and Deaths (1973–1980)

	Estimated Number of Injuries Treated in Hospital Emergency Rooms, 1980		*Number of Deaths, 1973–1980*	
Sport	*All Ages*	*Ages 5–14*	*All Ages*	*Ages 5–14*
Football	463,800	173,100	260	19
Baseball	442,900	121,700	183	40
Basketball	421,000	92,800	37	6
Soccer	94,200	37,800	11	6
Racquet sports	74,700	5,400	3	1
Volleyball	73,700	13,900	4	0
Wrestling[a]	67,500	20,000	23	2
Gymnastics	61,400	38,200	8	0
Ice hockey	36,400	10,800	10	2
Track and field	31,600	8,800	10	2
Golf[b]	18,800	4,600	28	14
Trampoline	6,100	2,900	13	6

Source: G.W. Rutherford, R.B. Miles, V.R. Brown, and B. MacDonald, *Overview of Sports-Related Injuries to Persons 5–14 Years of Age,* Washington, DC: U.S. Consumer Product Safety Commission, 1981.

Note: Injuries were estimated from the Consumer Product Safety Commission's National Electronic Injury Surveillance System. Deaths were identified from death certificates, newspaper clippings, consumer complaints, medical examiner reports, and NEISS data.

[a]Includes deaths from "rough-housing."

[b]Includes children playing with golf clubs, and spectators.

7 and 16 give examples of two approaches developed to assist in the systematic identification of options for injury prevention. Because of their importance, sports injuries will be used to illustrate approaches based on Haddon's ten basic strategies for preventing injury.[5-7]

The first strategy is to prevent the creation of the hazard in the first place, for example, by not manufacturing sports equipment that is apt to cause injury. This strategy might be applied to trampolines, an important source of spinal cord injuries. After the American Academy of Pediatrics recommended in 1977 that school use of trampolines be banned, there was a drop of more than 60 percent in the number of trampoline head and neck injuries treated in hospitals participating in the Consumer Product Safety Commission's National Electronic Injury Surveillance System (NEISS).[15]

The second strategy is to reduce the amount of hazard that is created, for example, reducing the height from which people can fall or jump, limiting the speed capability of snowmobiles, or limiting the speed of beginning skiers by providing slopes with only small vertical drops in relation to the lengths of the trails.[9] Exposure can be curtailed through shorter periods of play or by permitting hunting only on certain days. Reducing the number of players who participate in a particular sport is another example, illustrated by limiting participants to members of a specified age group.

The third strategy involves either preventing or reducing the likelihood of the release of a hazard. Examples include not allowing boxers to fight and designing hunting weapons that will not discharge inadvertently. In ancient times, the cessation of gladiatorial contests provides an additional example, as would the ending of bull fighting in Latin countries. Reducing the likelihood of the release of the hazard is often a more practical approach; an example is packing and grooming ski slopes to reduce hidden obstacles that might cause skiers to fall.

The fourth strategy is to modify the rate or spatial distribution of release of the hazard from its source. Examples include release bindings on skis, controlled release of dammed-up water to protect boaters downstream, and the use of shorter cleats on football shoes so that the foot can rotate easily without transmitting a sudden force to the knee. Changes in football rules have outlawed spearing and face-tackling; these techniques use the head as a primary contact point, and the forces on the head and neck are likely to exceed injury thresholds. Yet, more than one-third of high school football players in Minnesota continued to use these maneuvers a year after they were banned, and one player in five reported concussion symptoms during the playing season.[4]

The fifth strategy is to separate, in time or space, the hazard and its release from that which is to be protected. Starting avalanches during times when ski slopes are closed, an example of temporal separation, decreases the likelihood that avalanches will occur when skiers are on the slopes. Placing benches and other equipment farther from playing areas reduces the frequency of "out of bounds" injuries that commonly occur when players run into them.[3] Spatial separation is also illustrated by storing pistols used for target shooting at the shooting range rather than at home, and by providing paths for bicyclists, joggers, and people walking that are separate from roads for motor vehicles.

The sixth strategy is to separate the hazard from whatever is to be protected by interposing a material barrier. In many sports, the head, face, eyes, chest, or other body parts need to be protected from balls, bats, or other players. A review of sports-related injuries and deaths among people ages 5-14 revealed that 38 percent of the deaths involved baseball.[15] Being struck on the chest by the baseball with subsequent cardiac arrest appeared to be the predominant cause. This suggests a need for chest protection for young baseball players. Eye protection devices for racquetball and squash can prevent many eye injuries, the most common serious injury associated with such racquet sports.[10] Facial and dental injuries among hockey and football players have been substantially reduced by face masks.[2,14,17] Protective helmets are appropriate to many sports, such as football and horseback riding, where head injuries are a serious problem.

The seventh strategy is to modify the relevant basic qualities of the hazard. Illustrations include recent adoption of a softer ball in squash rather than the previously used hardball, padding the outer edge of racquets, and using balls large enough so that the bony socket of the eye affords some protection. The pointed ends of hockey sticks, once a major source of facial injuries, are now rounded to make them less injurious. Gymnasium walls should be designed without protrusions and either made of energy-attenuating materials or padded in areas where players can strike them. Breakaway goalposts and slalom poles that yield on impact are further examples.

The eighth strategy is to make that which is to be protected more resistant to damage from the hazard. Conditioning of the musculoskeletal system is an important means of reducing the likelihood of injury. Grouping school athletes by skills, physical fitness, and physical maturity rather than age has reportedly reduced injury rates.[16] Exercise and therapy to reduce osteoporosis are promising approaches of special relevance to older people participating in athletic and recreational activities.

The ninth strategy is to begin to counter damage already done. Athletes who may have sustained spinal cord injuries, for example, need to be carefully supported when they are moved in order to reduce the likelihood of paralysis. Football players with concussion symptoms should not be returned to play on the same day because of the potential for progressive neurological debilitation. One study found that most high school players who experienced loss of consciousness returned to play the same day.[4] Communication systems and readily available emergency and definitive care are clearly important but often inadequate, except in some major urban centers and in states with good emergency systems.

The tenth strategy is to stabilize, repair, and rehabilitate the injured person. Reconstructive surgery, physical and mental rehabilitation, and modification of the environment to accomodate the handicapped help to minimize adverse outcomes of serious injury.

These ten strategies and examples of illustrative tactics suggest the wide variety of measures that can reduce the likelihood and severity of injuries, as well as the severity of the consequences of injury once it has occurred. In choosing among potentially useful preventive measures, priority should be given to the ones most likely to effectively reduce injuries. In general, these will be measures that provide built-in, automatic protection, minimizing the amount and frequency of effort required of the individuals involved.[1,5,8,13]

Notes

1. Baker, S.P. "Childhood Injuries: The Community Approach to Prevention." *Journal of Public Health Policy* 2 (1981): 235-246.

2. Downs, J. "Incidence of Facial Trauma in Intercollegiate and Junior Hockey." *Physician and Sports Medicine* 7 (1979): 88.

3. Garrick, J., G. Collins, and R. Requa. "Out of Bounds in Football: Player Exposure to Probability of Collision Injury." *Journal of Safety Research* 9 (1977): 34-38.

4. Gerberich, S.G., J.D. Priest, J.R. Boen, C.P. Straub, and R.E. Maxwell. "Concussion Incidence and Severity in Secondary School Varsity Football Players." *American Journal of Public Health* 73 (1983): 1370-1375.

5. Haddon, W., Jr. "Advances in the Epidemiology of Injuries as a Basis for Public Policy." *Public Health Reports* 95 (1980): 411-421.

6. Haddon, W., Jr. "On the Escape of Tigers: An Ecologic Note." *American Journal of Public Health* 60 (1970): 2229-2234.

7. Haddon, W., Jr. "The Basic Strategies for Reducing Damage from Hazards of all Kinds." *Hazard Prevention* 16 (1980): 8-12.

8. Haddon, W., Jr., and S.P. Baker. "Injury Control." *Preventive and Community Medicine*, edited by D. Clark and B. MacMahon. Boston: Little, Brown and Company, 1981, pp. 109-140.

9. Haddon, W., Jr., A.E. Ellison, and R.E. Carroll. "Skiing Injuries: Epidemiologic Study." *Public Health Reports* 77 (1962): 975-991.

10. Karlson, T.A. *The Incidence of Hospital-Treated Facial Injuries*. Madison: University of Wisconsin, 1983.

11. Kraus, J.F., M.A. Black, N. Hessol, P. Ley, W. Rokaw, C. Sullivan, S. Bowers, S. Knowlton, and L. Marshall. "The Incidence of Acute Brain Injury and Serious Impairment in a Defined Population." *American Journal of Epidemiology* 119 (1984): 186-201.

12. Kraus, J.F., C.E. Franti, R.S. Riggins, D. Richards, and N.O. Borhani. "Incidence of Traumatic Spinal Cord Lesions." *Journal of Chronic Diseases* 28 (1975): 471-492.

12. Robertson, L.S. *Injuries: Causes, Control Strategies, and Public Policy*. Lexington, MA: Lexington Books, 1983.

14. Rontal, E., M. Rontal, K. Wilson, and B. Cram. "Facial Injuries in Hockey Players." *The Laryngoscope* 87 (1977): 884-894.

15. Rutherford, G.W., R.B. Miles, V.R. Brown, and B. MacDonald. *Overview of Sports-Related Injuries to Persons 5-14 Years of Age*. Washington, DC: U.S. Consumer Product Safety Commission, 1981.

16. Van Dusen, K. *A Model State Recreational Injury Control Program*. Atlanta: U.S. Department of Health and Human Services, Public Health Service, Centers for Disease Control, 1981.

17. Wilson, K., E. Rontal, and M. Rontal. "Facial Injuries in Football." *Transactions of the American Academy of Opthalmology and Otolaryngology* 77 (1973): 434-437.

18. World Health Organization. *Manual of the International Statistical Classification of Diseases, Injuries and Causes of Death*. Volume 1. Geneva: World Health Organization, 1977.

8 Non-Motor Vehicle Transportation

Although motor vehicle crashes are the leading cause of injury deaths, other forms of transportation are also significant. During the past half century, the death rate from all forms of transportation combined has declined only slightly, from about 31 to 24 per 100,000 population. While the overall death rate per mile of travel has shown a much larger decrease, it should be recognized that the human cost of traveling has changed very little during a period when deaths from injuries at home and in the workplace have declined substantially.

Major shifts in the mode of travel have resulted in large changes in transportation-related injury death rates — for example, a 60 percent increase in the aviation death rate and an 85 percent reduction in the death rate related to trains since 1930. Of particular interest are deaths in this country from plane crashes in World War II; more than 20,000 aviation deaths among military personnel occurred in the continental United States (i.e., excluding combat and other overseas military deaths), approximating the reduction in highway deaths during the same period (figure 8-1).[12-13]

The terms *travel* and *transportation* include not only business travel but also recreational driving, flying, and boating, the context in which the majority of transportation deaths occur. The number of deaths per person-mile of travel differs markedly by mode of travel (table 8-1). Among users of road vehicles, for example, there is more than a 100-fold difference between bus occupants and motorcyclists.

For air travelers, there is a 300-fold difference between general aviation (private or business aircraft) and scheduled noncommuter airlines. Passengers traveling by train and those on scheduled airlines have the lowest rates. Rates for boat travel are not available. Most deaths in the ICD category called "water transport" are drownings related to small boats, discussed in Chapter 13.

The mode of transport selected for shipment of freight is an important determinant of injury and death rates. The death rate per billion ton-miles varies a thousandfold among the various modes for which estimates are available (table 8-2). Highway transport of freight is associated with the highest rate, about 11 deaths per billion ton-miles for federally regulated carriers during 1963-1968. This was more than four times the rate for rail transport.[3,9] In recent years, heavy trucks have

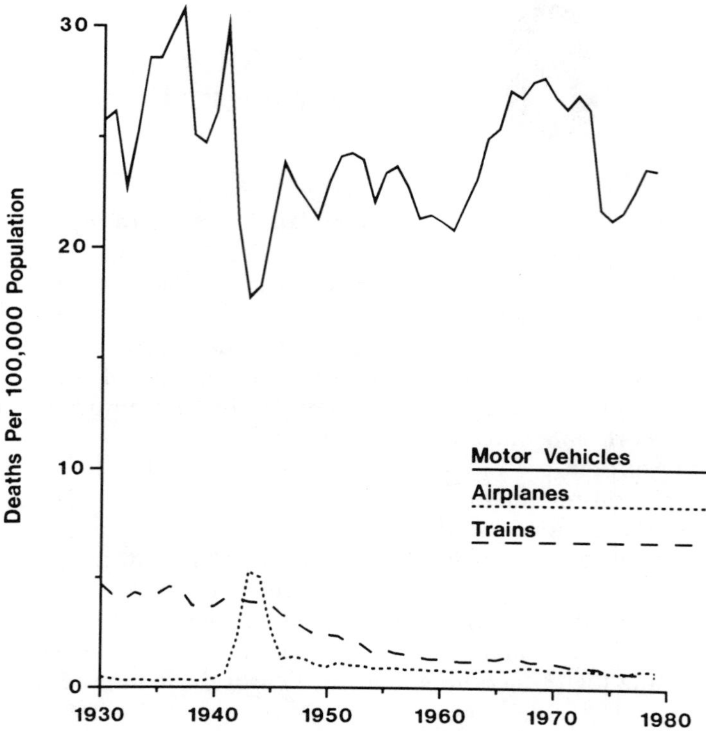

Figure 8-1. Death Rates from Motor Vehicles, Airplanes, and Trains by Year, 1930-1979

Table 8–1
Death Rates of Vehicle Occupants Per 100 Million Miles of Travel, by Type of Vehicle, 1978–1980

Vehicle	*Deaths per 100 Million Person-Miles of Travel*
Motorcycle	21
General aviation	14
Car	1.3
Bus	0.15
Passenger train	0.07
Scheduled plane	0.04

Sources: National Safety Council, Accident Facts—1979–1982 Editions, Chicago: National Safety Council, 1979–1982, and R.G. Snyder, "Survival in Airplane Crashes," *The UMTRI Research Review* 13 (1983):1–11.

Table 8–2
Surface Freight Transportation Fatality Rates, 1963–1968

Transport Mode	*Deaths Per Billion Ton-Miles*
Highway (federally regulated carriers)	10.9
Rail	2.5
Marine	0.31
Petroleum pipeline	0.01

Source: National Transportation Safety Board, *Special Study: Fatality Rates for Surface Freight Transportation, 1963–1968,* Report No. NTSB-STS-71-4, Washington, DC: National Transportation Safety Board, 1971.

been involved in more than 4,000 fatal crashes annually.[5] In some geographic areas or for certain types of freight, there may be little choice as to mode of transport. However, the large differences among modes in the *human* costs of freight transport should be a major factor in policy related to development and use of transportation systems.[3]

Railroads

Few of the 1,300 annual deaths related to trains involve passengers on the trains. Rather, the majority (about 60 percent) are occupants of motor vehicles, and about one-third are people on foot who are struck by trains. In addition, about 100 railroad employees are killed each year. Freight train conductors, brakemen, and flagmen have the highest on-duty death rates among railroad employees.[4,6] Passengers represent less than 1 percent of all deaths related to rail transport. Their death rate per 100 million person-miles of travel is estimated to be about one-twentieth the rate for passenger car occupants (table 8-1).

Collisions between trains and motor vehicles are discussed in Chapter 17, since virtually all of the deaths and injuries in such collisions are to motor vehicle occupants.

People unprotected by vehicles, such as pedestrians and motorcyclists, are at extremely high risk of death when struck by trains. Pedestrians killed by trains, who number about 400 annually, are predominantly adult males. The rate for Native Americans is 4 times the rate for blacks and 7 times the rate for whites. Death rates are also high in low-income areas.

Among Native Americans, the pedestrian-train death rate per 100,000 population is highest in remote rural areas, while among whites the rate is highest in the six largest cities. Since the rates described are population-based, the differences cannot be explained by the fact that Native Americans are more likely than whites to live in remote areas. Collection and analysis of state- or county-specific data on the characteristics of those killed (including acute and chronic alcoholism), the circumstances of death, amount of train mileage, and approaches to separating pedestrians from train tracks might explain some of the demographic differences in death rates and suggest ways to reduce the rates.

Unlike motor vehicle-train fatalities, which are most common from October through January, pedestrian-train fatalities are most common in summer and fall; the number in July and August is twice the number in January and February. It seems likely that the winter peak in deaths from motor vehicle-train collisions is related to weather conditions and increased hours of darkness, reducing the ability of drivers to make timely and appropriate decisions. The summertime peak in pedestrian deaths may reflect greater outdoor activity in warm months.

Trends in pedestrian-train fatality rates between 1968 and 1979 showed a 40 percent decline. (During this period, death rates from motor vehicle collisions with trains declined by 55 percent.) The tremendous forces involved when trains strike people on foot make it essential to reduce the potential for such events. Where trains or light rail vehicles pass through communities or other high-risk areas, physical barriers, vertical separation, or other measures are needed to keep pedestrians from the tracks. Rapid rail systems that allow passengers to wait for and get on or off trains without risk of falling onto the track illustrate effective means of separation.

Aviation

Airplane crashes are the eighth leading cause of unintentional injury death. They are also an important cause of occupational injury deaths among commercial air crew, flying instructors, test pilots, crop dusters, pipeline inspectors, and people who travel extensively on business. A census of occupational injury deaths in Maryland in 1978 determined that 5 percent resulted from airplane crashes.[1] The Bureau of Labor Statistics estimates that plane crashes cause more than one-tenth of all work injury deaths in the oil/gas extraction industry.[2] Almost 60 percent of *all* deaths of Navy officers are from plane crashes, private as well as military.[14] Death rates are not available for specific groups of civilians such as pilots of light aircraft, whose rates are probably high since 60 percent of all light aircraft can be expected to crash in a typical 20-year "lifetime."[11]

From 1977 to 1982, the number of deaths in plane crashes averaged about 1,600 each year (table 8-3). Of these, 82 percent were in general aviation crashes, while only 9 percent involved scheduled airline service. The fatal crash rate per 100,000 aircraft hours was about 25 times as great for general aviation as for scheduled airline service. Commuter and unscheduled commercial carriers had intermediate rates.[7] Not included in these figures are deaths in military aircraft, which average about 100 each year, according to NCHS mortality data (which may underestimate such deaths since details are missing from many death certificates).

General aviation deaths account for 5 out of 6 deaths in plane crashes. The following analyses of aviation mortality during 1977-1979 are restricted to the 3,188 deaths that were coded on NCHS tapes as related to noncommercial, nonmilitary aviation. Since the actual number of general aviation deaths in this period was about 4,000, the death rates calculated for general aviation are accordingly low. However, they help to provide a picture of this major group of fatal injuries.

General aviation death rates are highest for ages 25-54 and have a male:female ratio of almost 5:1. Whites and Native Americans have the highest rates (0.6 and 0.3 per 100,000 population, respectively), compared to 0.04 and 0.11 for blacks and Asians.

In contrast to most causes of injury, general aviation death rates increase with per capita income (figure 8-2). For the U.S. population as a whole, the death rate in high-income areas is almost double the rate in low-income areas. This difference would undoubtedly be greater if the analyses were based on individual income of the deceased, given the high cost of light aircraft ownership and use. The relationship to population density is even stronger, with death rates among residents of remote rural areas four times the rate in the largest cities.

Table 8–3
Aviation Deaths and Fatal Crashes Per 100,000 Aircraft Hours, 1977–1982

	Deaths			*Fatal Crashes*	
Type of Carrier	*No.*	*Average per year*	*Percent*	*No.*	*Rate per 100,000 hours*
Scheduled airline service	828	138	9	21	0.07
Scheduled commuter service	232	39	2	60	0.54
On-demand air taxis	620	103	7	231	1.2
General aviation	7,762	1,294	82	3,862	1.8
Total	9,442	1,574	100	4,174	

Source: National Transportation Safety Board, *Annual Report to Congress 1982,* Washington, DC: National Transportation Safety Board, 1983.

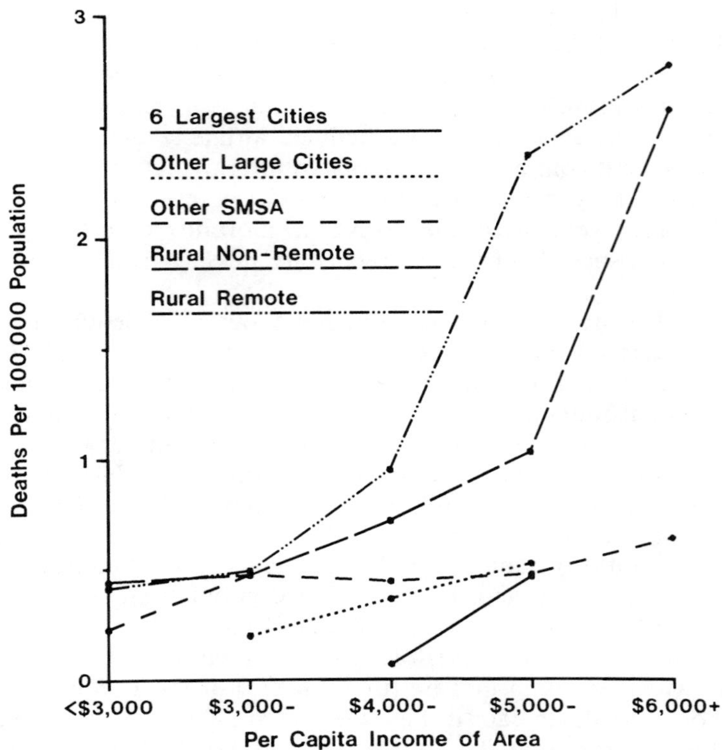

Figure 8-2. Death Rates from General Aviation Crashes by Per Capita Income and Place of Residence, 1977-1979

Among all injuries, general aviation deaths have one of the strongest associations with geographic factors. Death rates are highest in the western half of the United States (figure 8-3), reflecting the greater private ownership and use of light aircraft where the population and air traffic are of low density.

Alaska's death rate from general aviation is 12 per 100,000 population, 6 times the rate in the next highest state (Idaho) and 24 times the average for the United States. Of all unintentional injury deaths in Alaska, 16 percent result from airplane crashes (commercial as well as general aviation), compared to less than 2 percent nationally. In part, the high rates in Alaska reflect the fact that much of the travel is by noncommercial aircraft because of the lack of roads in many areas. It also seems likely that adverse weather conditions and very short days for much of the year contribute to the high aviation death rates in Alaska. The remoteness of many small communities probably influ-

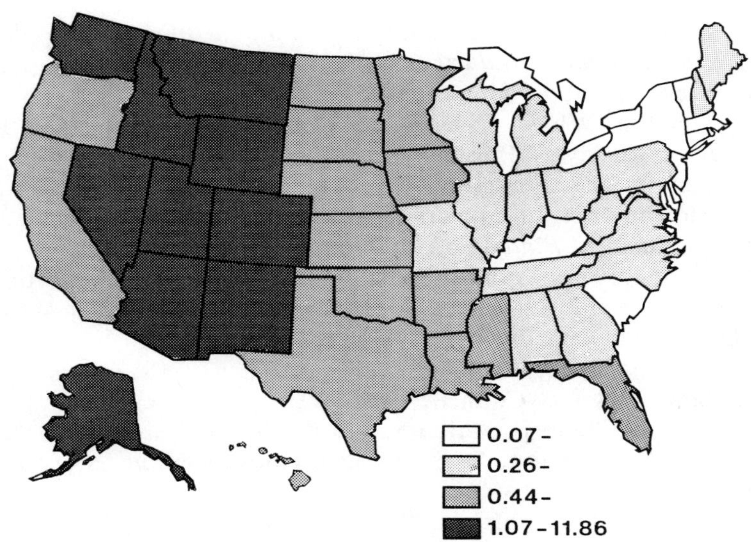

Figure 8-3. Death Rates from General Aviation Crashes by State, Per 100,000 Population, 1977-1979

ences death rates from all types of injuries through lack of speedy access to medical treatment.

Most efforts to reduce aviation deaths have focused on preventing crashes. Comparable attention should be given to preventing injuries when crashes occur, for, contrary to popular belief, most airplane crashes would be survivable in well-designed aircraft. Typically, plane crashes need not produce forces on their occupants in excess of their injury thresholds.

A substantial portion of serious injuries and deaths in general aviation as well as in scheduled airline service could be prevented through application of available knowledge and technology to seat designs and other structural components. In addition, crashworthy fuel systems, cabin furnishings that do not ignite easily or emit toxic gases, and better means of egress would reduce the large number of preventable deaths in postcrash fires.[8,10-11]

Notes

1. Baker, S.P., J.S. Samkoff, R.S. Fisher, and C.B. Van Buren. "Fatal Occupational Injuries." *Journal of the American Medical Association* 248 (1982): 692-697.

2. Bureau of Labor Statistics. *Occupational Injuries and Illnesses in the United States by Industry, 1981*. Washington, DC: United States Department of Labor, January 1983.

3. Haddon, W., Jr. "The Safety of the Automobile — An International Perspective." Presented at the Nordic Seminar on the Safety of the Automobile, Linkoping, Sweden, June 14, 1983.

4. Metropolitan Life Insurance Company. "Railroad Accident Fatalities." *Statistical Bulletin* 62 (July-September 1981): 4-7.

5. National Highway Traffic Safety Administration. *Fatal Accident Reporting System 1981*. Technical Report DOT HS-806-251. Washington, DC: U.S. Department of Transportation, 1983.

6. National Safety Council. *Accident Facts — 1982 Edition*. Chicago: National Safety Council, 1982.

7. National Transportation Safety Board. *Annual Report to Congress 1982*. Washington, DC: National Transportation Safety Board, 1983.

8. National Transportation Safety Board. *Safety Report — The Status of General Aviation Aircraft Crashworthiness*. Washington, DC: National Transportation Safety Board, 1980.

9. National Transportation Safety Board. *Special Study: Fatality Rates for Surface Freight Transportation, 1963 to 1968*. Report No. NTSB-STS-71-4. Washington, DC: National Transportation Safety Board, August 18, 1971.

10. Snyder, R.G. "Comparison of Automobile and Airplane Crashes: Implications for Preventing Injuries." *Proceedings of the American Medical Association Conference on Prevention of Disabling Injuries*. Chicago: American Medical Association, 1983.

11. Snyder, R.G. "Survival in Airplane Crashes." *The UMTRI Research Review* 13 (1983): 1-11.

12. United States Army, Office of Statistical Control. *Army Air Forces Statistical Digest — World War II*. Washington, DC: United States Army, 1945.

13. United States Marine Corps Historical Center, Reference Files. Subject: Marine Corps Casualties During World War II.

14. Withers, B.F., III. "Occupational Mortality in Naval Aviation." *U.S. Navy Medicine*, in press.

9 Machinery

Severe injury and death from fixed machinery in factories and mills were once problems of major proportions, but the incorporation of machine guards, fail-safe devices, and other types of automatic protection has greatly reduced this problem. By 1980, only 2 percent of all deaths from machinery were due to power presses, saws, or other woodworking and metal-working machines — that is, the machines that now commonly incorporate a variety of automatic protection devices (table 9-1).

Of some 1,500 machinery-related deaths annually, more than half involve farm equipment. In Georgia, the rate of tractor-related deaths among male farm residents is 24 per 100,000, which is higher than the national death rate for injuries related to road vehicles.[3]

Detailed analysis of death certificate information on about 4,500 farm machinery fatalities in the United States during 1975-1981 revealed that about three-fourths involved tractors. The major problems were tractor overturns, falling from and/or being run over by tractors, and entanglement by the power take-off shaft. Corn pickers, augers, and combines also caused a substantial number of deaths. Farm machinery operating on public roads was involved in about 200 deaths annually, including occupants of other vehicles.[5]

As in the case of tractors, deaths from cranes, forklifts, and bulldozers often involve overturns. In addition, electrocution is an important contributor to fatalities related to augers and cranes. Cranes were

Table 9–1
Deaths from Machinery Other than Transport Vehicles, 1980

Type of Machinery	*Number*	*Percent*
Agricultural machines	814	55
Cranes, forklifts, lifting machines	239	16
Earth moving machines	101	7
Mining and earth drilling machines	78	5
Metalworking and woodworking machines	33	2
Other or unspecified	206	14
Total	1,471	99[a]

Source: National Center for Health Statistics, unpublished data, 1980. Excludes deaths when driven or towed on the highway and deaths from electric current.

[a]Percents do not add to 100 due to rounding.

the most common type of nonroad land vehicle involved in deaths of Maryland workers.[1]

Age-specific farm machinery death rates differ markedly from rates for other machinery (figure 9-1). Deaths from nonfarm machinery peak at ages 20-24 and are rare among children. Farm machinery death rates, on the other hand, are *lowest* at ages 20-24; they are highest at ages 65-74, when deaths from other causes of occupational injury are uncommon. Farm machinery death rates are also high among young children; for ages 3-4 years, the number of these deaths in 1979 was almost the same as from poisoning by solids and liquids, and it approached the number from falls. This is remarkable, for virtually all young children are exposed at times to the possibility of poisoning or falling, whereas only 2 percent live on farms.[2] Circumstances of farm machinery deaths among young children include being run over by tractors and falling from tractors, on which they are often carried as passengers. Entanglement in augers and power take-off shafts also causes serious injuries to young children.[5]

Farm machinery death rates are highest in the north central states, whereas death rates from other machinery are generally highest in the mountain states (figure 9-2).

During the past 50 years, markedly different trends have characterized deaths from farm and other machinery. Between 1930 and 1980, the farm machinery death rate per 100,000 population increased by 44

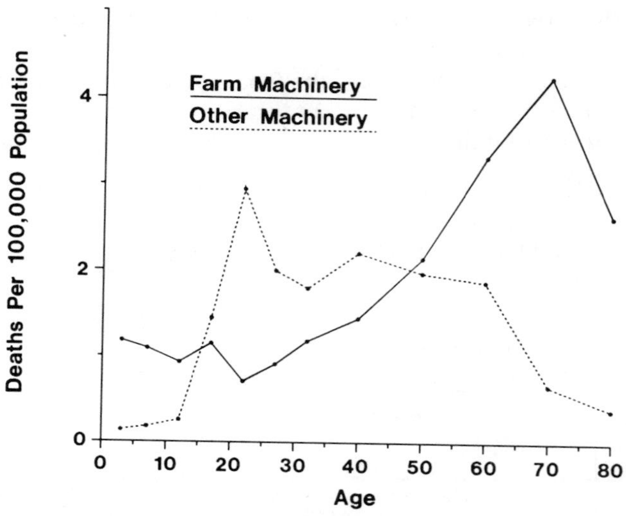

Figure 9-1. Death Rates from Farm and Other Machinery by Age, 1979

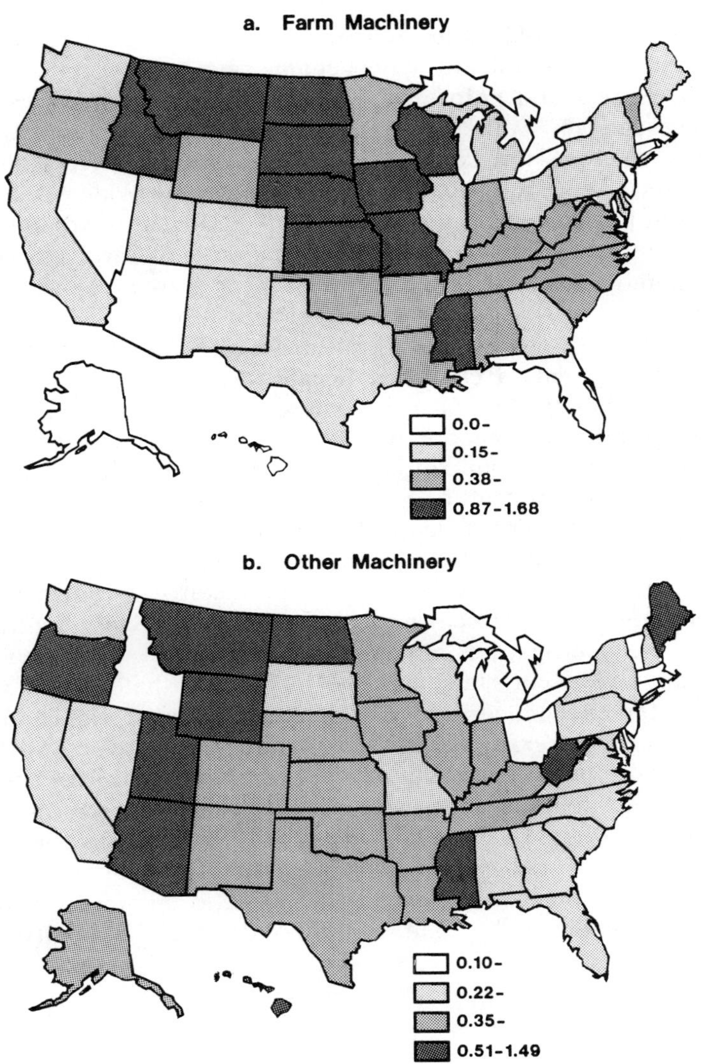

Figure 9-2. Death Rates from Farm and Other Machinery by State, Per 100,000 Population, 1979

percent (table 4-2). During the same period, the death rate from all other machinery *dropped* by almost 80 percent. This dramatic decrease involved not only fixed machinery but also deaths from elevators, which in 1930 surpassed deaths from farm machinery (348 vs. 314 deaths, respectively). Although the number of elevators has increased many fold, elevator-related deaths have become rare as stringent codes have been developed and enforced.* In contrast to road vehicles, home appliances, and most other consumer products sold in the United States, farm machinery is not covered by federal product safety standards. Employers of more than 10 farm employees must provide workers with equipment that meets Occupational Safety and Health Administration (OSHA) requirements, but the great majority of farm workers are family members or work on small farms and thus are not covered under OSHA.[1,4]

Prevention of deaths and injuries from machinery, especially farm machinery, presents a challenge because many of the events occur outdoors, rather than in factories where machine guarding and other forms of automatic protection have long been accepted. Many of those killed are working alone, often under difficult conditions and time pressures created by maturing crops and changes in the weather.

Despite improvements in machinery in recent years, further design changes are needed to provide automatic protection from death or dismemberment under a wide variety of predictable circumstances. For example, not only is it necessary to separate workers from cutting and grinding mechanisms, but also means are needed to clear machinery that is jammed by cornstalks or other material so that workers will not have to intervene. Tractors need rollover protection devices and power take-offs need integrated guards that cannot be removed. Along with forklifts and other vehicles that are apt to overturn, tractors need improved design to prevent backward and sideward overturns. Cranes and other equipment with long booms should be insulated or designed with fail-safe devices to preclude electrocution from contact with overhead wires. While it may never be possible to eliminate all injuries related to machinery, the major sources of death and disability deserve attention.

Notes

1. Baker, S.P., J.S. Samkoff, R.S. Fisher, and C.B. Van Buren. "Fatal Occupational Injuries." *Journal of the American Medical Association* 248 (1982): 692-697.

2. Bureau of the Census. "Farm Population of the United States: 1979." *Current Population Reports — Farm Population* 53 (1980): 8.

---

*Elevator deaths are now so uncommon that they are not separately coded; they are combined with the far more numerous deaths from forklifts and cranes.

3. Goodman, R.A., J.D. Smith, R.K. Sikes, D.L. Rogers, and J.L. Mickey. "An Epidemiologic Study of Fatalities Associated with Farm Tractor Injuries," submitted for publication.

4. Karlson, T.A., and J. Noren. "Farm Tractor Fatalities: The Failure of Voluntary Safety Standards." *American Journal of Public Health* 69 (1979): 146-149.

5. McKnight, R.H. "U.S. Agricultural Equipment Fatalities 1975-1981: Implications for Injury Control and Health Education." Baltimore, MD: Johns Hopkins University, unpublished doctoral dissertation, 1984.

10 Falls

Falls are the most common cause of nonfatal injury in the United States and the second leading cause of both spinal cord and brain injury, accounting for about one-fifth of these injuries.[15,16] Each year 1 person in 20 receives emergency room treatment because of a fall.[2]

Of all injuries, the one resulting in the largest number of hospital admissions is fracture of the hip (see Chapter 3), which occurs mainly as a result of falls. The primary cause of more than 200,000 hospital admissions each year, this injury is especially influenced by age, with people 65 years or older sustaining 84 percent of all hip fractures. On average, each such fracture requires 21 days of hospitalization in a short-stay hospital, almost double the average stay for *all* causes of hospital admission in this age group. A total of 3.6 million hospital days is required annually to treat hip fractures in the population age 65 or older.[11] These figures exclude the far greater number of days of nursing home care and do not convey the tragic changes in life style and loss of independence that commonly ensue.

In addition to producing substantial morbidity and disability, falls are a major cause of injury death, surpassed only by motor vehicles and firearms. Among unintentional injury deaths, only those from motor vehicles exceed falls. Each year about 13,000 deaths are attributed to falls. In addition, in an unknown number of deaths a fall initiates or contributes to the sequence of events leading to death but is not mentioned on the death certificate.[12] As a result, the total number of deaths related to falls may be far greater than that attributed to falls on death certificates. In King County, Washington, a review of deaths under the jurisdiction of the medical examiner's office revealed that in about half of those related to falls, the death certificate listed the fall as a contributory factor rather than as the underlying cause.[12] Only deaths for which falls are listed as the underlying cause of death are included in the following analyses and discussion.

Injuries from falls result from an abrupt dissipation of mechanical energy. As in motor vehicle crashes, the intensity of the forces on the body of a person who falls depends in part on the person's velocity at the moment of impact. In turn, the velocity is determined primarily by the height from which the person has fallen and whether the fall has been "broken," for example, by grasping a handrail or landing on shrubbery. The impact velocity may also be increased by other aspects of the dynamics of a fall, as when a person slips on ice and falls backward.

When a person falls, the impact forces decrease as the decelerative, or stopping, distance increases. This stopping distance depends on several things, including the energy-absorbing qualities of the structure that one falls onto or against, the thickness and energy-absorbing qualities of clothing, and the yield or compressibility of the part of the body on which the forces operate.

Increasing the area on which the forces operate is also an important means of reducing injuries from falls. Falling against a narrow, sharp, or pointed structure focuses the forces and increases the chance of injury, whereas a wider contact area distributes the forces less harmfully over a larger portion of the body, with less likelihood of injury.

The implications of these basic determinants of fall injuries are still generally unrecognized, in spite of the pioneering work of Hugh De Haven.[5,9,10] His classic study of people who survived falls from great heights showed that under appropriate conditions the human body can withstand very high deceleration forces without significant injury. The study also demonstrated that injury severity in falls is largely determined by the characteristics of the environment, including the impact surface and what is beneath it.

The place where injury occurred is specified for about two-thirds of all fatal falls. In the majority of cases where the place of injury is specified, the injury occurs at home. This proportion is highest among young children and lowest at ages 15-19 (figure 10-1).

Except for the more than 300 falls per year in which the death certificate mentions industrial sites and mines, it is not possible to identify work-related falls in the national mortality files. A review of all fatal occupational injuries in 1978 in Maryland found that 9 percent were due to falls, a proportion surpassed only by vehicle-related deaths and shootings.[1] National estimates by the Bureau of Labor Statistics for companies employing more than 10 workers also indicate that 9 percent of work-related injury deaths are from falls. In these national estimates, only road vehicles and industrial vehicles cause a greater proportion of occupational deaths[4] (see Chapter 16).

About 1,800 fatal falls are known to occur each year in residential institutions such as nursing homes. Studies conducted in such facilities for the elderly reveal high rates of falls and fall injuries, including hip fractures.[8,12] In view of the advanced age and imperfect health of many nursing home residents, a large number of falls with serious sequelae should be anticipated in these institutions. Because of the prolonged disability and the high cost of such injuries to the individual, the family, and society, much could be gained from measures to reduce both the

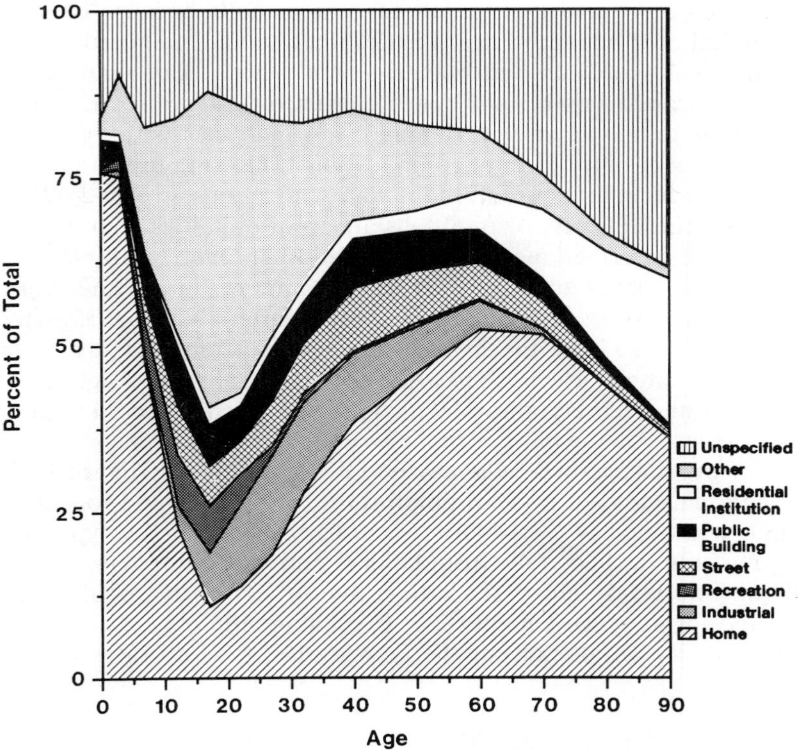

Figure 10-1. Places Where Fatal Falls Occurred by Age, 1977-1979

incidence and severity of fall injuries in institutions designed to house the elderly.

Age and Sex

Almost 30 percent of all deaths from falls occur among people age 85 or older, although this age group makes up only 1 percent of the population. More than half of all fall deaths involve people 75 or older, who comprise only 4 percent of the population. The importance of the problem is illustrated by comparing fall deaths among the elderly with motor vehicle occupant deaths among teenage males, who are well known to be at high risk of death in motor vehicle crashes. There are more deaths from falls among people 85 or older than there are motor vehicle occupant deaths among males ages 18-19 (3,800 versus 3,000), and the death rate per 100,000 population is more than twice as high.

The elderly have high death rates from falls because of several concomitants of advanced age: greater likelihood of falling due to various medical problems and impairment of vision, gait, and balance; increased fragility of certain bones caused by osteoporosis, a loss of bone mass that is greater in females and increases with age;[6,14] and greater susceptibility to fatal complications following injury.

The circumstances of fatal falls vary with age (figure 10-2). During childhood the majority of fatal falls are from buildings or other structures or are described merely as "from another level." Fatal falls from buildings, ladders, and scaffolds are prominent during the working years. Falls on stairs are relatively important after about age 35. Among the elderly, who have the highest death rates from *all* types of falls, the circumstances are not specified for most falls. The age and sex pattern of unspecified falls, which comprise two-thirds of all fatal falls, closely resembles the pattern for falls on the same level, suggesting that most of the unspecified falls may be falls on one level (figure 10-3).

The male:female ratio of death rates for all ages and for all types of falls combined is 1.2:1. The ratio varies, however, by type of fall, ranging from 22:1 for falls from ladders and scaffolds to about 1:1 for falls on one level. These sex ratios, like others in this book, are not adjusted for age (see Chapter 3). At each age the male death rate for each category of fall exceeds the female rate. If death rates were age-

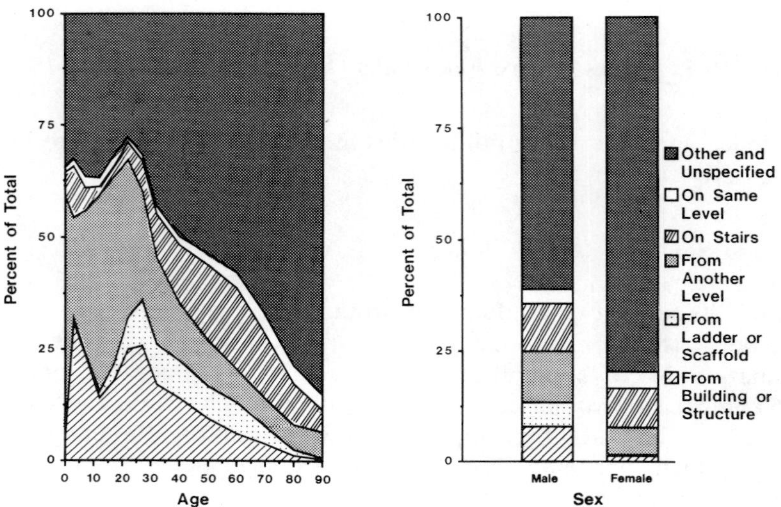

Figure 10-2. Percent of Fall Deaths by Age and Type, and by Sex and Type, 1977-1979

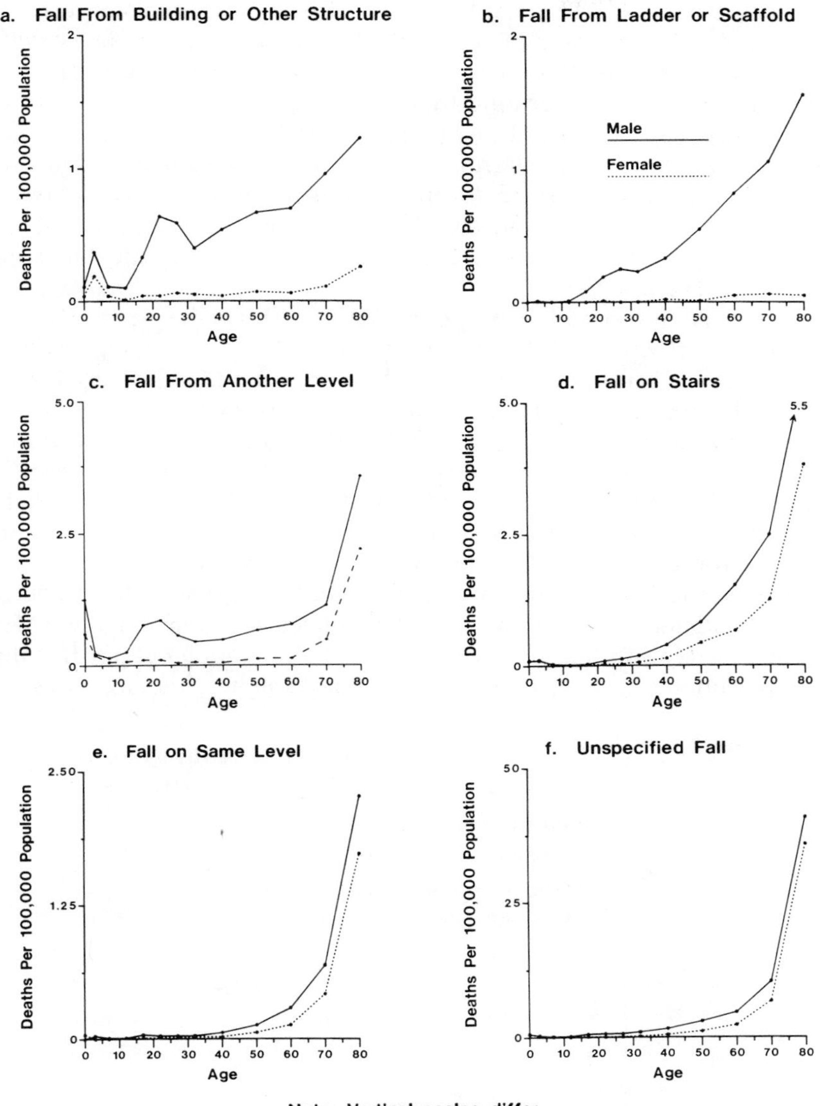

Figure 10-3. Death Rates from Falls by Age, Sex, and Type, 1977-1979

adjusted, the male:female ratio for falls on one level would be slightly greater than 1. However, the larger proportion of elderly females in the total female population causes the unadjusted death rate for females to equal the rate for males in the case of falls on one level and actually to exceed it in the case of unspecified falls. The higher age-specific death rates among males contrast with their lower age-specific fracture rates (figure 10-4), suggesting that falls among males are, on the average, more severe than among females, involving greater heights and/ or more head injuries. Differences between the sexes in use of alcohol may also be involved, since severe injuries are more likely to involve alcohol than are minor injuries. At least among pedestrians, falls resulting in head injuries are frequently associated with alcohol while other falls are not.[17]

The age-associated increase in fracture rates is especially pronounced for fractures of the hip (figure 10-4). After age 75, hip fractures in both sexes outnumber all other fractures combined as a cause of hospitalization. Among females, the rate of hip fractures at age 85 and older is 10 times the rate at ages 65-74. Although males have lower hip fracture rates, they show almost as great a rate of increase with increasing age. For both sexes, the hospitalization rate for all fractures excluding those of the hip is about three times as high for ages 85 and older as for ages 65-74. These new analyses of previously unpublished data from the National Hospital Discharge Survey show that fractures are a significant problem among elderly males as well as females. Most scientific attention has been given to fractures among elderly females, who outnumber elderly males and also have higher fracture rates.

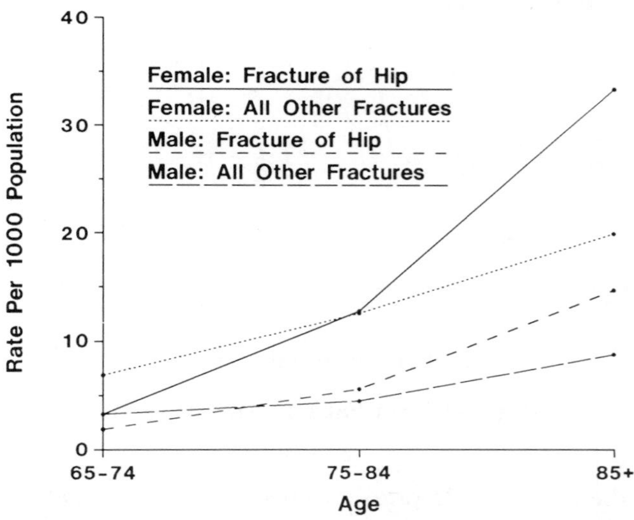

Figure 10-4. Short-Stay Hospital Discharge Rates for Fracture of the Hip and All Other Fractures by Age and Sex, for Ages 65 and Older, NCHS Hospital Discharge Survey, 1980

It must be remembered that the rates shown in figure 10-4 represent only those for hospitalized fractures. For both sexes, advanced age substantially increases the likelihood of hospital admission following minor fractures. On the other hand, age would not greatly influence the probability of admission following hip fractures, almost all of which result in hospital admission.

Children are also at high risk of fall injury, but their death rate is low. Based on Massachusetts data, about one-tenth of all children ages 1-3 require emergency room treatment each year for falls, with the highest incidence at age 1. Falls on stairs account for one-eighth of the childhood falls treated in emergency rooms and one-fourth of the hospital admissions. Most hospital admissions for falls among children involve falls from another level, such as a roof, porch, stairs, or dressing table[7,19] — reflecting the greater impact forces in falls from heights.

Each year about 150 children younger than 5 years old are killed in falls, primarily falls from another level, from buildings or other structures, or on stairs (figure 10-5). During childhood, fatal falls from

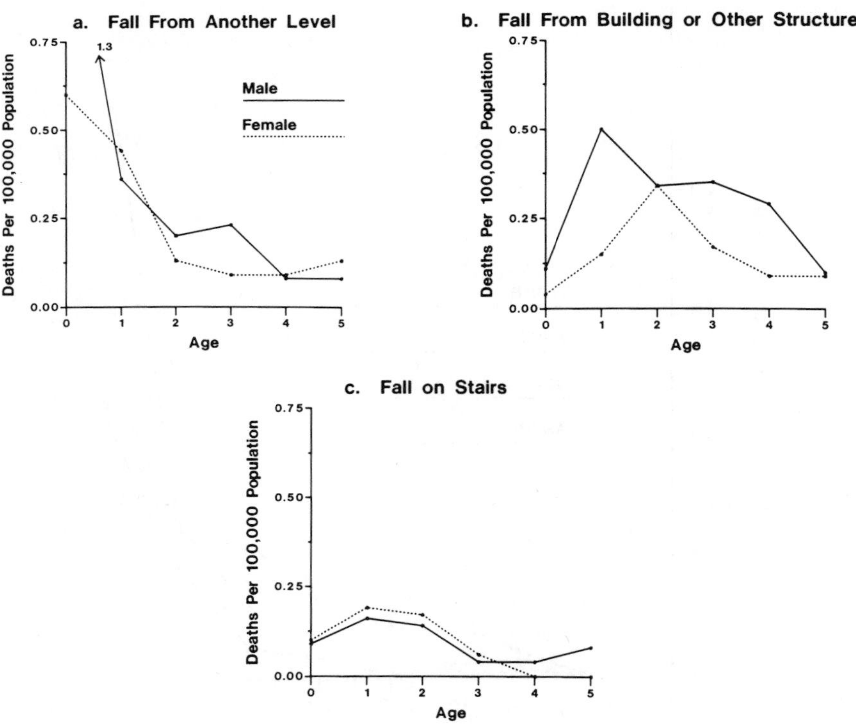

Figure 10-5. Death Rates from Falls by Age, Sex, and Type, for Ages 0-5, 1977-1979

buildings and on stairs are most common at age 1 for boys and ages 2-4 for girls, whereas other fatal falls from a different level (e.g., bed or chair) are most common during the first year of life for both sexes (figure 10-5). These differences may reflect differing developmental patterns of childhood activity and suggest the need for research on the relationships between age, sex, degree of supervision, and the role of the physical environment in childhood injury.

Race and Per Capita Income

Racial patterns of fall mortality differ substantially from racial patterns of other injury deaths. For all falls among all ages combined, the death rate is more than 50 percent higher among whites than blacks and Native Americans, and almost four times the rate for Asians. Until about age 70, however, the death rate from falls is higher among blacks than whites (figures 10-6 and 10-7). The higher rate among elderly whites is consistent with the greater prevalence of osteoporosis and the higher rate of fracture of the hip for whites.[6,20]

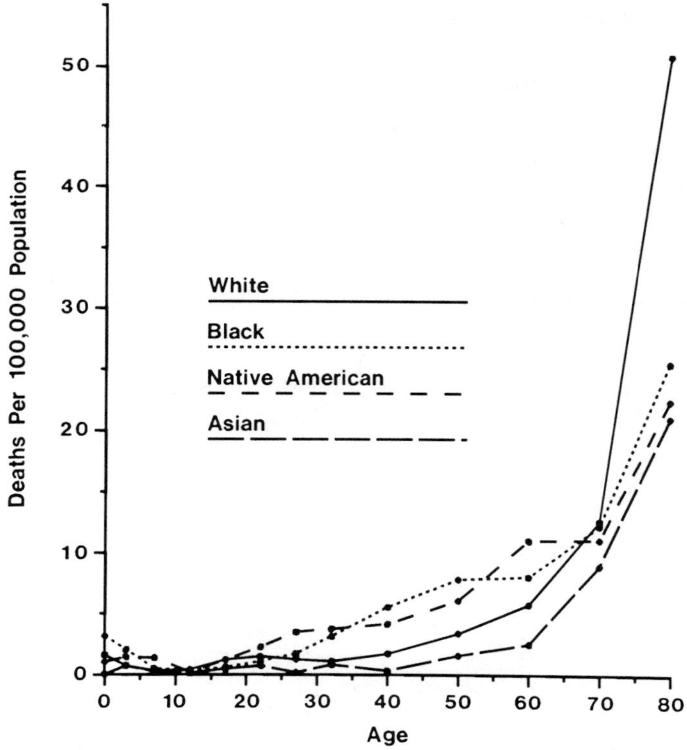

Figure 10-6. Death Rates from Falls by Age and Race, 1977-1979

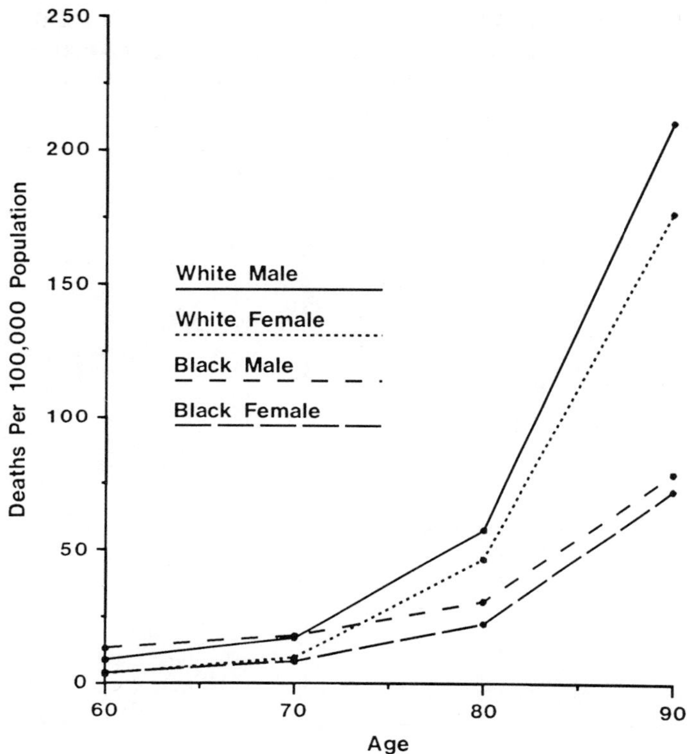

Figure 10-7. Death Rates from Falls by Age, Sex, and Race, for Ages 60 and Older, 1977-1979

The racial pattern varies with the type of fall. For falls on one level, which predominantly involve the elderly, the death rate is three times as high among whites as blacks. For falls from buildings or other structures, the death rate is 67 percent higher among blacks than whites. In considering such comparisons, it must be remembered that the circumstances are not specified for the majority of falls.

Of all injuries, falls show the least relationship to per capita income of the area of residence (figure 4-9). While this is true of both whites and blacks, the death rates among Native Americans and Asians in low-income areas are about twice the rates in high-income areas.

Urban/Rural and Geographic Differences

For all falls combined, there is little difference between death rates in cities and rural areas. For specific kinds of falls, however, substantial urban/rural differences are apparent (figure 10-8). Falls from buildings or other structures and falls on stairs occur disproportionately in large cities. In cities where many families live in high apartment buildings,

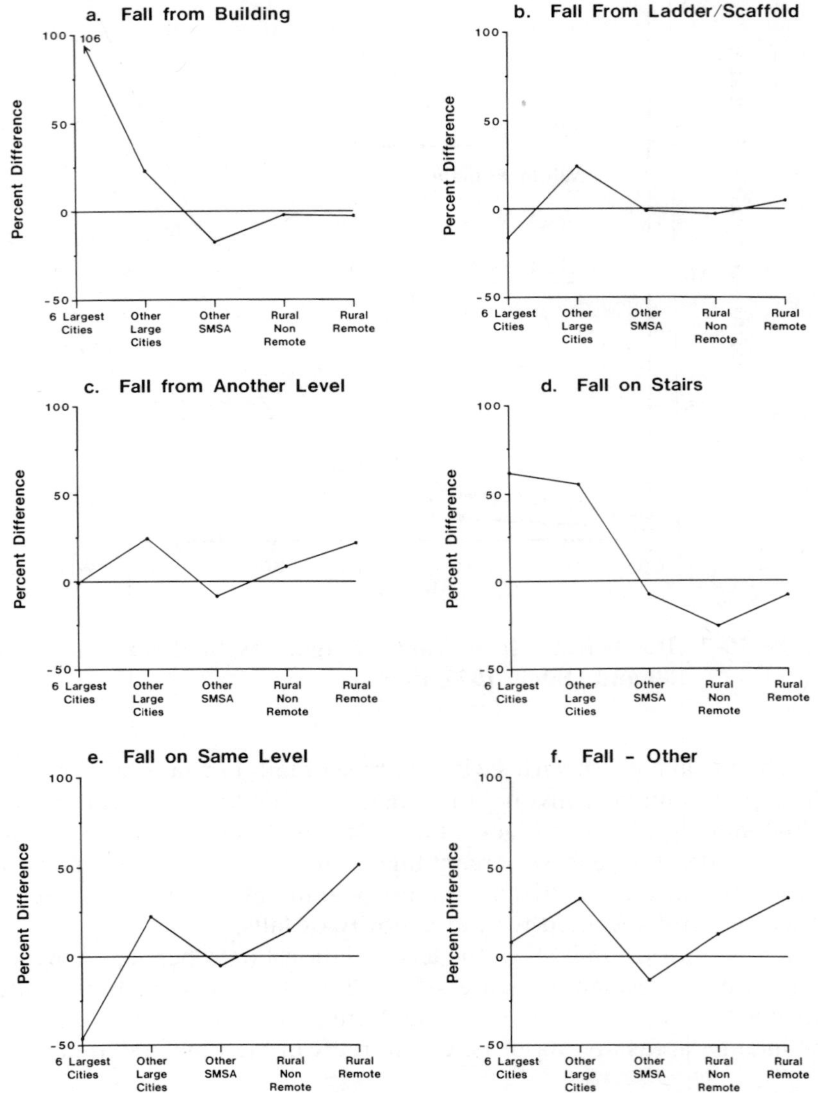

Figure 10-8. Percent Difference from the Average Death Rates from Falls by Type and Place of Residence, 1977-1979

children appear to be at special risk of being killed in falls from buildings. In recognition of this problem, the New York City Board of Health requires landlords to provide window guards for apartments in which children age 10 or younger are living.[18]

There is considerable geographic variation in death rates from falls, with northern states generally having higher death rates than southern states (figure 4-12). This is true in summer as well as winter, suggesting that the phenomenon is not explained by the longer, colder, and icier northern winters.

Since overall death rates from falls are largely determined by the high rates among elderly whites, state-specific rates were calculated for whites only, subdivided into two broad age groups (figure 10-9). Among people younger than 65, whose deaths from falls frequently involve working males who fall on stairs or from heights, the death rates do not show a strong North-South pattern. In fact, rates for this age group are highest in the West. For whites age 65 or older, death rates tend to be higher in the northern states. The exceptions to this pattern may be due to differences among states in the age distributions of their populations. In Alaska, for example, which has a low death rate from falls among ages 65 and older, the median age of this group is low compared to the rest of the United States. However, the generally higher rates in the northern half of the country appear not to be explained by the age mix of the 65-and-older population, since even age-adjusted rates for this age group are high in northern states.[13]

Given the seriousness of the problem of falls among the elderly, further exploration of the geographic differences would be worthwhile. Some of the differences could be due to variations in describing and coding deaths, so such research should include comparisons of state practices regarding the certification of the cause and manner of deaths from late complications of injury.

Historical Trends

The trend in death rates from falls from 1968 to 1979 has been downward. While the overall death rate decreased by 37 percent, this decrease was not uniform across age groups (figure 10-10). There was little change among ages 15-24. The greatest decrease (68 percent) was among children younger than one year; this was very close to the 64 percent decrease for this age group from all unintentional injuries.

During the past two decades, there has been an important shift in the sex ratio for fall deaths among elderly whites. In 1960, the female rate was about 20 percent higher than the male rate for ages 75 and

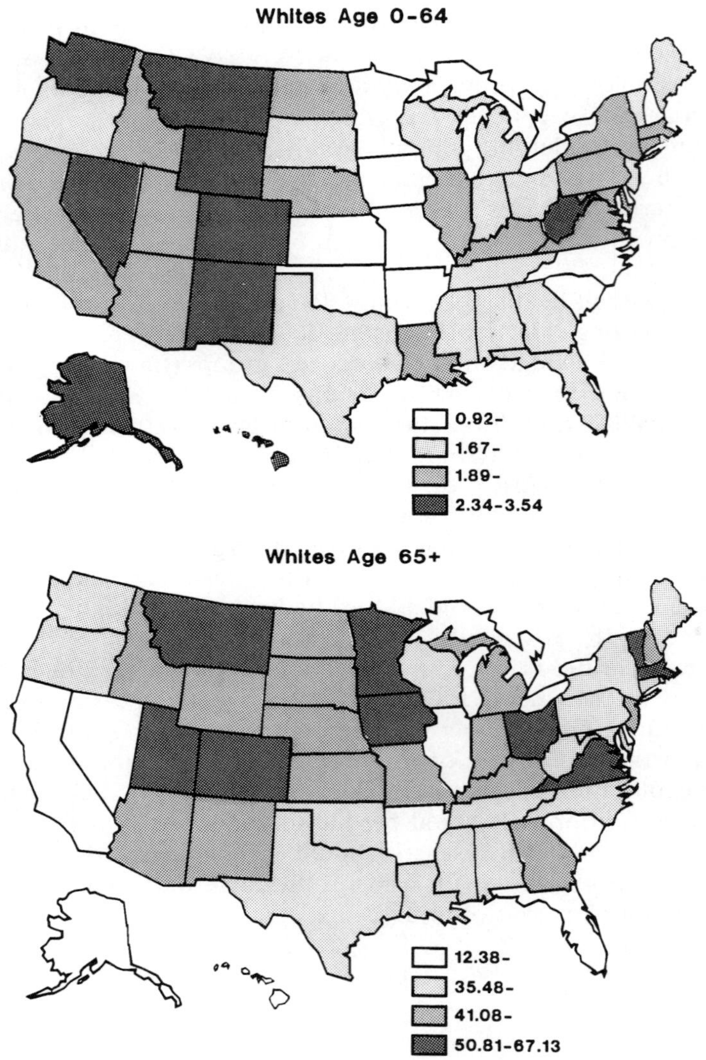

Figure 10-9. Death Rates from Falls by State and Age for Whites, Per 100,000 Population, 1977-1979

older.[13] By 1979, it was about 20 percent lower than the male rate. This shift occurred because the death rate from falls in the elderly declined more for females than for males between 1960 and 1979. During the 1968-1979 period, the decrease was 59 percent for females

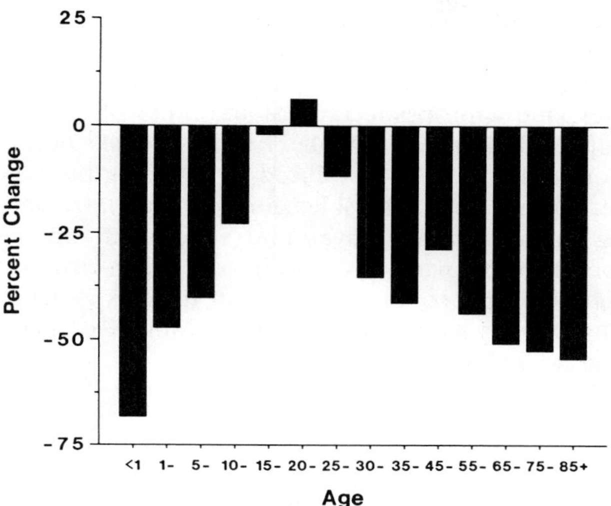

Figure 10-10. Percent Change in Death Rates from Falls by Age, Based on 1968-1979 Trend

and 43 percent for males among ages 75 and older. For age groups younger than 65, there was little difference between the sexes in the percent change.

The shift in the sex ratio for fall mortality may result from an improved ability of the medical care system to prevent fatal complications following injury. Consistent with this hypothesis is the fact that among the elderly who die following falls, a greater proportion of males have fallen on stairs or from heights and thus could be expected to have sustained more severe injuries, on average, than females. Further, the ratio of moderate to severe injury among people with fractures is higher in females and increases with age in both sexes.[3] Reductions in injury mortality probably have been greatest for less severe injuries that usually are not immediately fatal. Specific studies are needed, however, to explore the complex relationships between age, sex, height of fall, severity of injury, and survival patterns.

In general, preventive efforts have emphasized the behavioral aspects of falls, despite the difficulty of changing relevant behaviors such as hurrying, shuffling, or thrill seeking. Often ignored has been the potential benefit from modifying the environment. Particular attention needs to be given to the design of private homes, where most fall injuries occur, nursing homes and other facilities for the elderly where the population is at especially high risk of fall injury, and playgrounds. In these and many other places, falls should be anticipated and the potential for serious injury reduced or eliminated. Good lighting and visual clues, walking surfaces that provide adequate friction and are free of irregularities, and appropriate railings and other physical barriers are among the means of preventing falls. Even when falls occur, the likelihood of injury can be greatly reduced by reducing the height of falls (playground slides built into hillsides, for example) or by placing energy-attenuating surfaces under playground equipment, on the floors of nursing homes, below windows, and in other high-risk areas. One of the most ignored opportunities to prevent injuries is the rounding of likely contact points such as table edges, cabinet corners, and stair edges to spread impact forces.

Notes

1. Baker, S.P., J.S. Samkoff, R.S. Fisher, and C.B. Van Buren. "Fatal Occupational Injuries." *Journal of the American Medical Association* 248 (1982): 692-697.

2. Barancik, J.I., B.F. Chatterjee, Y.C. Greene, E.M. Michenzi, and D. Fife. "Northeastern Ohio Trauma Study: I. Magnitude of the Problem." *American Journal of Public Health* 73 (1983): 746-751.

3. Bauer, G.C.H. "Epidemiology of Fracture in Aged Persons — A Preliminary Investigation in Fracture Etiology." *Clinical Orthopaedics* 17 (1960): 219-225.

4. Bureau of Labor Statistics. *Occupational Injuries and Illnesses in the United States by Industry, 1981*. Washington, DC: United States Department of Labor, January 1983.

5. De Haven, H. "Mechanical Analysis of Survival in Falls from Heights of Fifty to One Hundred and Fifty Feet." *War Medicine* 2 (1942): 539-546.

6. Engh, G., A.J. Bollet, G. Hardin, and W. Parson. "Epidemiology of Osteoporosis II. Incidence of Hip Fractures in Mental Institutions." *The Journal of Bone and Joint Surgery* 50A (1968): 557-562.

7. Gallagher, S.S., B. Guyer, M. Kotelchuck, J. Bass, F.H. Lovejoy, Jr., E. McLoughlin, and K. Mehta. "A Strategy for the Reduction of Childhood Injuries in Massachusetts: SCIPP." *The New England Journal of Medicine* 307 (1982): 1015-1019.

8. Gryfe, C.I., A. Amies, and M.J. Ashley. "A Longitudinal Study of Falls in an Elderly Population: I. Incidence and Morbidity." *Age and Ageing* 6 (1977): 201-210.

9. Haddon, W., Jr. "Advances in the Epidemiology of Injuries as a Basis for Public Policy." *Public Health Reports* 95 (1980): 411-421.

10. Haddon, W., Jr., E.A. Suchman, and D. Klein. *Accident Research: Methods and Approaches*. New York: Harper and Row, 1964.

11. Haupt, B.J., and E. Graves. *Detailed Diagnoses and Surgical Procedures for Patients Discharged from Short-Stay Hospitals: United States, 1979*. DHHS Publication No. (PHS) 82-1274-1. Washington, DC: U.S. Department of Health and Human Services, 1982.

12. Hongladarom, G.C., W.F. Miller, J.M. Jones, D. Sandison, K. Van Dusen, B.D. Ford, and C.J. Colfer. *Analysis of the Causes and Prevention of Injuries Attributed to Falls*. Olympia, WA: Office of Environmental Health Programs, Department of Social and Health Services, 1977.

12. Iskrant, A.P., and P.V. Joliet. *Accidents and Homicide*. Cambridge, MA: Harvard University Press, 1968.

14. Johnson, R.E., and E.E. Specht. "The Risk of Hip Fracture in Postmenopausal Females With and Without Estrogen Drug Exposure." *American Journal of Public Health* 71 (1981): 128-144.

15. Kraus, J.F., M.A. Black, N. Hessol, P. Ley, W. Rokaw, C. Sullivan, S. Bowers, S. Knowlton, and L. Marshall. "The Incidence of Acute Brain Injury and Serious Impairment in a Defined Population." *American Journal of Epidemiology* 119 (1984): 186-201.

16. Kraus, J.F., C.E. Franti, R.S. Riggins, D. Richards, and N.O. Borhani. "Incidence of Traumatic Spinal Cord Lesions." *Journal of Chronic Diseases* 28 (1975): 471-492.

17. Merrild, U., and S. Bak. "An Excess of Pedestrian Injuries in Icy Conditions: A High-Risk Fracture Group — Elderly Women." *Accident Analysis and Prevention* 15 (1983): 41-48.

18. Spiegel, C.N., and F.C. Lindaman. "Children Can't Fly: A Program to Prevent Childhood Morbidity and Mortality from Window Falls." *American Journal of Public Health* 67 (1977): 1143-1147.

19. Statewide Childhood Injury Prevention Program. "Target Injuries to Young Children." *SCIPP Reports* 4, Boston, MA: Department of Public Health, Division of Family Services, Spring 1983.

20. Trotter, M., G.E. Broman, and R.R. Peterson. "Densities of Bones of White and Negro Skeletons." *The Journal of Bone and Joint Surgery* 42A (1960): 50-58.

11 Firearms

Firearms account for one-fifth of all injury deaths and are second only to motor vehicles as a cause of fatal injury. In 1980, shootings caused almost 34,000 deaths (table 11-1). Shootings are the sixth leading cause of fatal unintentional injury for all ages combined, and the third leading cause at ages 10-19. Two out of three homicides and four out of seven suicides are caused by firearms, as are virtually all deaths from "legal intervention" (see Chapter 3). Also an important source of work-related fatalities, firearms are an especially serious hazard to law enforcement agents as well as taxi drivers, storekeepers, and others whose jobs make them likely targets for armed robberies.[2]

In general, there are few reliable sources of data on nonfatal firearm injury. One population-based study in Northern California found that only motor vehicle crashes and falls surpassed shootings as a cause of spinal cord injury.[6] Reflecting the severity of firearm-related injury, the death rate among patients hospitalized because of head injuries is many times higher for gunshot wounds than for any other type of injury.[5] The best available national estimate of nonfatal firearm injuries from NHIS is 155,000 gunshot injuries in 1972. The estimate is based on a relatively small sample with correspondingly large potential for error.[7]

Some of the similarities and differences between intentional and unintentional firearm deaths will be pointed out in this section. Additional details on firearm suicide and homicide can be found in Chapters 5 and 6.

Table 11–1
Firearm Deaths as a Percent of All Injury Deaths, by Major Category, 1980

Category	*Firearm Deaths*	*All Deaths*	*Percent Firearm*
Unintentional	1,955	105,718	2
Suicide	15,404	26,869	57
Homicide	15,522	23,967	65
Legal intervention	303	311	97
Undetermined and other	629	3,686	17
Total	33,813	160,551	21

Source: National Center for Health Statistics, unpublished data, 1980.

Age and Sex

The death rate from unintentional shootings is highest for males ages 13-17 (figure 4-4). Females show a less pronounced increase than males during the teen and young adult years. For all ages combined, the female death rate is only one-sixth the male rate. Similarly, for homicide and suicide by firearm, the female rate is about one-fifth the male rate (figure 3-4).

Race and Per Capita Income

Death rates from unintentional shootings are highest among Native Americans: 2.2 per 100,000, compared to 1.2 for blacks, 0.8 for whites, and 0.1 for Asians. When examined by 5-year age groups, the rate peaks sharply among whites at ages 15-19, whereas among blacks the rate remains high until the mid-thirties (figure 11-1). Black males ages

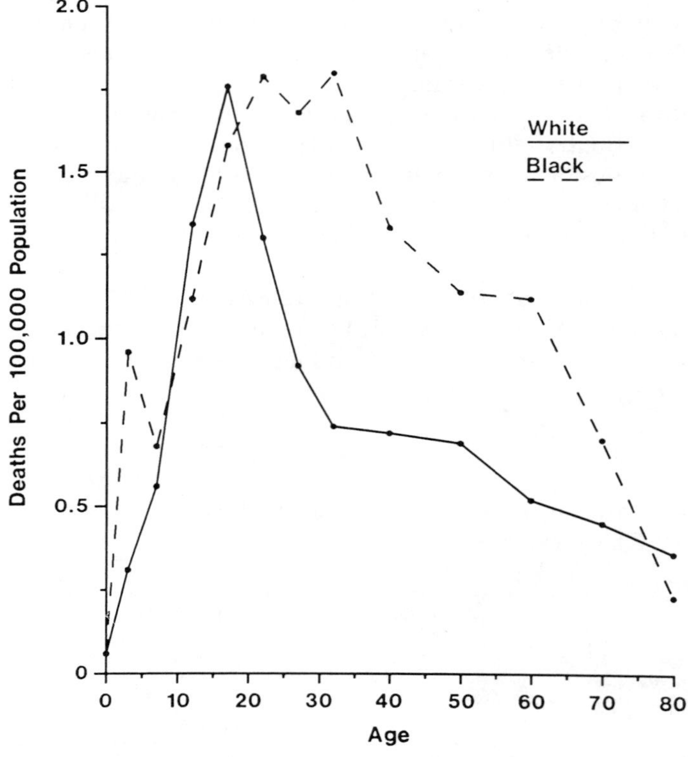

Figure 11-1. Death Rates from Unintentional Firearm Injury by Age and Race, 1977-1979

1-4 have a high death rate (1.5), more than three times the rate for black females or white males.

Death rates are highest in low-income areas, where they are almost identical for whites and blacks. For the population as a whole, the association between high death rates and low per capita income is stronger than for any other cause of unintentional injury. This association is not evident for large cities, but it is seen in other SMSAs and in rural nonremote counties (figure 11-2). In rural remote counties (not shown), the death rate is especially high in both low-income and high-income counties; many of the latter are in Alaska.

For suicide and homicide, the correlation between firearm death rates and per capita income is not as strong as for unintentional injuries (figure 11-3). Among whites, for example, the rate for unintentional firearm deaths is ten times as high in areas of low per capita income as in high-income areas. The comparable ratio is 2:1 for firearm suicides and homicides.

Urban/Rural and Geographic Differences

The death rate in remote rural areas from unintentional shootings is seven times the rate in the largest cities (figure 11-4). For homicides, the trend is in the opposite direction. Consistent with the high death

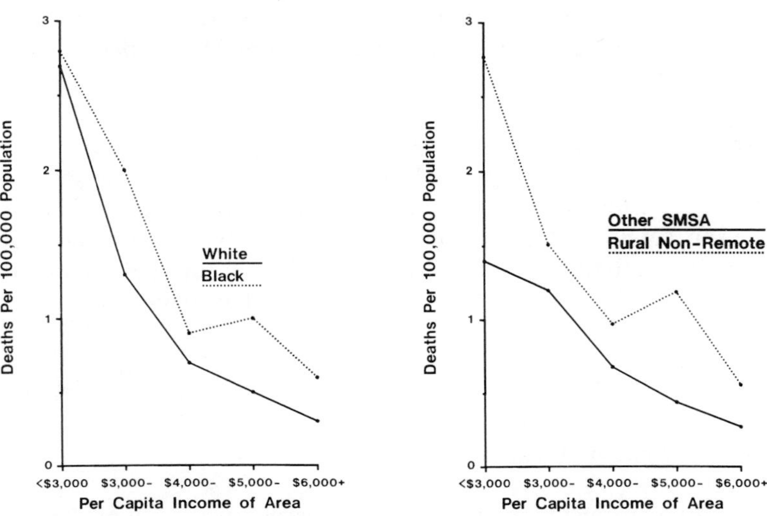

Figure 11-2. Death Rates from Unintentional Firearm Injury by Per Capita Income and Race, and by Per Capita Income and Place of Residence, 1977-1979

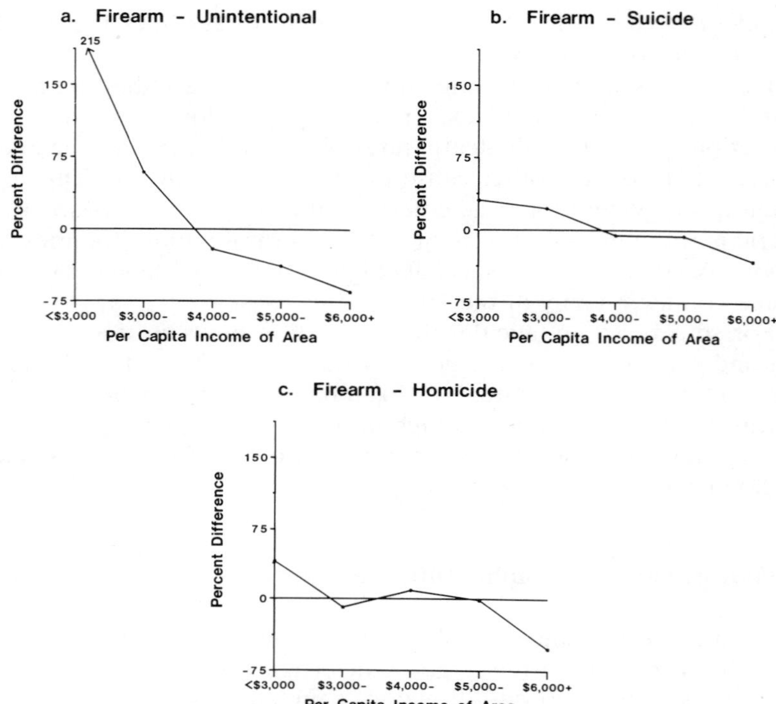

Figure 11-3. Percent Difference from the Average Death Rates from Firearms by Per Capita Income of Area of Residence for Unintentional Deaths, Suicides, and Homicides, 1977-1979

rates from unintentional shootings in rural areas, the regions with the highest rates are generally the South and northern mountain states (figure 11-5). This pattern generally resembles the geographic pattern for firearm suicides (figure 5-9). Death rates from firearm homicides are also high in the South but are relatively low in some of the northern mountain states (figure 6-9), where death rates from unintentional shootings are high.

Season and Type of Weapon

Unintentional firearm deaths exhibit a pronounced seasonal pattern, with one-fourth occurring in November and December, the primary

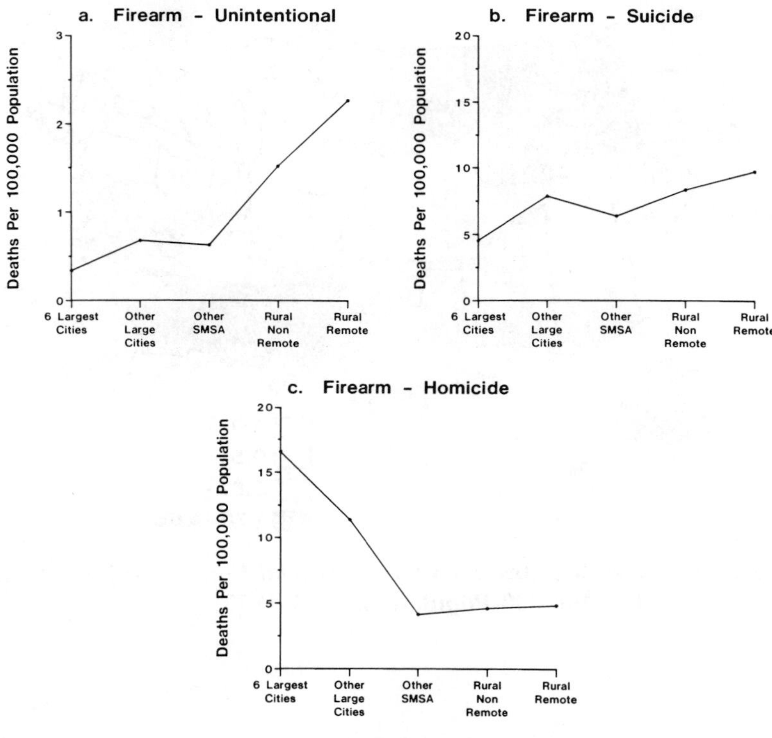

Figure 11-4. Death Rates from Firearms by Place of Residence for Unintentional Deaths, Suicides, and Homicides, 1977-1979

hunting season in most areas (figure 4-15). Unfortunately, ICD codes do not distinguish deaths that occur in connection with hunting.

The best information on the type of weapon involved in homicides comes from police investigations. According to the Federal Bureau of Investigation, almost 80 percent of firearm homicides are by handguns (figure 11-6).[4] Comparable police data are not available for suicides and unintentional shootings.

Death certificates do not indicate the type of firearm in the case of 4 out of 5 firearm homicides and 2 out of 3 firearm suicides and unintentional deaths. A bias toward recording long guns, while leaving the weapon unspecified in the case of handguns, is suggested by the fact that among the relatively few firearms specified on homicide death certificates, the number of shotguns exceeds the number of handguns. (Therefore, although handguns predominate among weapons *men-*

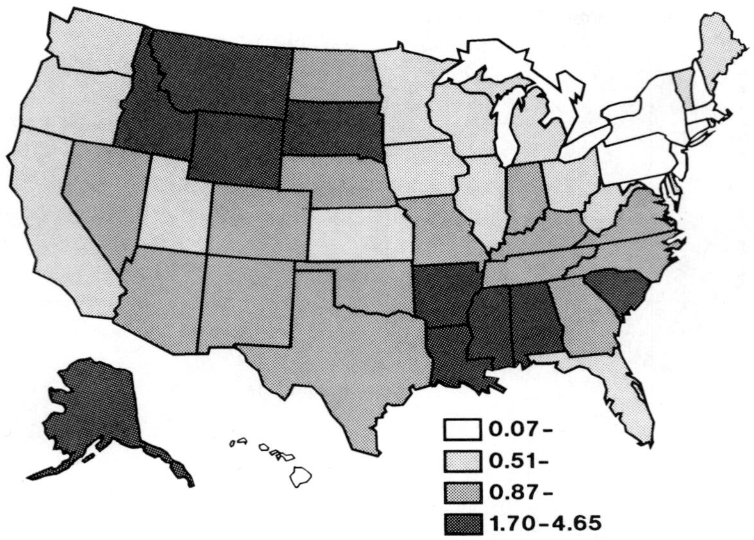

Figure 11-5. Death Rates from Unintentional Firearm Injury by State, Per 100,000 Population, 1977-1979

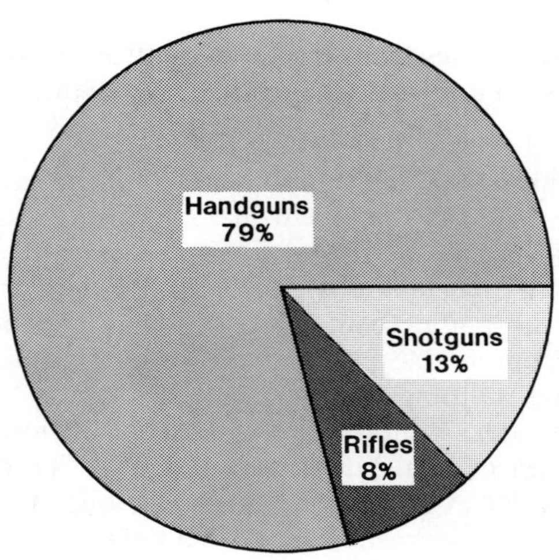

Figure 11-6. Percent of Firearm Homicides by Type of Weapon, FBI, 1981

tioned in suicides and unintentional firearm deaths, currently available national death certificate data should not be used to estimate their overall contribution to deaths from firearms.)

Historical Trends

From 1930 to 1980, the death rate from unintentional firearm injury decreased by about two-thirds. Firearm suicide and homicide rates decreased substantially during World War II and then increased, so there was little net change (figures 5-10 and 6-10).

Trend analysis of unintentional firearm death rates during 1968-1979 reveals an overall decline of 29 percent. The smallest decrease occurred for ages 5-14; otherwise the decline was fairly consistent among the age groups (figure 11-7). During the same period, death rates from

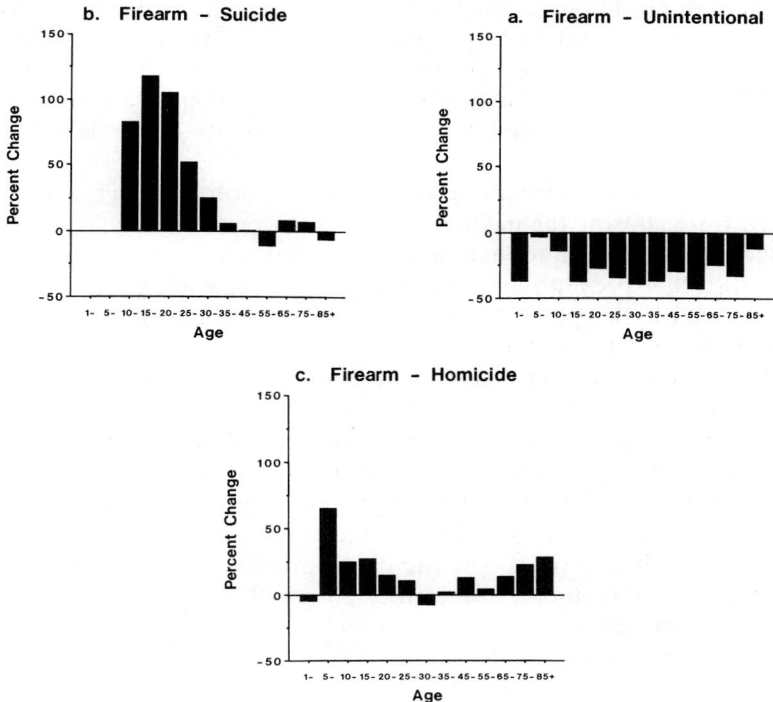

Figure 11-7. Percent Change in Death Rates from Firearms by Age for Unintentional Deaths, Suicides, and Homicides, Based on 1968-1979 Trend

firearm suicides increased by 30 percent overall and approximately doubled in age groups younger than 25. For firearm homicides, there was a 21 percent increase, with the largest increase among 5-9 year olds.

The gradual decline in unintentional shooting deaths during the past half-century has been slightly greater than for unintentional injuries as a whole, 66 percent versus 59 percent (table 4-2). This may reflect increasing urbanization and general improvements in the economic status of the population. The very high rural:urban ratio of death rates from firearms and the exceptionally strong correlation with low per capita income are consistent with such speculation.

Firearm injuries and deaths, intentional as well as unintentional, can be prevented through application of a broad spectrum of approaches. Potentially effective measures include reducing weapons and ammunition through limitations on production or importation. Efforts to keep guns from young children and to prevent handgun possession by criminals are likely to have only limited success if widespread ownership by the general public is permitted. The common tendency to focus on gun purchases by potential criminals ignores the difficulty of regulating the sale and distribution of a widely available commodity, as well as the fact that most homicides are committed by relatives and acquaintances.

The motives and circumstances of many shootings suggest possible benefit from altering the incentives (e.g., making cash unavailable) and disincentives (e.g., illuminating convenience stores and other likely targets). Other preventive possibilities include providing high-risk employees with bullet-proof barriers or clothing and altering the characteristics of weapons and ammunition.[1,3,8,9]

The type of firearm involved in shooting deaths is important for policy related to injury prevention. Handguns are readily concealed, a characteristic that makes them easier to use to kill people intentionally, although it is not essential to their usefulness in target practice, hunting, or even home protection, which is the major reason given for handgun ownership. It was noted earlier that the trend over time in homicides has been largely determined by firearm homicides (figure 6-10). In fact, the shape of the homicide curve since about 1970 has been dictated by *handgun* homicides alone, with relatively little change in death rates from rifles and shotguns.[9]

Notes

1. Baker, S.P., and P.E. Dietz. "The Epidemiology and Prevention of Injuries." In *The Management of Trauma*, edited by G.D. Zuidema,

R.B. Rutherford, and W.G. Ballinger, II. Philadelphia: W.B. Saunders Company, 1979.

2. Baker, S.P., J.S. Samkoff, R.S. Fisher, and C.B. Van Buren. "Fatal Occupational Injuries." *Journal of the American Medical Association* 248 (1982): 692-697.

3. Baker, S.P., S.P. Teret, and P.E. Dietz. "Firearms and the Public Health." *Journal of Public Health Policy* 1 (1980): 224-229.

4. Federal Bureau of Investigation. *Uniform Crime Reports in the United States, 1981*. Washington, DC: U.S. Government Printing Office, August 26, 1982.

5. Jagger, J., J.I. Levine, J.A. Jane, and R.W. Rimel. "Epidemiologic Features of Head Injury in a Predominantly Rural Population." *Journal of Trauma* 24 (1984): 40-44.

6. Kraus, J.F., C.E. Franti, R.S. Riggins, D. Richards, and N.O. Borhani. "Incidence of Traumatic Spinal Cord Lesions." *Journal of Chronic Diseases* 28 (1975): 471-492.

7. National Center for Health Statistics. *Persons Injured and Disability Days by Detailed Type and Class of Accident, United States, 1971-1972*. Rockville, MD: U.S. Department of Health, Education, and Welfare, 1976.

8. Robertson, L.S. *Injuries: Causes, Control Strategies, and Public Policy*. Lexington, MA: Lexington Books, 1983.

9. Teret, S.P., and G.J. Wintemute. "Handgun Injuries: The Epidemiologic Evidence for Assessing Legal Responsibility." *Hamline Law Review* 6 (1983): 341-350.

12 Burns and Fire Deaths

Burns and fires are surpassed only by motor vehicle crashes, falls, and drownings as a cause of unintentional injury death. In recent years they have caused about 6,000 deaths annually. This figure does not include deaths related to arson or "suspicious circumstances," estimated at 500 annually, which are included with homicides or deaths of undetermined intent. In addition, deaths associated with post-crash fires are counted among deaths from motor vehicle and airplane crashes.

More than a million burn injuries each year require medical attention or restriction of activity.[15] Of these, about one-third are treated at hospital emergency departments. The 90,000 patients admitted to hospitals each year with burns require over a million days of hospital care, or an average of 12 days per admission.[10] For severely burned patients, such as those who need skin grafting, lengthy hospitalizations and multiple admissions are often necessary. Disability, disfigurement, and emotional problems are common sequelae.

Burns are usually caused by thermal energy. They may also result from exposure to certain chemicals, electricity, ultraviolet radiation, and ionizing radiation. This chapter focuses on thermal energy burns, which occur when heat reaches the body in amounts or at rates that exceed the body's ability to dissipate the heat. Included among deaths attributed to fires are those resulting from exposure to the toxic by-products of combustion. In housefires and other conflagrations, the great majority of deaths are actually due to carbon monoxide poisoning.

However, until recently mortality data did not differentiate between fire deaths from combustion products and those from burns. In 1980, of all deaths from housefires (i.e., conflagrations in private dwellings, including trailers), 66 percent were attributed to carbon monoxide or unspecified fumes, 28 percent to burns, and 4 percent to falls or building collapse. The remaining 2 percent were unspecified.

Housefires

Housefires cause three-fourths of all deaths from fires and burns (table 12-1). Death rates are highest among young children and the elderly

Table 12–1
Primary Causes of Fire and Burn Deaths, 1980

	Number	*Percent of Total*
Housefire (conflagration)	4,509	75
Conflagration, other building	292	5
Other uncontrolled fire	66	1
Controlled fire	66	1
Ignition of clothing	311	5
Ignition of highly flammable material	105	2
Ignition of bedclothes	53	1
Other or unspecified fire	420	7
Hot liquid or steam	161	3
Other or unspecified hot substance	33	1
Total	6,016	101[a]

Source: National Center for Health Statistics, unpublished data, 1980.
[a]Percents do not add to 100 due to rounding.

(figure 12-1), in part because of their difficulty in escaping from burning buildings. In addition, young and old people have higher case-fatality rates than people of intermediate ages with burn injuries of comparable extent and severity.[4] In the case of housefires, however, the relationship

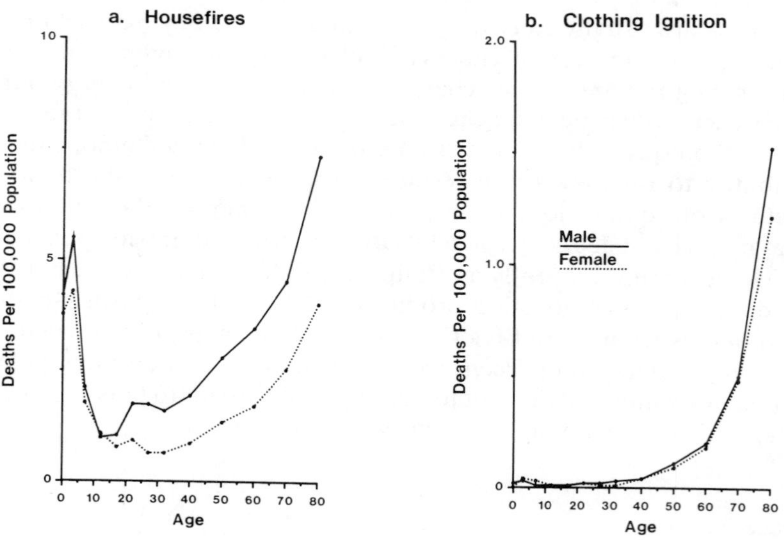

Figure 12-1. Death Rates from Housefires and Clothing Ignition by Age and Sex, 1977-1979

between age and ability to survive injury is less important than for other burns, since housefire deaths usually involve either carbon monoxide poisoning or incineration, which are rapidly lethal events at any age.

The male:female ratio for housefire deaths is 1.6 to 1, less than for most injury deaths (figure 3-4). Among children, the greatest sex difference is at ages 2-3 (figure 4-5g), when boys also have the highest rates for nonfatal burns from playing with matches.[5] About 2 percent of residential fire deaths are attributed to children playing with matches, cigarette lighters, and other ignition sources.[16]

Cigarettes are the leading cause of fatal housefires, about half of which are started by smoldering cigarettes that ignite upholstered furniture or mattresses.[3] Heating equipment is the second leading ignition source.[16]

Among blacks and Native Americans, housefire death rates are more than twice the rate for whites. In both groups, the rates are high among young children (figure 12-2). Among Native Americans they

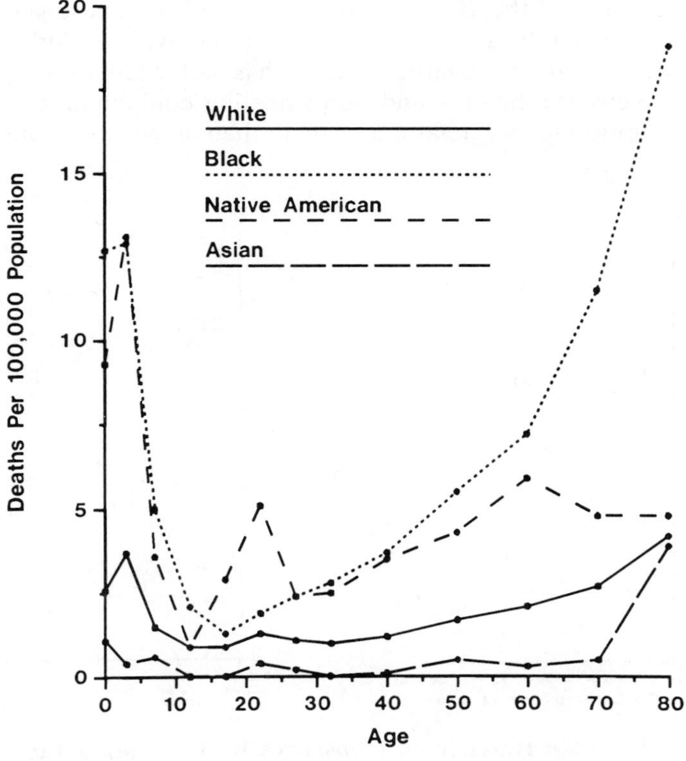

Figure 12-2. Death Rates from Housefires by Age and Race, 1977-1979

peak again at ages 15-24, while the rates for blacks increase throughout the adult years. The racial differences in housefire death rates diminish in higher-income areas (figure 12-3).

For both races, death rates are more than twice as high in areas of low per capita income. As might be expected, ignition sources vary with income. A Baltimore study found that although cigarettes were the primary ignition source at all income levels, the proportion of fires ignited by faulty heating or electrical systems was greatest in low-income areas.[14]

Housefire death rates for whites show little variation with place of residence, while for blacks the rates are about twice as high in rural areas. These urban-rural differences probably reflect not only economic disparities, but also differences in housing materials and heating methods, the likelihood of fires being detected, and, especially in remote areas, the availability and response time of fire equipment.

There is a pronounced geographic pattern in housefire deaths, with high death rates in the East, especially the Southeast, and low rates in the western half of the United States (figure 12-4). These geographic patterns are generally similar for whites and nonwhites. Although the high death rate in the southern states has not been thoroughly researched, kerosene heaters and other heating equipment are a more common ignition source in fatal fires there than in the rest of the United

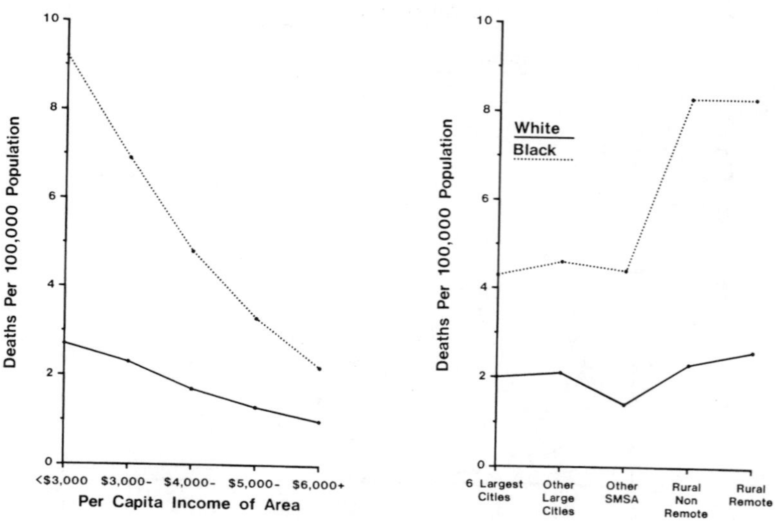

Figure 12-3. Death Rates from Housefires by Per Capita Income and Race, and by Place of Residence and Race, 1977-1979

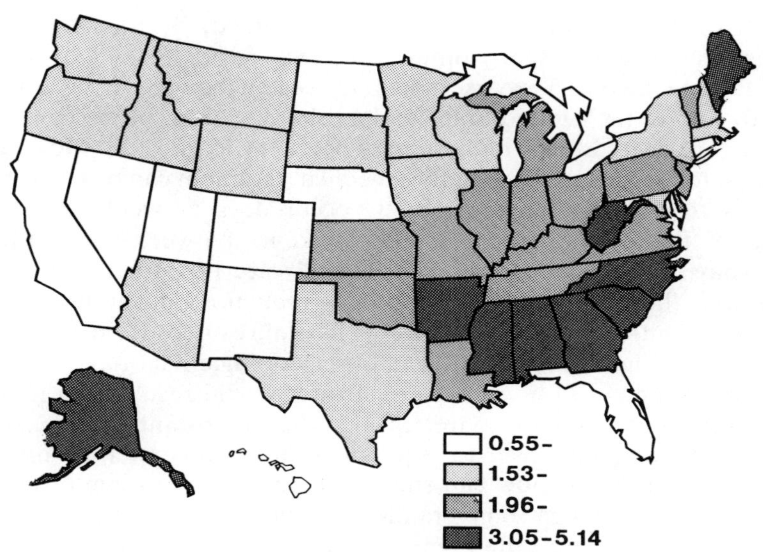

Figure 12-4. Death Rates from Housefires by State, Per 100,000 Population, 1977-1979

States.[16] The availability and use of wood for building materials and fuel also probably play a role in regional differences.

The majority of housefire deaths occur during December-March, when the weather is cold, the hours of darkness long, and heating and lighting systems most utilized. Deaths are more than three times as common in January as in July (figure 4-15i). Weekends are disproportionately represented (figure 4-14e), consistent with evidence of high blood alcohol concentrations in about half of the adults who die in housefires.[9,14] The association between cigarette and alcohol use is important because intoxication increases the likelihood that a lighted cigarette will fall unnoticed onto a chair or bed and remain undetected. After smoldering, often for several hours, fire erupts and may then spread very rapidly. Typically, deaths from cigarette-initiated housefires occur between midnight and 6:00 A.M.

Injuries from housefires and other conflagrations, while the major cause of death, account for only a small fraction of hospital admissions for burns — about 4 percent of the burn admissions in New York State.[7] The fatality rate among patients hospitalized for burns from conflagrations is higher than for burns from other causes; about 12 percent of patients admitted with burns from conflagrations died during their first hospitalization, compared to 3 percent of other burn patients (table 12-

2). If deaths prior to admission were included, the fatality rate for housefires would be many times greater.

During the past 50 years, there has been an increase in the housefire death rate in the United States, while the rate from burns from other causes has decreased by more than 85 percent (figure 12-5). Most deaths related to housefires occur before medical treatment can be given, while deaths from other burns generally occur days or weeks later. This suggests that a major factor in the difference between the two trends may have been advances in the medical care of burned patients. In addition, there may have been greater reductions in the incidence of clothing ignitions and scalds than of housefires because of changes in clothing,[13,21] ignition sources, and other etiologic factors.

Improvement in housefire death rates would result from reducing the ignition potential of cigarettes and other important ignition sources such as heating and electrical equipment in low-income housing. Most brands of cigarettes now can smolder long enough to ignite furniture and bedding, although some brands self-extinguish more rapidly.[12] Much can be done to reduce the flammability of materials and the toxicity of their combustion products. Also important are building designs that inhibit the spread of fires and provide adequate escape routes. Smoke detectors and sprinkler systems that automatically extinguish fires could reduce housefire deaths as well as those in hotels, offices, airplanes, and other settings.

Table 12–2
Leading Causes of Hospital Admissions for Burns, New York State, 1974–1975

	Number of First Admissions	*Percent of Total*	*Deaths per 100 Admissions*
Hot liquids	1,654	29	1.2
Clothing ignition	583	10	10.6
Gasoline	367	6	2.7
Automotive	354	6	0.6
Chemicals	342	6	1.5
Grease	305	5	0.3
Conflagrations	213	4	11.7
Stoves	192	3	2.6
Other	1,781	31	2.6
Total	5,791	100	3.0

Source: G. Feck, M.S. Baptiste, and C.L. Tate, Jr., *An Epidemiologic Study of Burn Injuries and Strategies for Prevention,* Atlanta: U.S. Department of Health and Human Services, Public Health Service, Centers for Disease Control, 1978.

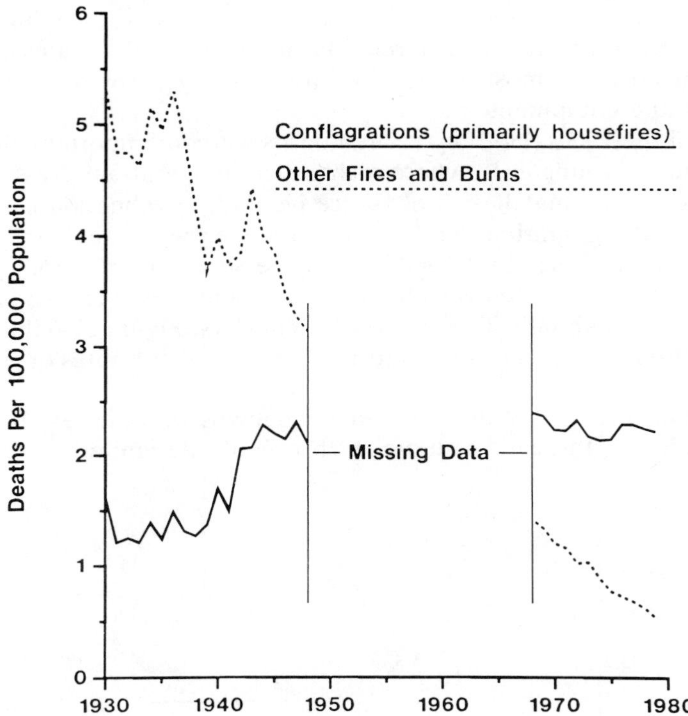

Figure 12-5. Death Rates from Conflagrations and from Other Fires and Burns by Year, 1930-1979

Other Burns

Death from clothing ignition, although second to housefires as a cause of burn mortality, today is relatively uncommon. Only 5 percent of all deaths related to fires and burns are caused by clothing ignition. About three-fourths of these occur among people age 65 or older. There is little sex difference in clothing ignition deaths, which now are rare among children (figure 12-1).[21]

Death rates from clothing ignition are extremely low among Asians: 0.03 per 100,000, compared to 0.14, 0.21, and 0.26 among whites, Native Americans, and blacks, respectively. For each of the last three racial groups, death rates are several times as high in low-income areas as in high-income areas. These findings for fatal burns are consistent with clothing burn injury rates, which one study found to be highest in low-income census tracts. The relationship between burn rates and per capita income was most pronounced for clothing burns related to appliances and equipment.[2]

Until the 1960s, clothing-related burns were an important cause of death among young girls, whose nightgowns and bouffant dresses were easily ignited by matches, fires, space heaters, or other sources.[18] Although clothing ignition deaths were combined with other fire deaths in national statistics until 1968, they were so common among young girls that the death rate from all flame burns and fires (including housefires) was substantially higher for girls than boys. Figure 12-6 illustrates the sex difference prior to the mid 1960s in burn death rates of children ages 5-9.

During the 1960s, dresses and nightgowns became less bouffant (thus reducing the ease with which they could be ignited), pants and

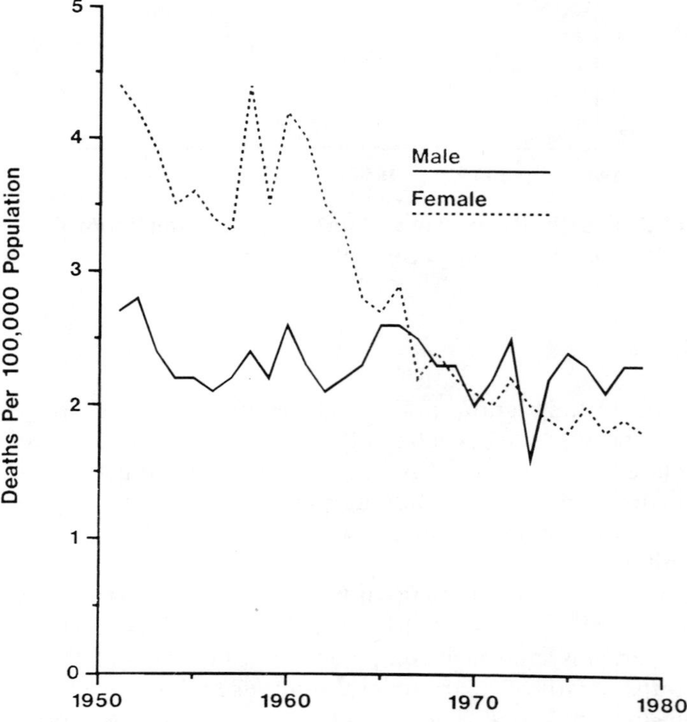

Figure 12-6. Death Rates from All Fires and Burns by Year and Sex, for Ages 5-9, 1951-1979

other tight-fitting clothing became popular among girls and women, the use of some highly flammable materials for clothing decreased, and burn survival rates improved.[4,21] During the same decade, the female excess in total burn deaths disappeared. In 1968, the first year for which national mortality data specific to clothing ignition burns became available, 40 girls and 11 boys ages 5-9 died following ignition of clothing. By 1980, the corresponding numbers were 1 and 0. For all ages combined, the trend in clothing ignition deaths between 1968 and 1979 produced a decrease of 71 percent among males and 82 percent among females, with the largest reductions among ages 0-14.

Although death rates have improved, nonfatal burns resulting from clothing ignition are still a matter of concern because they are often severe and potentially disfiguring. Cases admitted to hospitals have a fatality rate surpassed only by housefires (table 12-2). Because of the close proximity of clothing, which in the case of some fabrics may actually melt and stick to the body, clothing-related burns tend to be deeper and more extensive than nonfatal burns from many other sources.[2]

Burns from scalds and other contact with hot substances result in about 200 deaths each year, or 3 percent of all deaths from fires and burns. About 80 percent are caused by hot liquids or steam. Caustic or corrosive substances and hot objects cause the remainder. Scalds from hot liquids cause about 30 percent of all hospital admissions for burns (table 12-2). Thus, although the case-fatality ratio is low, scalds are a major source of burn morbidity and associated costs. This is especially true for children ages 0-4, who accounted for 45 percent of all admissions for hot liquid scalds in New York State.[1] Hot beverages, notably coffee, are a major cause of scalds to young children.

For all ages combined, hot water, including tap water in bathtubs and showers, is the leading source of scalds and of all hospital admissions for burns. The relative importance of various burn sources changes with age (figure 12-7). Hot liquids are the most important cause of hospitalized burns among children and the elderly. For most ages, clothing ignition is the second leading cause of burns resulting in hospital admission.

In the 15-24-year-old age group, the largest number of burn admissions in New York State were related to automobiles. Crashes caused more than one-fourth of such burns. Steam from radiators was also a frequent cause. The low ratio of deaths to injuries shown in table 12-2 for automotive burns is partly because a large proportion of deaths in post-crash fires occur at the scene of the fire; such cases that did not involve hospitalization were not included in the study.[8]

Substantial decreases have occurred in deaths from scalds and other

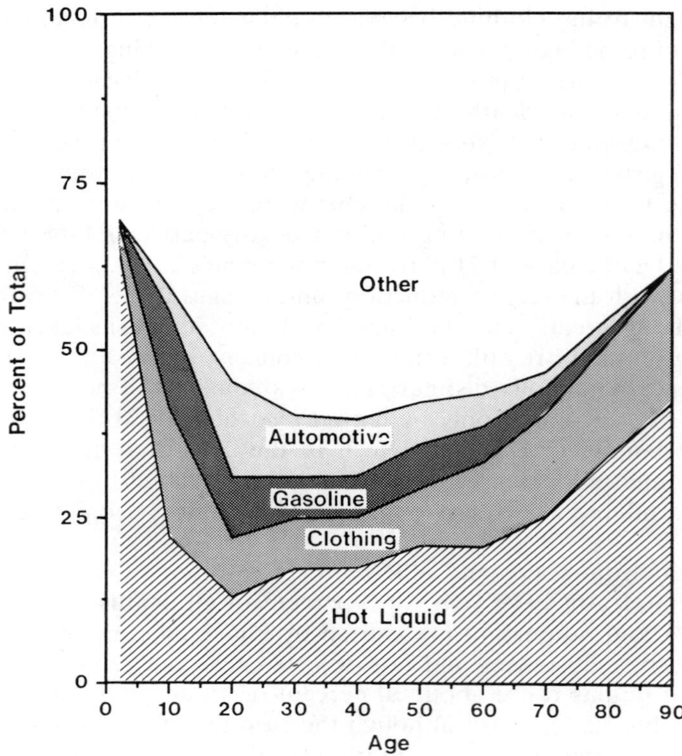

Figure 12-7. Percent of Hospital Admissions for Burns by Age and Cause, New York State Burn Study, 1974-1975

burns by hot substances. From 1968 to 1979, death rates from scalds decreased by about three-fourths for ages 0-19 and by almost half for all ages combined. Deaths resulting from ignition of highly flammable substances such as gasoline have also decreased by about two-thirds.

Probably the greatest potential for preventing scalds lies in modifying hot water systems. Although it is not uncommon for the temperature of tap water in homes and public buildings to be 160° F (71°C) or more, first degree burns can result from about 30 seconds of exposure to water above 130° F (54° C). More severe burns result from longer exposures or from higher temperatures. Consequently, hot water heaters and systems should be designed or modified so that people do not come in contact with water hotter than 130°F. This is especially important in bathtubs and showers, where large areas of the skin are exposed to water.[1,6-8]

Explosions

Explosions, electric current, and lightning are discussed in this chapter because all three may involve burns. None has been the subject of a population-based study. Explosions have killed about 350 people annually in recent years. These deaths primarily involve explosive gases; they exclude explosions involving tanker trucks and other road vehicles, as such deaths are counted with motor vehicle deaths. Most of the deaths occur on industrial sites (29 percent) or in homes (32 percent); only 2 percent occur in mines. As with many work-related injuries, the male:female ratio is high, about 7:1.

Among the states with high death rates (figure 12-8), several have many oil or gas fields, coal mines, or grain storage elevators.[17] Louisiana has the highest death rate from explosions (0.6), about 3 times the national average. Overall, the death rate from explosions during 1968-1979 decreased by about half.

Electric Current

Of the 1,100 deaths from electric current each year, about one-third occur in the home and one-fourth on industrial sites or farms. Death rates are highest among young adult males and then decline sharply (figure 12-9). The overall male:female ratio of 17:1 is one of the highest for all injury deaths. For deaths related to home wiring the ratio is 5:1, compared to 29:1 for other deaths from electricity, most of which are probably work-related.

Deaths from electric current are also unusual in their racial distribution. The death rate among whites is almost twice the rate among blacks, possibly reflecting employment patterns and availability of electricity. For both whites and blacks, the death rate in low-income counties is about twice the rate in high-income counties.

In rural areas the death rate from electric current is 3 times the rate in large cities. Higher rates in rural counties are seen for all income and racial groups. Oklahoma has the highest death rate, followed by other midwestern and southern states (figure 12-8). In general, the Pacific and northeastern states have the lowest rates. The pattern is very similar to that for explosions.

Like the geographic pattern, the pronounced seasonal variation in deaths from electric current suggests that further research on the epidemiology of these injuries would be of value. Following a seasonal distribution that appears to be a less exaggerated version of the pattern for lightning, deaths from electric current occur predominantly in the

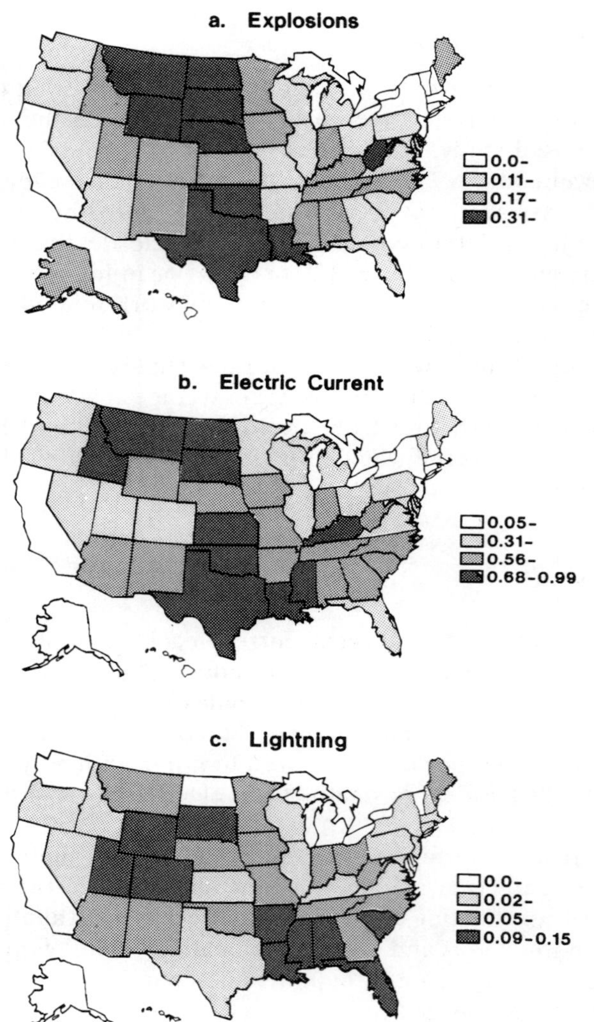

Figure 12-8. Death Rates from Explosions, Electric Current, and Lightning by State, Per 100,000 Population, 1977-1979

summer (figure 4-15).[20] The summertime peak may be partly related to seasonal patterns in construction work, since many electrocutions involve contact with overhead wires by cranes or other equipment. It may also be related to farm work, where electrocutions sometimes occur when long sections of irrigation pipe touch overhead wires while being

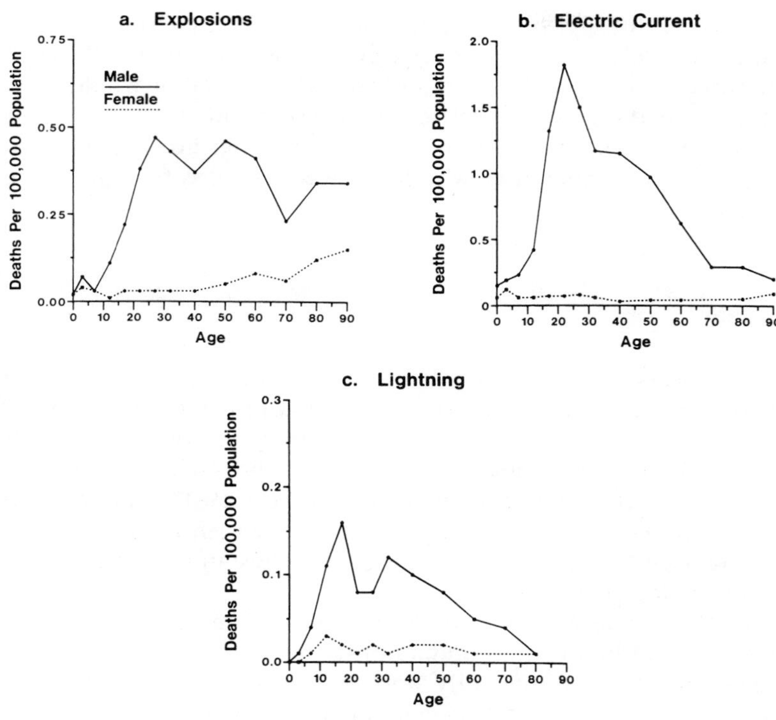

Figure 12-9. Death Rates from Explosions, Electric Current, and Lightning by Age and Sex, 1977-1979

repositioned.[11] Other factors that may contribute to the summertime peak include greater use of outdoor electrical equipment, which may be less likely to be grounded than equipment used indoors, and a tendency for people to perspire, which markedly lowers the skin's resistance to electric current. In addition, rainfall in late spring and summer, leading to moister earth, may increase electrical hazards. The importance of the problem warrants further research on the circumstances of electrocution and contributing factors, many of which could be altered.

As with other hazards, efforts to prevent electrical injuries and deaths should by no means be limited to providing workers and consumers with relevant information. Countermeasures include burying transmission lines or otherwise placing them out of reach and designing irrigation pipes that fold or separate into pieces that are too short to reach power lines. Improving insulation on crane booms and other equipment likely to be used near electrical wires, electrically shielding their cables and controls, using electronic sensors that would preclude contact with dangerous electrical fields or conductors, reducing the voltage, and installing ground fault interruptors are a few more examples of approaches that would reduce exposure to lethal doses of electricity.

Lightning

Lightning kills about 100 people each year in the United States, more than the average annual number of deaths attributable to any single type of "natural disaster." As with other injury-producing events, being struck by lightning is most common in certain high-risk groups. The rate of deaths from lightning is highest at ages 10-19, and it is 6 times as high among males as females. About one-fifth of all deaths from lightning occur on farms. Death rates are highest in southern and mountain states (figure 12-8).

Deaths are most common during the summer, when people are likely to be outdoors and thunderstorms are most common. Two-thirds of all deaths occur in June, July, and August (figure 4-15). Most involve people who are in open fields or on the water and/or are touching metal equipment, such as antennae. Deaths related to recreation are most apt to involve golfers, fishermen, and campers.[19]

During the past 50 years, the death rate from lightning has shown one of the largest decreases of all injuries (table 4-2). While part of the reported decrease is because deaths from fires ignited by lightning are no longer included with lightning deaths, the number of such deaths is now small. Probably much of the decrease reflects improvements in electrical systems and decreases in the farm population.

Notes

1. Baptiste, M.S., and G. Feck. "Preventing Tap Water Burns." *American Journal of Public Health* 70 (1980): 727-729.

2. Barancik, J.I., and M.A. Shapiro. "Pittsburgh Burn Study. Pittsburgh and Allegheny County, Pennsylvania, 1 June 1970-15 April 1971." Washington, DC: U.S. Consumer Product Safety Commission, May 1976.

3. Birky, M.M., B.M. Halpin, Y.H. Caplan, R.S. Fisher, J.M.

McAllister, and A.M. Dixon. "Fire Fatality Study." *Fire and Materials* 4 (1979): 211-217.

4. Bull, J.P. "Revised Analysis of Mortality Due to Burns." *The Lancet* 2 (1971): 1133-1134.

5. Consumer Product Safety Commission, Bureau of Epidemiology. "Annual Report of Flammable Fabric Data, Fiscal Year 1975." Washington, DC: U.S. Consumer Product Safety Commission.

6. Feck, G., and M.S. Baptiste. "The Epidemiology of Burn Injury in New York." *Public Health Reports* 94 (1979): 312-318.

7. Feck, G., M.S. Baptiste, and C.L. Tate, Jr. "Burn Injuries: Epidemiology and Prevention." *Accident Analysis and Prevention* 11 (1979): 129-136.

8. Feck, G., M.S. Baptiste, and C.L. Tate, Jr. *An Epidemiologic Study of Burn Injuries and Strategies for Prevention.* Atlanta: U.S. Department of Health and Human Services, Public Health Service, Centers for Disease Control, 1978.

9. Halpin, B.M., J.J. Dinan, and O.J. Deters. *Fire Problems Program-Assessment of the Potential Impact of Fire Protection Systems on Actual Fire Incidents.* Laurel, MD: The Johns Hopkins University Applied Physics Laboratory, October 1977.

10. Haupt, B.J., and E. Graves. *Detailed Diagnoses and Surgical Procedures for Patients Discharged from Short-Stay Hospitals: United States, 1979.* DHHS Publication No. (PHS) 82-1274-1. Washington, DC: U.S. Department of Health and Human Services, 1982.

11. Helgerson, S.D., and S. Milham, Jr. "Irrigation Pipes and Electrocutions in Washington State: A Life Threatening Hazard for Agricultural Workers." State of Washington Department of Social and Health Services, unpublished manuscript, 1983. (Portions of this paper appear in S. Milham, "Irrigation-Pipes — Associated Electrocution Deaths — Washington," *Morbidity and Mortality Weekly Report* 32 (1983): 169-171.)

12. McLoughlin, E. "The Cigarette Safety Act." *Journal of Public Health Policy* 3 (1982): 226-228.

13. McLoughlin, E., N. Clarke, K. Stahl, and J.D. Crawford. "One Pediatric Burn Unit's Experience with Sleepwear-Related Injuries." *Pediatrics* 60 (1977): 405-409.

14. Mierley, M.C., and S.P. Baker. "Fatal House Fires in an Urban Population." *Journal of the American Medical Association* 249 (1983): 1466-1468.

15. National Center for Health Statistics. "Persons Injured and Disability Days by Detailed Type and Class of Accident, United States: 1971-1972." Rockville, MD: U.S. Department of Health, Education, and Welfare, 1976.

16. National Fire Data Center. *Fire in the United States: Deaths, Injuries, Dollar Loss and Incidents at the National, State and Local Levels*. Washington, DC: U.S. Government Printing Office, 1978.

17. National Materials Advisory Board. *Prevention of Grain Elevator and Mill Explosions*. Washington, DC: National Academy Press, 1982.

18. Oglesbay, F.B. "The Flammable Fabrics Problem." *Pediatrics* 44 (1969 Supp.): 827-832.

19. Weigel, E.P. "Lightning: The Underrated Killer." *National Oceanic and Atmospheric Administration Magazine* 6 (1976).

20. Wright, R.K., and J.H. Davis. "The Investigation of Electrical Deaths: A Report of 220 Fatalities." *Journal of Forensic Sciences* 25 (1980): 514-521.

21. Young, G.S., and S.P. Baker. "Recent Trends in Childhood Burn Deaths." Paper presented at the Annual Meeting of the American Public Health Association, 1978.

13 Drowning

Drowning is the third most common cause of unintentional injury death for all ages and ranks second for ages 5-44. Among Native Americans and Asians, only deaths from motor vehicles exceed drownings as a cause of unintentional death. Drowning is classified by the ICD into two major groups. The larger group, numbering about 6,000 deaths each year, includes drownings not related to boats. The smaller group, about 1,200 annually, involves boats, primarily small recreational craft. Because drownings related to boats are categorized as "water transport" deaths, they are often excluded from drowning statistics. A third group of drownings, about 500 each year, is included with motor vehicle-related deaths and not separately identified in NCHS mortality statistics. Suicidal drownings and drownings of undetermined intent add another 1,000 deaths annually to the toll.

National data detailing the circumstances of nonboat drownings are limited. A survey of news reports that identified three-fourths of all nonboat drownings in 1971 indicated that one-fourth were swimmers; four out of five who drowned while swimming were not at designated swimming areas. About one-third, including about 500 children under age 5, were people who fell into water. Drownings from scuba diving (58), skin diving (31), and surfing (13) together accounted for less than 2 percent of the total.[3] A complete census of the 133 Maryland drownings in the same year revealed that although sailing and ocean swimming are common sports in the state, only 1 person drowned while sailing and 1 while swimming in the ocean.[1]

Details on recreational (noncommercial) boating deaths are available from the U.S. Coast Guard. Although some recreational boating deaths result from falls, burns, crushing, or other mechanisms, about 90 percent result from drowning. In 1980, about 1,200 drownings involved recreational boats. Almost 60 percent of the boats were less than 16 feet long and the majority were open motorboats (table 13-1A). Capsizing or falling overboard caused almost two-thirds of the deaths (table 13-1B). In 20 percent of all deaths, the boats had too few personal flotation devices (PFDs) or none at all. In contrast, only 5 percent of all boats involved in incidents reported to the Coast Guard had insufficient PFDs.[7]

Table 13–1
Recreational Boat Fatalities by Type of Boat and Event, 1980

(A) Type of Boat	*Deaths*	*Percent*
Open motorboat	720	53
Canoe/kayak	146	11
Rowboat	118	9
Sailboat	66	5
Cabin motorboat	63	5
Other	67	5
Unknown	180	13
Total	1,360[a]	101[b]

(B) Event	*Deaths*	*Percent*
Capsizing	536	39
Falling overboard	346	25
Collision:		
other vessel	69	5
fixed object	90	7
floating object	25	2
Swamping/flooding/sinking	123	9
Struck by boat or propeller	12	1
Fire/explosion	9	1
Other	79	6
Unknown	71	5
Total	1,360[a]	100

Source: Coast Guard, *Boating Statistics 1980,* COMDTINST M16754.1B Washington, DC: U.S. Department of Transportation, 1981.

[a]1,193 of these 1,360 deaths were due to drowning.

[b]Percents do not add to 100 due to rounding.

Age and Sex

The overall death rate from drowning is highest at ages 1 and 18. For drownings not related to boats, the rate is highest among children ages 1-2, a fact not previously reported because rates are usually calculated for broader age groups rather than by single year of age (figure 13-1). In the 1-4 age group, about 85 percent of drownings result from falling into water; baths and playing in water account for about 5 percent each.[3] Every year, about 250 children ages 1-4 drown in swimming pools, predominantly home pools. This is about one-third of all drownings in this age group.[4]

The male:female ratio of drowning rates is about 12:1 for those related to boats and 5:1 for others. Male drowning rates peak at age 2, decline until age 10, and then sharply rise to the maximum at age 18 (figure 13-2). Among females, the death rate is highest at age 1, then decreases sharply and does not rise again. The contrast between males and females in drowning rates after age 10 is a striking example

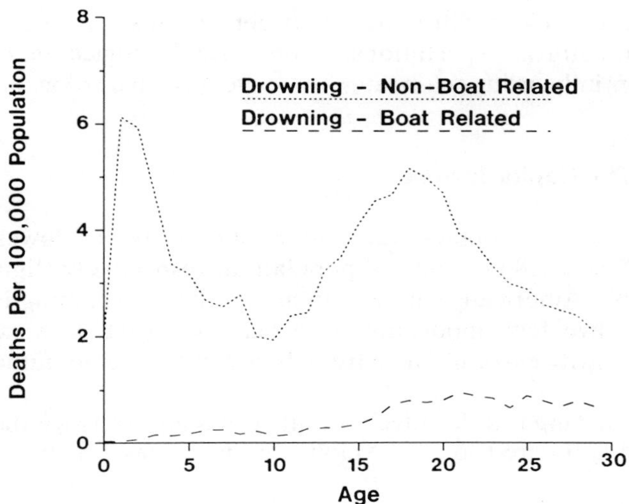

Figure 13-1. Death Rates from Boat and Non-Boat Related Drowning by Age, for Ages 0-29, 1977-1979

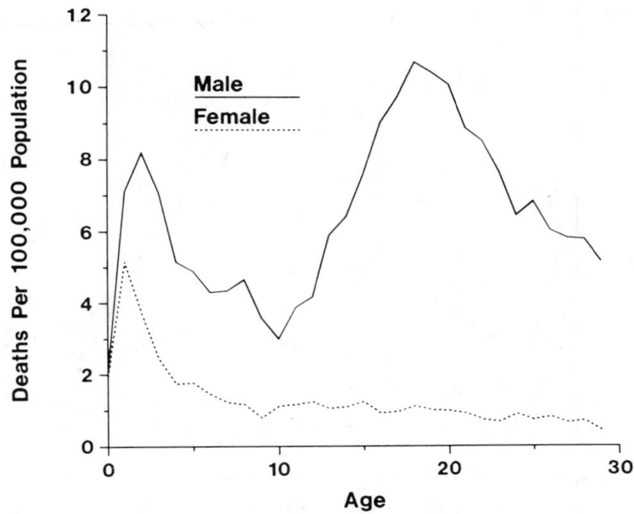

Figure 13-2. Death Rates from Drowning by Age and Sex, for Ages 0-29, 1977-1979

of the effect of likely differences between the sexes in exposure, superversion, cultural expectations, alcohol use, biological makeup, and other factors influencing death rates from potentially hazardous activities.

Race and Per Capita Income

Drowning rates are highest for Native Americans and lowest among Asians, 8.5 and 1.8 per 100,000 population, respectively (figure 13-3). Some Native Americans who live in areas where swimming is uncommon may have few opportunities to learn to swim. Others may be exposed to swift currents or extremely low water temperatures, as in Alaska.

The drowning rate for blacks of all ages is almost twice the rate for whites, 5.4 compared to 2.9. Among children ages 1-4, the pattern is

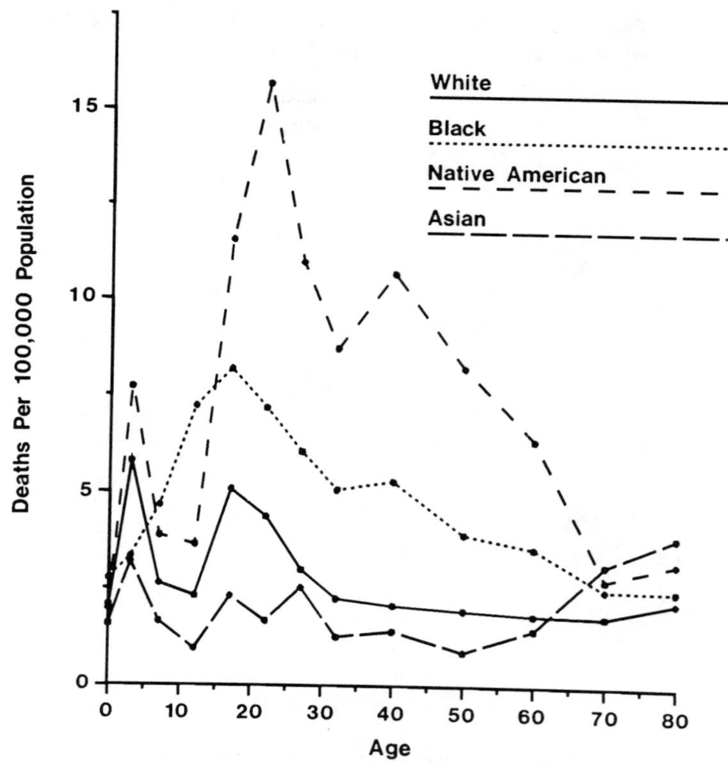

Figure 13-3. Death Rates from Drowning by Age and Race, 1977-1979

reversed, with the rate for whites almost twice the rate for blacks. This difference, which in Maryland is associated with more swimming pool drownings among white children,[1] is an additional example of the influence of the physical environment on racial differences in injury death rates.

Drowning rates vary inversely with the per capita income of the area of residence, decreasing from 5.6 to 2.2 as the per capita income increases. Similar effects occur for both types of drowning (figure 13-4). An exception is that boat-related drowning rates increase slightly in areas of very high per capita income, where boat ownership is likely to be more common.

Urban/Rural and Geographic Differences

Drowning rates are highest among residents of rural areas, especially among blacks (figure 13-5). The regional differences shown on the maps reflect many other factors, including climate (figure 13-6). Rates for drownings that do not involve boats are generally highest in southern and western states. Alaska has the highest rate (10 per 100,000), which

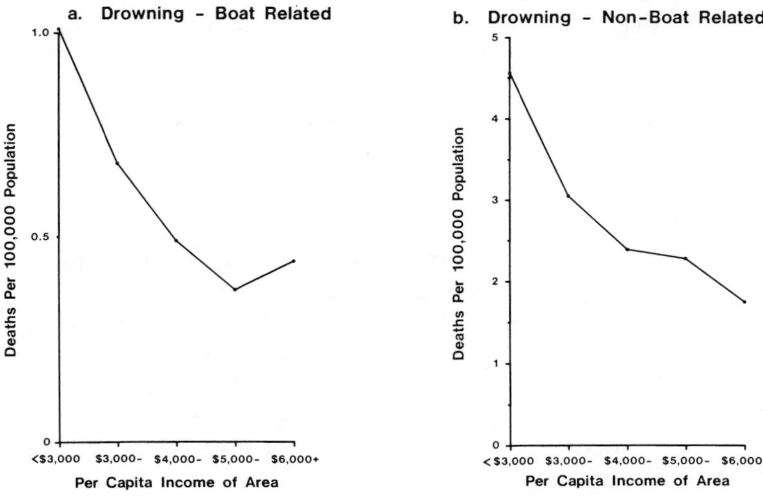

Figure 13-4. Death Rates from Boat and Non-Boat Related Drowning by Age and Per Capita Income of Area of Residence, 1977-1979

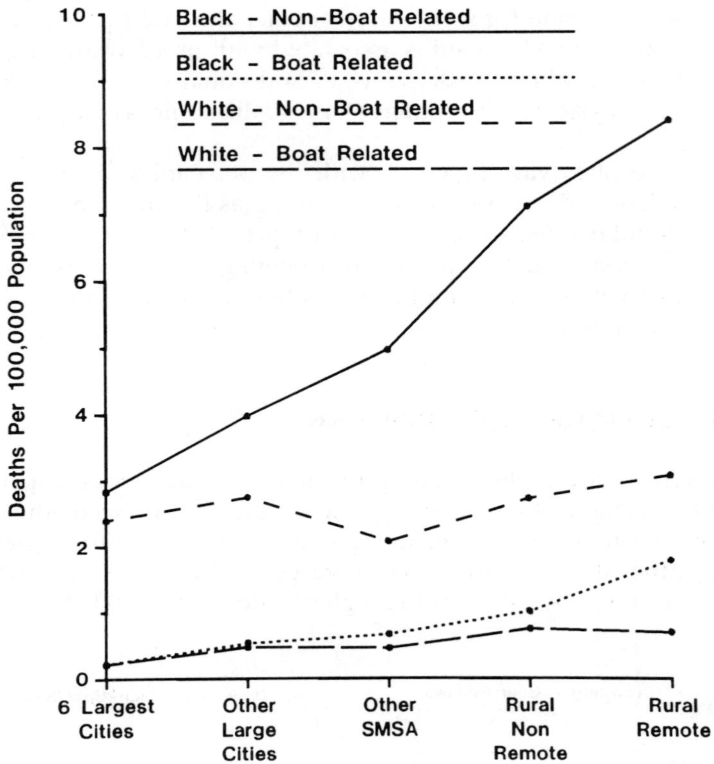

Figure 13-5. Death Rates from Boat and Non-Boat Related Drowning by Place of Residence and Race, 1977-1979

is double the rate in the next highest state, Louisiana. A major factor in the extremely high rate in Alaska is the very low water temperature, which reduces the chance of survival. In addition, fishing and other occupational exposure is common in Alaska. In warm climates, regional differences may reflect the amount of swimming in hazardous places and the prevalence of swimming pools. The latter would especially influence rates among young children, who account for the majority of drownings in home pools.[4]

Drownings involving boats occur most often in lakes and ponds (table 13-2). The highest rates are in the South and Northwest. Overall, the pattern is similar to other drownings, except for California and several southwestern states, which have low rates for drownings involving boats and high rates for other drownings. The rate in Alaska

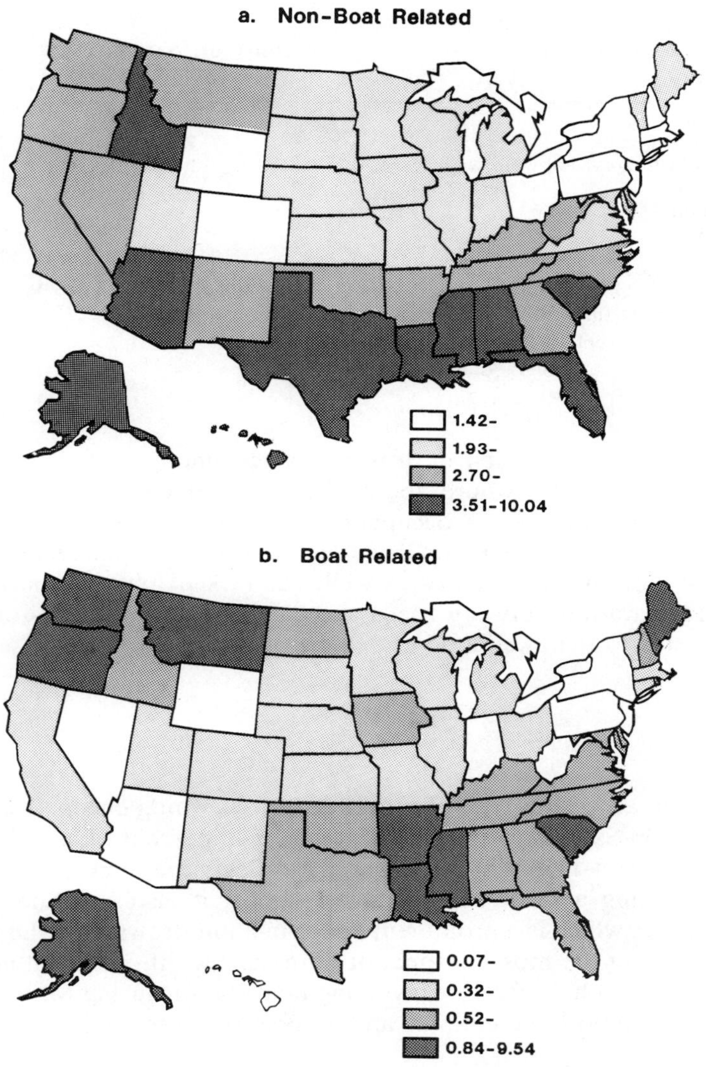

Figure 13-6. Death Rates from Boat and Non-Boat Related Drowning by State, Per 100,000 Population, 1977-1979

is 9.5, almost 5 times the rate in Louisiana, which has the second highest rate.

The high drowning rate in Louisiana is of particular interest because analyses of data for motor vehicle-related deaths reveal that Louisiana

Table 13–2
Recreational Boat Fatalities by Type of Body of Water, 1980

Body of Water	*Number*	*Percent*
Lake/pond/reservoir	688	51
River/stream/creek	365	27
Bay/harbor/intercoastal waterway	200	15
Great Lakes	69	5
Ocean/gulf	34	3
Unknown	4	0
Total	1,360[a]	101[b]

Source: Coast Guard, *Boating Statistics 1980,* COMDTINST M16754.1B, Washington, DC: U.S. Department of Transportation, 1981.

[a]1,193 of these 1,360 deaths were due to drowning.

[b]Percents do not add to 100 due to rounding.

is second only to Florida in drowning rates among motor vehicle occupants. In Florida, where about 75 motor vehicle occupants drown each year, the number of occupant drownings per 100 million vehicle miles is three times the national average. In both Louisiana and Florida, and probably in other states as well, the lack of physical barriers or spatial separation between roads and canals or other bodies of water contributes to the likelihood of vehicle occupant drownings.

Temporal Variation

More than any other type of injury death, drowning occurs disproportionately on Saturdays and Sundays, when 40 percent of all drownings occur (figure 4-14). While this pattern reflects the increase in recreational boating and swimming on weekends, it also is influenced by alcohol use, which is a prominent factor in adult drownings.[1] Drowning is also among the most seasonal of injuries. Two-thirds of all nonboat drownings and half of those involving boats occur during May through August when both recreational and occupational use are highest (figure 4-15).

Historical Trends

During the past half century, the rate for deaths usually categorized as "drowning" (i.e., excluding those involving boats) has decreased by more than half (figure 13-7). Most of this decrease occurred between 1930 and 1950. In contrast, the rate for "water transport" deaths (boat-related deaths, which are primarily drownings) has changed very little. Increases in recreational boat usage may have counteracted improve-

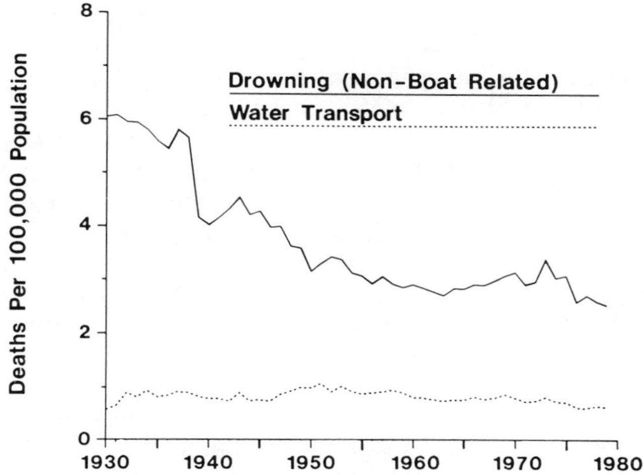

Figure 13-7. Death Rates from Water Transport and Non-Boat Related Drowning by Year, 1930-1979

ments in boats, flotation devices, boating practices, and rescue capability that occurred during these decades.

The percent changes in drowning rates calculated from 1968-1979 trendlines show an overall reduction of 20 percent. The largest decreases in age-specific drowning rates were for ages 5-19 (figure 13-8).

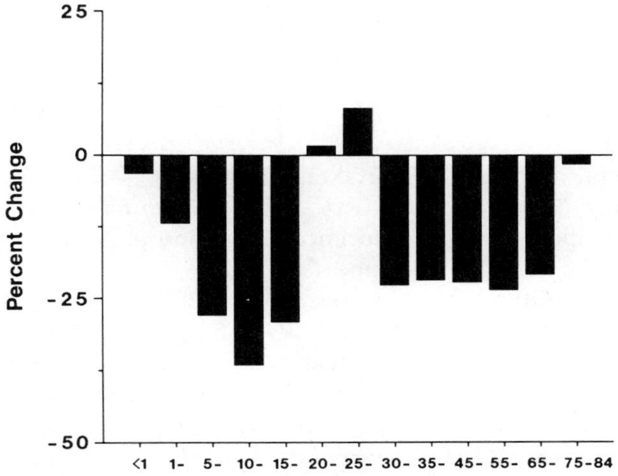

Figure 13-8. Percent Change in Death Rates from Drowning by Age, Based on 1968-1979 Trend

The increase in death rates among ages 20-29 was predominantly due to an increase of more than 40 percent in nonboat drownings among females. Despite this increase, drowning rates for young females were still only one-tenth of the male rates at the end of this period.

Between 1958 and 1968, the drowning rate among children ages 1-4 increased by 16 percent.[2] Drownings among children in this age group continued to increase until about 1974, then decreased slightly. While the reason for this trend is not known, the rapid increase in home pools to an estimated 4 million in 1977 underscores the need for "childproof" swimming pools.[4] The effectiveness of designs that separate young children from home swimming pools is suggested by data from two Australian cities where swimming pools are equally common. In Canberra, where childproof fences were required around home swimming pools, the drowning rate for children was found to be one-ninth the rate in Brisbane, where such fences were not required.[5]

In addition to childproof swimming pools, drowning prevention involves a variety of other strategies.[1] Training in water survival should include not only swimming, floating, and boating skills, but also the use of essential equipment such as helmets for kayaking and whitewater rafting, PFDs for all boaters, and parkas with flotation capabilities for cold water boating. Research is needed on the relationships between swimming training, survival skills, perception of swimming ability, and the likelihood of drowning.[6]

Other preventive measures include changing the speed capabilities and designs of small boats and improving ability to locate and rescue people at risk of drowning. The important role of alcohol in drownings, including those related to boats, must be taken into consideration in planning and choosing preventive strategies.

Notes

1. Dietz, P.E., and S.P. Baker. "Drowning — Epidemiology and Prevention." *American Journal of Public Health* 64 (1974): 303-312.

2. Metropolitan Life Insurance Company. "Accidental Drowning." *Statistical Bulletin* 53 (June 1972): 6-8.

3. Metropolitan Life Insurance Company. "Accidental Drownings by Age and Activity." *Statistical Bulletin* 58 (May 1977): 3-5.

4. Metropolitan Life Insurance Company. "Swimming Pool Drownings." *Statistical Bulletin* 58 (July-August 1977): 4-6.

5. Pearn, J., and J. Nixon. "Are Swimming Pools Becoming More Dangerous?" *The Medical Journal of Australia* 2 (1977): 702-704.

6. Schuman, S.H., J.R. Rowe, H.M. Glazer, and J.S. Redding.

"Risk of Drowning: An Iceberg Phenomenon." *Journal of the American College of Emergency Physicians* 6 (1977): 129-143.

7. United States Coast Guard. *Boating Statistics 1980*. Technical Report COMDTINST M16754.1B. Washington, DC: U.S. Department of Transportation, 1981.

14 Asphyxiation by Choking and Suffocation

Deaths ascribed to mechanical suffocation and asphyxiation by foreign materials in the respiratory tract account collectively for 40 percent of all deaths coded as unintentional injury among children younger than one year.

The category "aspiration of food" includes not only asphyxiation by solid food but also the presence in the respiratory tract of regurgitated food. The latter phenomenon, which may occur in the terminal phases of dying from a variety of causes, accounts for three-fourths of all deaths coded as asphyxiation by food in the first year of life and half of such deaths among older children.[2]

The ICD (and hence NCHS mortality data) does not differentiate between asphyxiation by regurgitated food and by food entering the airway while eating. Therefore, the analyses presented here include all deaths coded in this general category, referring to them as "aspiration of food." Some cases of sudden infant death syndrome (SIDS, or "crib death"), which annually causes more than 3,500 deaths among children ages 1-3 months, may erroneously be categorized as asphyxiation, but this practice is changing as SIDS becomes better recognized.

Age and Sex

Death rates from airway obstruction by food and by other foreign materials are highest among children and the elderly (figure 14-1). Among children younger than one year, the great majority of deaths attributed to these causes occur in the first 6 months (figure 14-2).

The number of childhood deaths from choking on solid food is estimated at about 75 per year. Most occur before age 4, with the highest incidence in children less than 2 years old.[2] The probability that a product will cause fatal choking depends on whether it is likely to be put into the mouth and also on its size, shape, and consistency. Fatal choking in children typically involves round products; pieces of hot dog predominate among obstructing foods, and candies, nuts, and grapes are the others most commonly recorded.[1,2] Especially prominent among the nonfood items reported are round or pliable objects such as un-

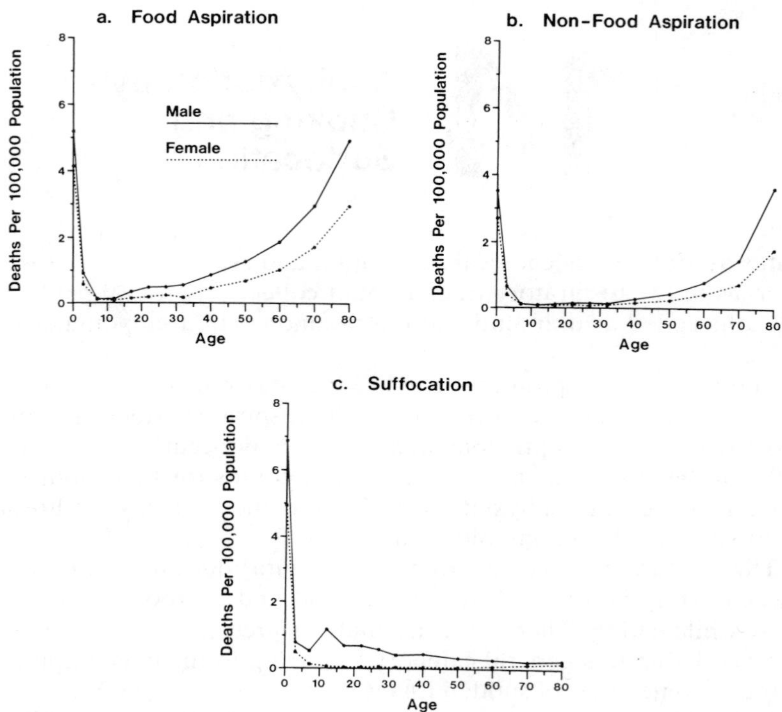

Figure 14-1. Death Rates from Food and Non-Food Aspiration and Suffocation by Age and Sex, 1977-1979

dersized infant pacifiers, small balls, and uninflated or underinflated balloons.

The highest death rates from choking on food or nonfood materials are among people age 75 or older. About 200 such deaths occur annually in residential institutions such as nursing homes and extended care facilities. The term *cafe coronary*, often used to describe adult deaths from food in the airway, reflects both the suddenness of onset and the fact that many deaths occur in restaurants, where both alcohol use and social inhibitions (such as possible reluctance to remove unchewable food from the mouth in public) probably play a role. Among cases where the place of death is given on the death certificate, more than half occur at home and only one-tenth in public places. These figures indicate the need for widespread ability to deal with this emergency.

Among adults other than the elderly, airway obstruction is most

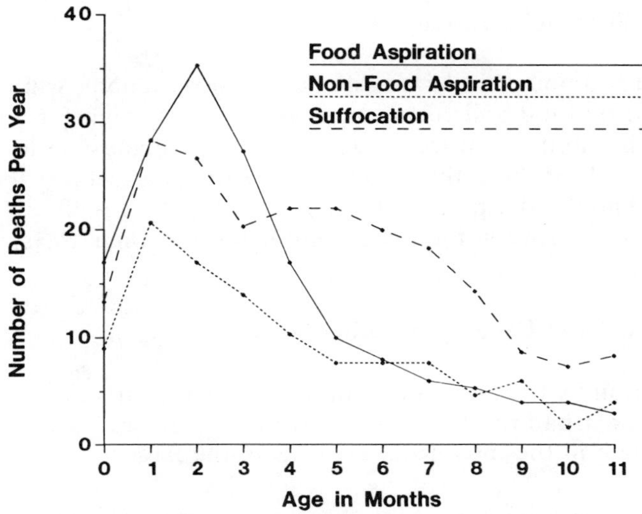

Figure 14-2. Average Number of Deaths Per Year from Food and Non-Food Aspiration and Suffocation by Month of Age, for Ages 0-11 Months, 1977-1979

often caused by a large piece of meat. Alcohol intoxication and, less commonly, sedative or hypnotic drugs are also important contributing factors. Among the elderly, poor dentition and diseases affecting motor coordination or mental function may be predisposing conditions.[4]

Deaths categorized as "mechanical suffocation" include asphyxiation when the mouth and nose are covered (as with plastic), entrapment in an airtight enclosed space such as a refrigerator or storage tank, unintentional hanging, and being covered by fallen earth or other materials. The last-mentioned problem causes a large number of deaths (141 in 1980) and is especially important among males ages 10-14, whose death rate from suffocation exceeds that for any other group except infants.[3] Suffocation is the fourth most common cause of unintentional injury death among males ages 10-14. The male:female ratio of suffocation rates is about 20:1 at this age, whereas for all ages combined it is about 4:1.

A 20-year review of suffocation and strangulation deaths among California children examined the specific events in relation to age. Crib strangulations and wedgings between crib mattress and frame were most common at 6-8 months of age. Entrapment in refrigerators occurred primarily among children ages 2-7 years. Suffocation by fallen earth at construction sites occurred most often at ages 8-12 years.[3]

Race and Per Capita Income

Death rates among blacks are similar to those among whites for asphyxiation by food and suffocation, and twice as high for airway obstruction by nonfood objects. Death rates are highest in low-income areas for each of these three causes of death (figure 14-3). For suffocation and nonfood aspiration there is a twofold to threefold difference in death rates between the lowest and highest income areas.

Urban/Rural and Geographic Differences

Asphyxiation by food or objects in the respiratory tract does not show a consistent urban/rural pattern. The rates from suffocation are four times as high in the most rural areas as in the largest cities.

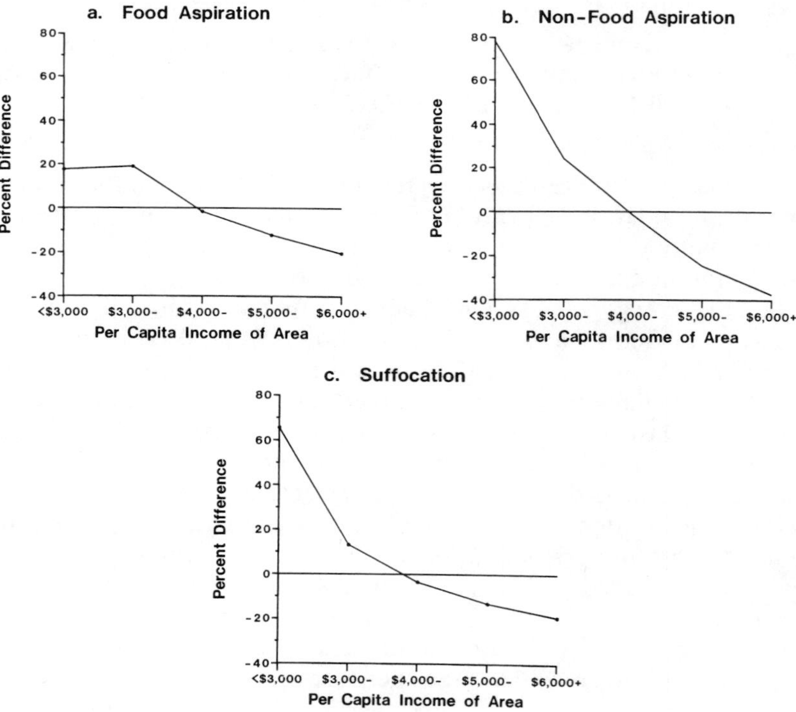

Figure 14-3. Percent Difference from the Average Death Rates from Food and Non-Food Aspiration and Suffocation by Per Capita Income of Area of Residence, 1977-1979

Regional patterns in rates of food-related deaths, which are highest in the South and West, may be partly due to variations in the certification of death when post-mortem examination reveals regurgitated food in the respiratory tract.[2] Airway obstruction by nonfood is most common in the South (figure 14-4).

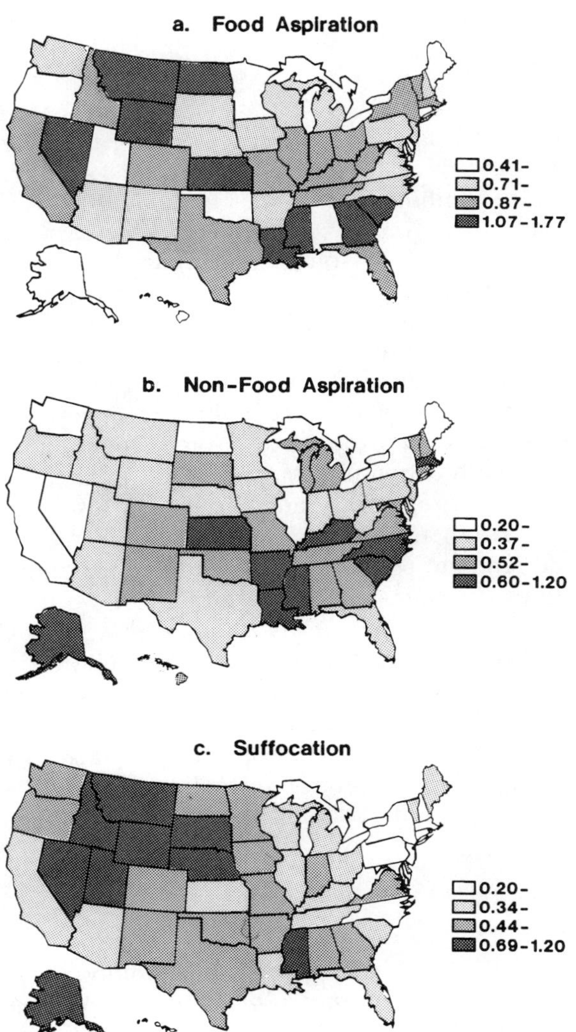

Figure 14-4. Death Rates from Food and Non-Food Aspiration and Suffocation by State, Per 100,000 Population, 1977-1979

Season and Day of Week

There is little variation by month or day of week in deaths from suffocation or from choking on nonfood materials. Choking on food is slightly more common on weekends, probably because of association with alcohol use.[4]

Historical Trends

During 1968-1979, death rates increased among the elderly from suffocation and from aspirating food or nonfood materials, especially the last. For all ages combined, trendlines calculated for this period indicated that death rates from nonfood chokings increased by 29 percent, while suffocation and food aspiration decreased by 48 percent and 25 percent, respectively.

Changing practices in coding SIDS deaths have contributed to the reductions of about 85 percent since 1968 in deaths during the first year of life that are coded either to aspiration of food or to suffocation. There have been decreases of about 20-40 percent among children ages 1-4 in deaths coded to all three causes. Some reduction in refrigeration entrapment and suffocation may have resulted from redesign of refrigerators or state laws regarding their disposal.[3] Research is needed to determine the extent to which changes in death rates reflect CPSC regulations designed to reduce choking and strangulation by children's products such as pacifiers, small toys, and cribs.

Preventive measures include the thoughtful design and packaging of all products likely to be used by or near young children, with attention to their size, shape, consistency, and likelihood of separating into hazardous pieces. Manufactured foods such as hot dogs and hard candies should be designed to avoid or minimize the characteristics associated with fatal choking.[1,2] In addition, information about the foods that are hazardous to young children should be widely disseminated.

Notes

1. Baker, S.P., and R.S. Fisher. "Childhood Asphyxiation by Choking or Suffocation." *Journal of the American Medical Association* 244 (1980): 1343-1346.

2. Harris, C.S., S.P. Baker, G.A. Smith, and R.M. Harris. "Childhood Asphyxiation by Food: A National Analysis and Overview." *Journal of the American Medical Association,* in press.

3. Kraus, J.F. "The Epidemiology of Suffocation Deaths in Infants and Children, California, 1960-1981," submitted for publication.

4. Mittleman, R.E., and C.V. Wetli. "The Fatal Cafe Coronary: Foreign-Body Airway Obstruction." *Journal of the American Medical Association* 247 (1982): 1285-1288.

15 Poisoning

Poisoning results from either brief or long-term exposure to a chemical agent. In general, this book addresses only acute poisonings. The mechanism of injury depends on the chemical agent itself and on whether it is injected, ingested, inhaled, or absorbed through the skin. Basic preventive approaches, comparable to those for preventing other injuries, include eliminating or reducing the manufacture or sale of an agent, reducing the length of exposure or the concentration of the poison to sub-injurious doses, preventing access to the substance, changing its chemical formulation, and providing appropriate emergency and therapeutic measures.

Poisoning causes about 11,000 deaths each year in the United States, almost all of them among adults. About half of all poisoning deaths are ruled suicidal (table 15-1).

Included with unintentional poisonings are an unknown number of deaths in which the intent of the person was not obvious. Both intentional and unintentional poisoning will be discussed in this chapter, since the agents are often the same, the intent may not be known, and preventive measures are sometimes similar.[5] In general, data from hospitals and poison control centers are not categorized by the presumed intent of the person.

Table 15–1
Poisoning Deaths, 1980

	Unintentional	*Suicide*	*Undetermined*	*Total*
Barbituric acid or derivatives	155	498	65	718
Antidepressants and tranquilizers	251	754	140	1,145
Opiates (heroin, methadone, etc.)[a]	322	[b]	[b]	322
Other or unspecified drugs and medications	1,764	1,509	621	3,894
Alcohol	385	[b]	[b]	385
Other or unspecified solids or liquids	212	274	67	553
Motor vehicle exhaust	611	1,998	177	2,786
Other or unspecified gases or vapors	631	420	70	1,121
Total	4,331	5,453	1,140	10,924

Source: National Center for Health Statistics, unpublished data, 1980.

[a]Excludes 629 deaths of drug-dependent persons; ICD coding rules require that such deaths be coded as ICD 304 rather than with injury deaths.

[b]Not separately identifiable.

About a quarter of a million people are admitted to hospitals each year for treatment of poisoning.[6] Poison control centers report on about 125,000 nonfatal poisonings annually,[4] but this represents only a small portion of poison ingestions. About 60 percent of all calls to poison centers involve children younger than 5 years, although this age group constitutes only 1 percent of all fatal poisonings. Only a small proportion of all poisoning deaths are reported to poison control centers, since death often occurs without help having been sought.

Carbon Monoxide

Carbon monoxide (CO) in motor vehicle exhaust is the most prominent single agent among all unintentional and suicidal poisoning deaths (table 15-1). Because its affinity for hemoglobin is far greater than that of oxygen, CO can kill very quickly by precluding the uptake of oxygen by red blood cells. Colorless and odorless, CO may produce unconsciousness with little or no warning. These characteristics increase the deadliness of CO, whether in motor vehicle exhaust or housefires, or in other circumstances where it is not properly dissipated, diluted, or separated from people.

Unintentional poisoning by motor vehicle exhaust sometimes occurs when people are working in enclosed garages or when fumes seep into working or living quarters connected to garages. Occasionally exhaust fumes enter a vehicle while it is moving. Most often, fatal poisoning occurs when cars are parked with the engine running to provide heat for the occupants; defects in the exhaust system and car body then allow fumes to enter.[2] Suicidal poisoning usually takes place in a garage or involves connecting the exhaust system to the occupant compartment of a vehicle.

The death rate from unintentional poisoning by motor vehicle exhaust rises very sharply to a peak at age 15-24, then declines rapidly (figure 15-1). Among males, it increases again after age 70, which suggests that the elderly may succumb more easily to respiratory depression, or that some suicides may be included among deaths certified as "accidental." Suicide by motor vehicle exhaust, which is about three times as common as unintentional poisoning by this means, has a striking age pattern, especially among females, for whom the death rate peaks in the 45-54 age group (figure 3-3).

There is little difference between whites and blacks in rates of unintentional deaths from motor vehicle exhaust. The suicide rate, however, is 10 times as high for whites (1.1 compared to 0.1 per 100,000). This white:black ratio, which is greater than for any other major injury

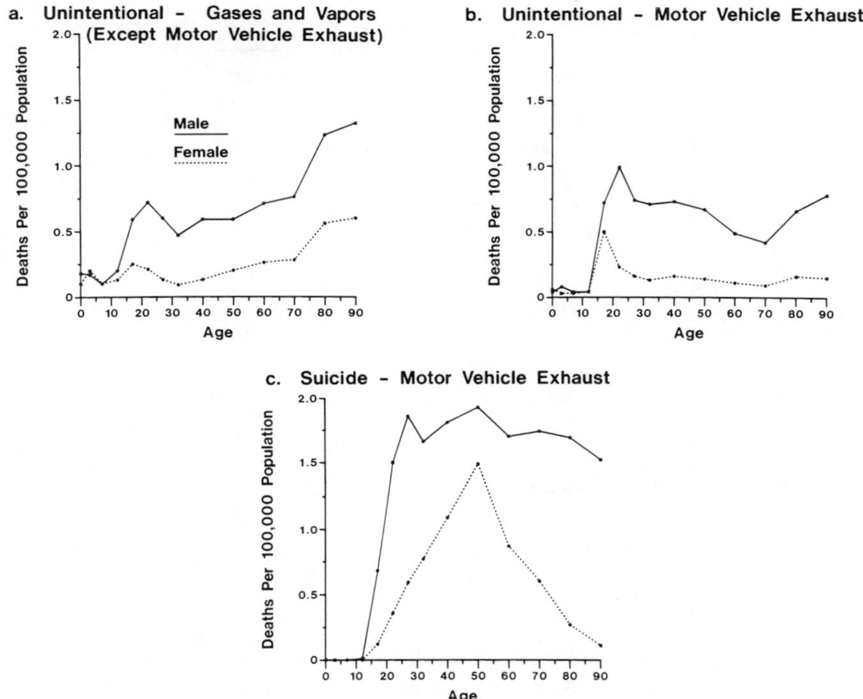

Figure 15-1. Death Rates from Unintentional and Suicidal Poisoning by Gases and Vapors by Age and Sex, 1977-1979

group except general aviation crashes, remains even when variations in per capita income or place of residence are taken into account.

Death rates from unintentional poisoning by motor vehicle exhaust are high in low-income areas, a fact possibly related to deterioration of old vehicles, a major factor in these poisonings. The death rate from suicide by vehicle exhaust increases elevenfold (from 0.14 to 1.60) as per capita income of area residents increases. Among all means of committing suicide, motor vehicle exhaust shows the most dramatic association with per capita income, an association that is consistent for all urban/rural groups.

Motor vehicle exhaust death rates are highest in rural areas in the case of unintentional poisoning, whereas suicide rates are highest in areas of intermediate urbanization (figure 15-2). For both suicide and unintentional deaths, rates tend to be high in northern states, where garages may offer more opportunity for this means of suicide and where

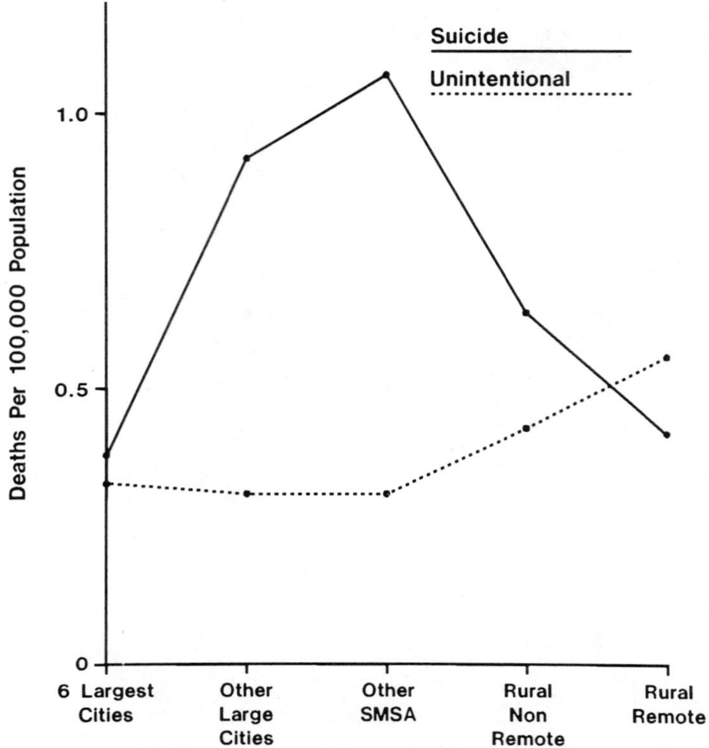

Figure 15-2. Death Rates from Unintentional and Suicidal Poisoning by Motor Vehicle Exhaust by Place of Residence, 1977-1979

the colder climate increases the use of car heaters (figure 15-3). The role of cold weather is further illustrated by the fact that deaths from unintentional poisoning by motor vehicle exhaust are three times as common in January and February as in June and July (figure 4-15).

Between 1930 and 1980, the death rate from unintentional poisoning by gases and vapors dropped by 72 percent, due mainly to reductions in poisoning by domestic gas. Since 1947, poisonings by domestic gas and by motor vehicle exhaust have been distinguished from one another in the national mortality data for "poisoning by gases and vapors." Between 1947 and 1980 there was a 96 percent decrease in unintentional deaths from gas piped to homes, with the steepest drop during the 1950s (figure 15-4). In addition to increased use of electric stoves, coal gas (which had a higher carbon monoxide content) was gradually replaced

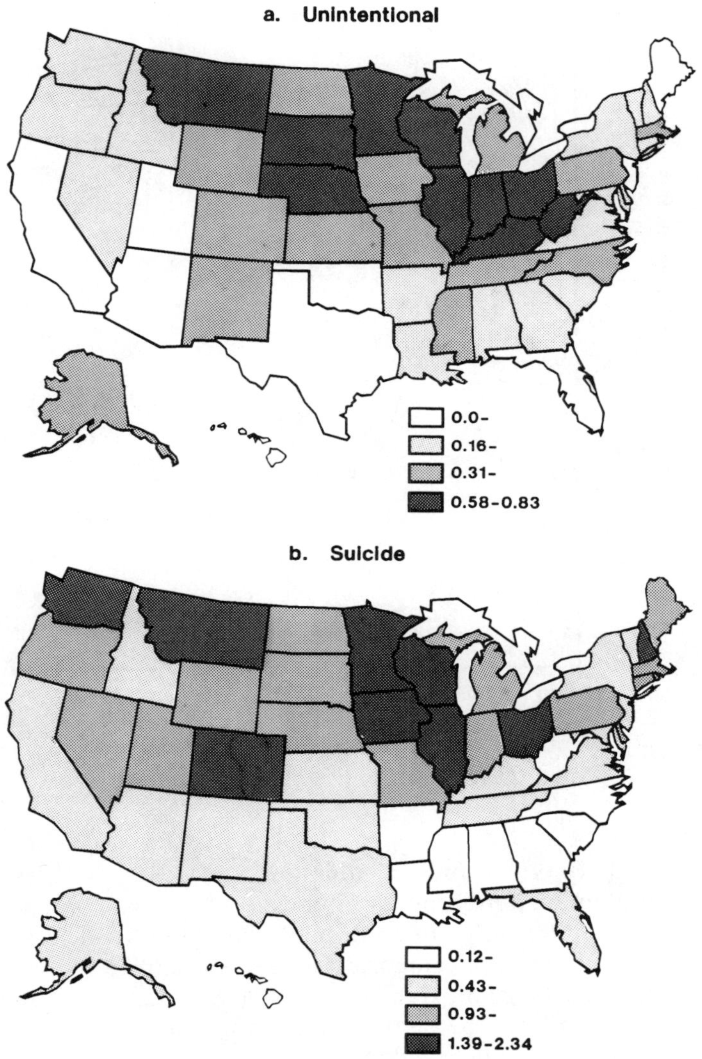

Figure 15-3. Death Rates from Unintentional and Suicidal Poisoning by Motor Vehicle Exhaust by State, Per 100,000 Population, 1977-1979

by natural gas as a fuel for cooking. Natural gas does not contain concentrations of carbon monoxide likely to cause fatal poisoning if the gas is emitted from a stove, other appliance, or gas line without

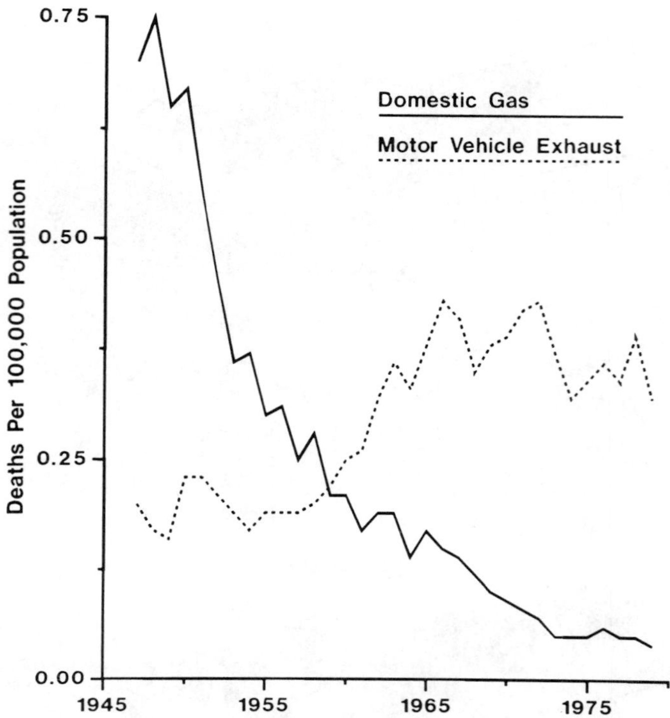

Figure 15-4. Death Rates from Unintentional Poisoning by Domestic Piped Gas and Motor Vehicle Exhaust by Year, 1947-1979

being ignited. By 1980, only 61 unintentional deaths and 23 suicides were attributed to poisoning by domestic piped gas, which in 1947 caused about 1,000 unintentional deaths and 1,200 suicides. Similar dramatic changes in both categories of deaths occurred in England and Wales as the carbon monoxide content of piped gas was reduced.[1,5]

From 1955 to 1965 the death rate from unintentional poisoning by motor vehicle exhaust doubled. Since then it has remained fairly constant, and in recent years there have been about 700 deaths annually. Measures to prevent entry of carbon monoxide into the passenger compartment (for example, by reducing the rusting-through of cars and exhaust systems, locating tailpipes appropriately, and inspecting older vehicles to identify hazardous defects) would do much to reduce these deaths. Some cars have been designed with fans that automatically maintain a slight flow of air into the passenger compartment whenever the ignition is on, an approach that should prevent the build-up of exhaust gases.

Opiates

Substances classified as "drugs and medications" cause more than 80 percent of all fatal poisonings by solids and liquids. Of the drugs specifically identified, the most common are opiates, barbiturates, and psychotherapeutic drugs (primarily antidepressants and tranquilizers) (table 15-1). Many more poisonings by these agents are undoubtedly included in the large numbers of fatal poisonings by unspecified agents.

Fatal poisoning by opiates is predominantly the result of heroin overdose. The majority of heroin deaths are not classified with unintentional deaths, since a 1971 coding change in the ICD requires that cases involving drug dependence be classified as "natural" rather than "accidental" deaths. In 1975, a peak year for heroin deaths, 1,031 deaths were classified as due to "opiates and synthetic analogues,"* 53 as intravenous narcotism, and 1,358 as the natural consequence of drug dependence. Deaths in the latter category are not included in our analyses but elsewhere have been shown to follow the same time trends as unintentional opiate poisoning.[8] The two groups probably overlap substantially, since whether a heroin overdose is coded as "accidental" or as a "natural death due to drug dependence" depends on the information available to the medical examiner or coroner as well as on the data recorded on the death certificate. Opiate poisoning is such a large component of fatal poisoning, especially in peak years of heroin use, that an understanding of these coding problems is important.

Death rates from unintentional poisoning by opiates are especially high for males (the sex ratio is 4:1) and for ages 20-34 (figure 15-5). A comparable but less pronounced peak at ages 20-34 is seen for poisonings by other and unspecified substances and may represent the inclusion of many opiate poisonings among unspecified poisonings.

The death rate among blacks is about twice the rate among whites, reflecting the racial composition of large cities, where the death rate from opiate poisoning is especially high. In cities of a million or more, the death rate is 25 times the rate in the most rural areas. When place of residence is taken into consideration, little difference between blacks and whites is seen in death rates from opiate poisoning (figure 15-6).

Opiate poisoning is one of the few causes of death for which mortality is higher in areas of high income (figure 15-7). Among large cities as well as in the remainder of SMSAs, those with high per capita income have rates several times as high as in places with low income.

---

*Methadone is a synthetic analogue of morphine, heroin a natural derivative of opium. Deaths from these substances cannot be distinguished in vital statistics data, but a survey of nonsuicide narcotic deaths in four major U.S. cities revealed that 96 percent were due to heroin.[7]

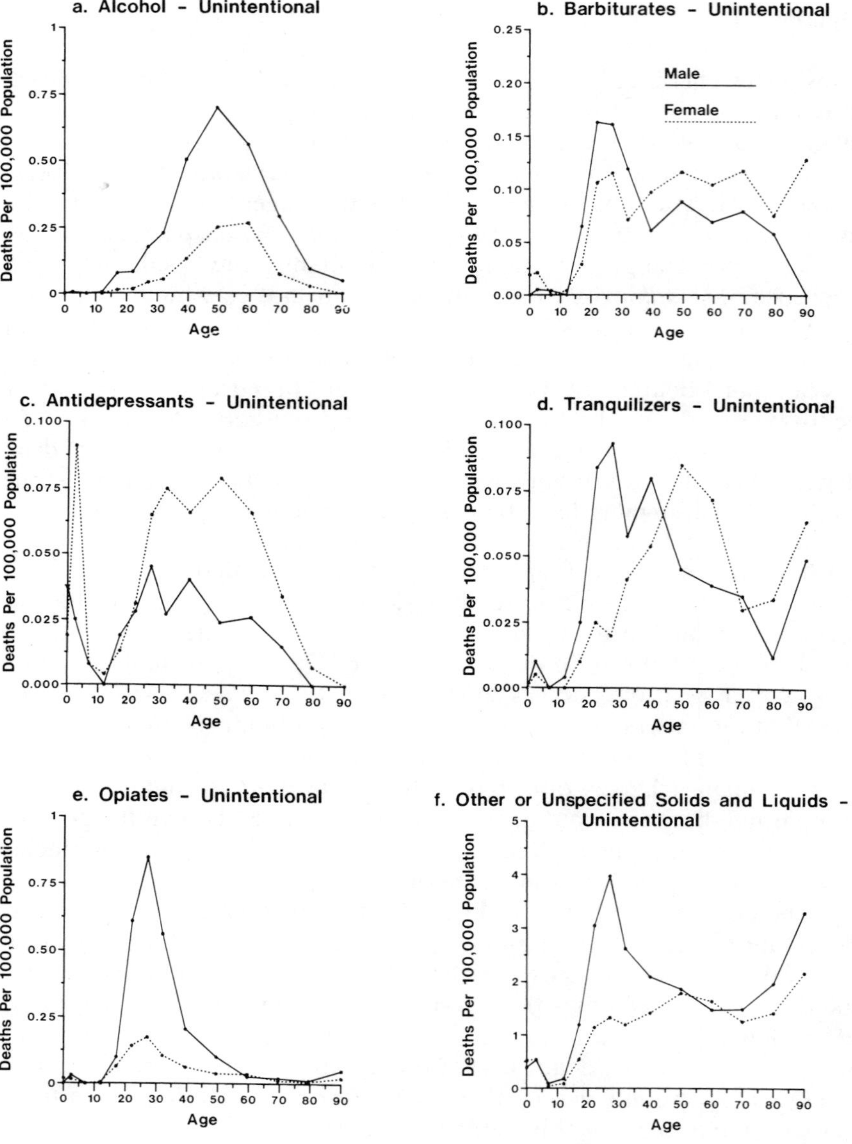

Figure 15-5. Death Rates from Poisoning by Solids and Liquids by Age, Sex, Type of Drug, and Intent, 1977-1979

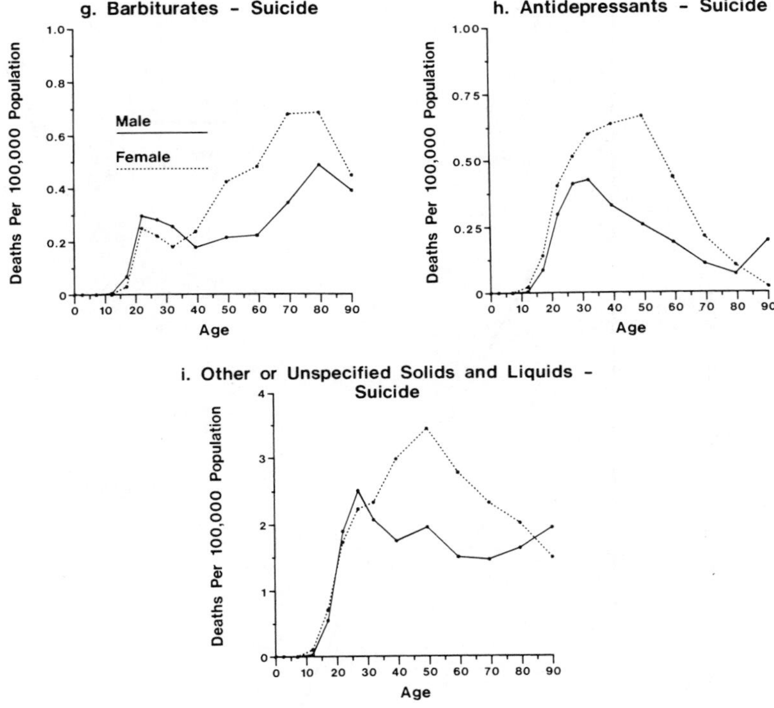

Figure 15–5 *(continued)*

Since 1970, fluctuations in opiate poisoning mortality in the United States appear to have coincided with variations in the flow of heroin into the country. When the heroin supply was interrupted in 1972 and again in 1976, there were corresponding decreases in heroin-related mortality.[8]

Other Drugs

In the case of both fatalities from unintentional drug poisoning and drug poisonings reported to poison control centers, about one-third of all cases involve either barbiturates, antidepressants, tranquilizers, or

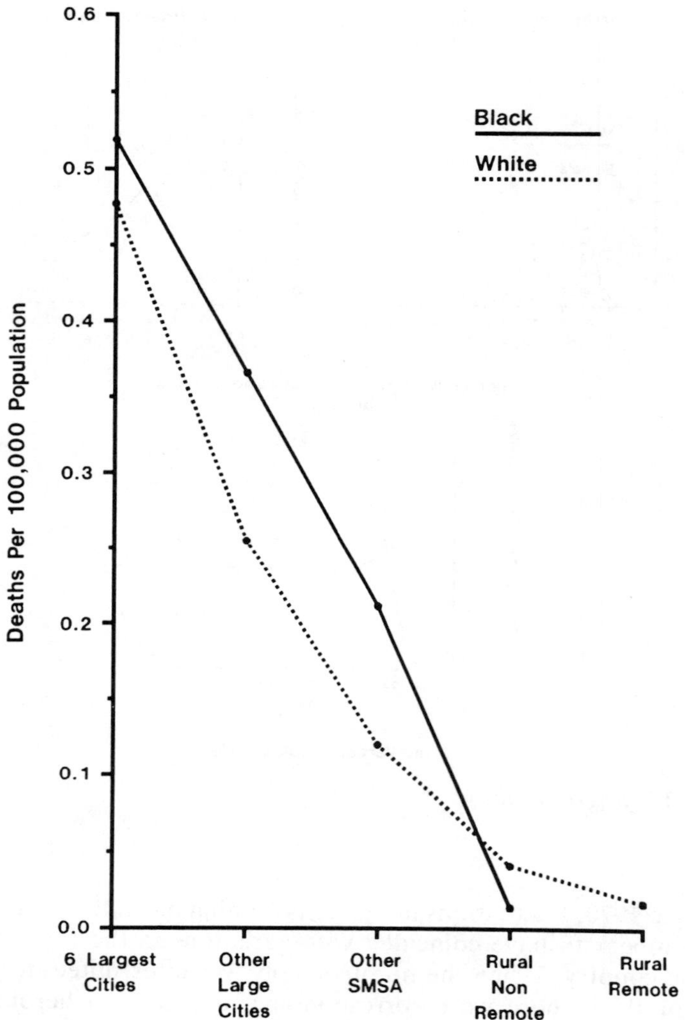

Figure 15-6. Death Rates from Unintentional Opiate Poisoning by Place of Residence and Race, 1977-1979

nonaspirin analgesics. Among teenagers admitted to Maryland hospitals, aspirin and its substitutes, benzodiazepines, alcohol, and antidepressants are the most common agents involved. Most cases of teenage poisoning are categorized as suicide attempts. Female teenagers have higher rates than males. The sex difference is especially great for aspirin poisoning.[9]

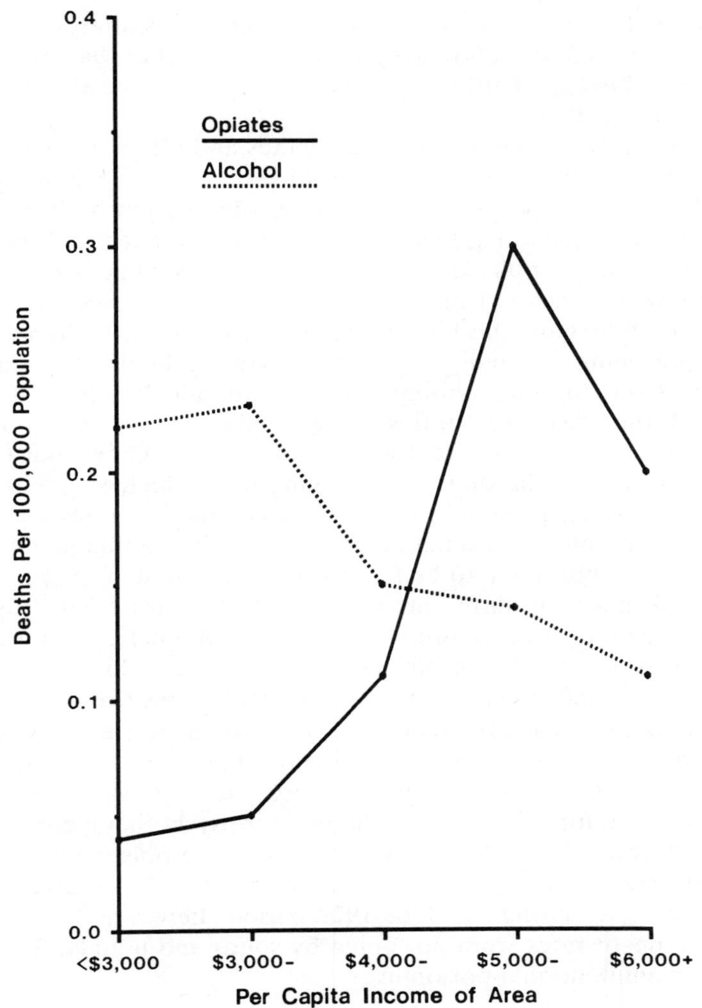

Figure 15-7. Death Rates from Unintentional Poisoning by Opiates and Alcohol by Per Capita Income of Area of Residence, 1977-1979

Barbiturate poisoning deaths show a peak at ages 20-29 for both sexes (figure 15-5). Beginning at about age 35, females have higher rates than males from both unintentional poisoning and suicide. Rates of suicide by barbiturates increase again after age 40 among females and after age 60 among males. Similarly, tranquilizers have higher unintentional death rates among females than males after age 40. Female death rates from antidepressants are much higher than male rates for almost all ages, a pattern not seen for any other cause of unintentional injury death.

There is little difference between whites and blacks in death rates from unintentional poisoning by barbiturates and psychotherapeutic drugs. In contrast, the suicide rate among whites from barbiturates is five times the rate among blacks; from psychotherapeutic drugs, it is twice the rate among blacks. In general, drug poisoning deaths do not show strong or consistent relationships with per capita income.

Urban areas have the highest death rates from virtually all types of drug poisoning. For poisoning by barbiturates, the urban:rural ratio is 4:1 or more for unintentional deaths and suicides. For all drugs combined, the urban:rural ratios are approximately 3:1.

Geographic patterns differ for the various types of poisoning (figure 15-8). California is the only state ranking in the highest group in all categories of drug poisoning excluding alcohol. The rates for many other states are based on small numbers of deaths, so that many of the differences are not likely to be statistically significant.

Several markedly different trends in death rates from drugs occurred during the 1970s (figure 15-9). The most dramatic was for opiate poisoning, reflecting the heroin poisoning epidemics discussed above. The greatest proportional increase was in death rates from antidepressants, which quadrupled between 1968 and 1979. Simultaneously, deaths from barbiturates rose slightly and then dropped; by 1979, the death rate from barbiturates was about one-third the 1970 rate. Comparable trends occurred for suicides, with the rate for psychotherapeutic agents increasing fivefold over the 12-year period, while poisoning by barbiturates decreased by 80 percent. In general, the various trends balanced one another, so during the 1968-1979 period there was little overall change in death rates from poisoning by solids and liquids, for either suicide or unintentional poisoning.

Alcohol

Alcohol use often accompanies or precipitates poisoning by drugs or carbon monoxide, decreasing protective inhibitions and awareness of hazards and acting additively or synergistically with other poisons. Alcohol may also prove fatal by itself when consumed in sufficient quantities. About 400 deaths annually are attributed to poisoning by alcohol.

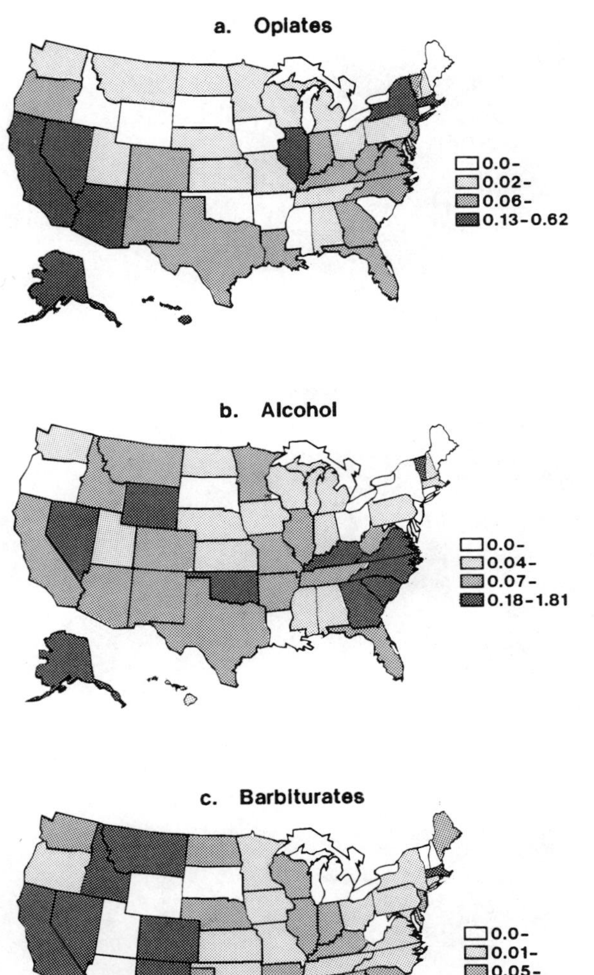

(continued)

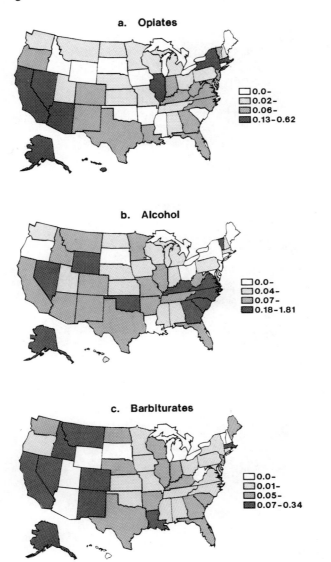

Figure 15-8. Death Rates from Unintentional Poisoning by Type of Drug and from Suicidal Poisoning by All Solids and Liquids by State, Per 100,000 Population, 1977-1979

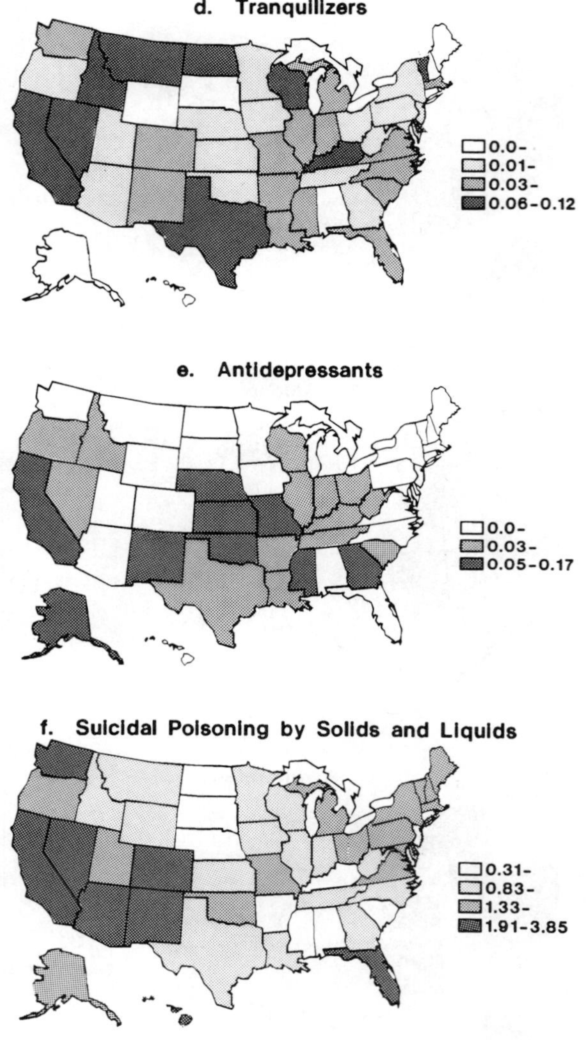

Figure 15–8 *(continued)*

(In addition, about 4,000 deaths each year are attributed to acute or chronic alcoholism. If the many effects of chronic, heavy use were included, the total number of deaths due to alcohol poisoning would be even greater.)

The death rate from acute alcohol poisoning among males is three

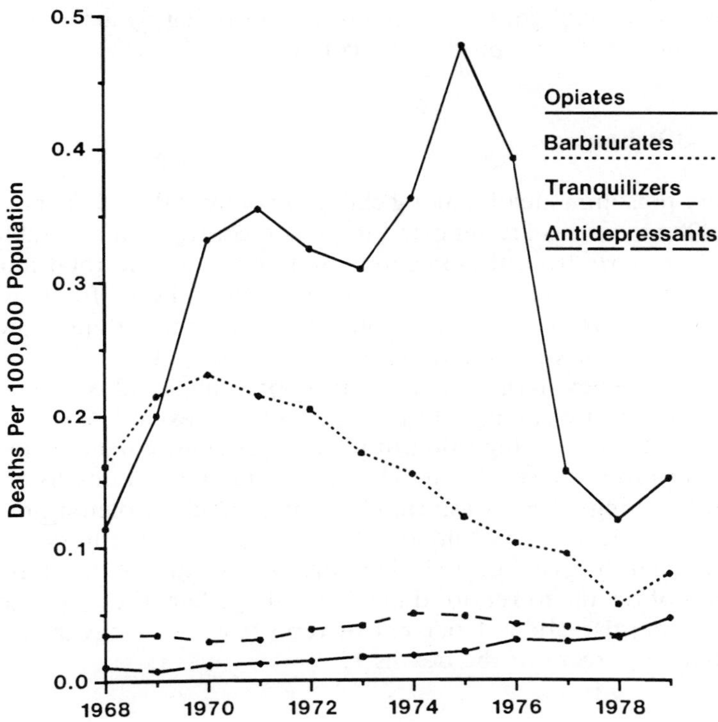

Figure 15-9. Death Rates from Unintentional Poisoning by Type of Drug and Year, 1968-1979

times the female rate, with a peak at about age 50 for both sexes (figure 15-5). Death rates are more than three times as high among blacks and Native Americans as among whites. For Asians, on the other hand, the rate is one-sixth the rate for whites.

Death rates from alcohol poisoning are highest in low-income areas. This is in marked contrast to poisoning by opiates, which show the reverse pattern (figure 15-7).

Hospitalizations related to alcohol show contrasting racial patterns among Maryland teenagers: admission rates for alcohol poisoning were twice as high in 1979-1982 among whites as among blacks.[9] Death rates from alcohol poisoning are especially high in some southern states (figure 15-8), with the rate in North Carolina more than 10 times the national rate. Virginia and West Virginia have the second and third highest rates. Research is needed to examine the effect of differing alcohol control policies and laws in these and other states on the amounts and types of alcohol consumption and on poisoning by alcohol (or by contaminants of illicitly produced alcohol).

Childhood Poisoning

For every poisoning death among children younger than 5 years, more than 1,000 ingestions are reported to poison control centers (table 15-2). While reports from these centers underestimate the total number of poisonings, they provide information on the relative frequency of ingestions that are of sufficient concern to warrant calling a poison control center. Forty percent of reports and 62 percent of deaths involve medicines. The next largest number of reports (about 12,000 per year) is for ingestion of cleaning and polishing agents, excluding petroleum products and caustics. Ingestion of plants is another common cause of reports but rarely causes death. The largest numbers of deaths in 1980 resulted from ingestion of aspirin (12 deaths) and petroleum products (9 deaths) (table 15-3).[4] Childhood poisonings by antidepressants and cardiovascular drugs are of special importance because of the extremely high ratio of deaths to reported incidents. Together, these two groups of drugs comprise about 1 percent of reported poisonings in this age group but 13 percent of the deaths.[4]

Table 15–2
Reported Poisonings and Fatal Poisonings Among Children Ages 0–4, 1979–1980

	Cases Reported to Poison Control Centers		*Deaths*	
Agent	*Number*	*Percent*	*Number*	*Percent*
Aspirin (salicylates)	6,144	4	20	13
Antidepressants	442	[a]	12	8
Cardiovascular drugs	1,427	1	7	5
Other medicines	56,483	35	55	36
Petroleum products	4,513	3	22	15
Pesticides/fertilizers	8,403	5	8	5
Cleaning/polishing agents	23,766	15	6	4
Mushrooms, toadstools	1,161	1	2	1
Other plants, berries, seeds	19,243	12	1	1
Other solids/liquids	38,225	24	18	12
Total (2 years)	159,807	100	151	100

Source: Food and Drug Administration, unpublished data.
[a]Less than 0.5%

Table 15–3
Causes of Fatal Poisoning Among Children Ages 0–4, 1960 and 1980

Agent	*1960*	*1980*
Aspirin	144	12
Lead	78	2
Petroleum products	48	9
Caustics/cleaning agents	23	7
All other solids and liquids	152	43
Total	445	73
Death rates per 100,000 population	2.2	0.5

Source: National Center for Health Statistics, unpublished data.

Since 1960, poisoning deaths among children younger than 5 years have decreased dramatically. The rate for poisoning by solids and liquids was 2.2 per 100,000 in 1960 and 0.5 in 1980 (table 15-3). Between 1960 and 1980, the number of deaths from lead poisoning dropped from 78 to 2. Deaths from kerosene and other petroleum products dropped from 48 to 9, while those from aspirin dropped from 144 to 12 (14, if aspirin substitutes are included).

An especially steep decline in childhood poisoning death rates occurred after childproof packaging was required on all drugs and medications beginning in 1973. The 50 percent decrease in poisoning by all drugs and medications in the first three years (1973-1976) was substantially greater than the decrease in poisonings by other solids and liquids, most of which were not required to be packaged in childproof containers (figure 15-10).[10] During 1968-1979, the period analyzed for most causes of death in this book, the 80 percent decline in poisoning death rates for children ages 1-4 exceeded that for any other major cause of childhood injury death.

Although childhood poisoning is not a major problem in terms of the number of deaths, it is worthy of special attention. When nonfatal cases are considered, the number of children and families affected each year is very large. Deaths and illnesses from poisoning can be further reduced by attention to the formulation, packaging, and use of poisonous agents.[3] Dramatic reductions in childhood poisoning deaths have resulted from changes in products (for example, reductions in the lead content of paint), packaging (such as childproof or single-dose packages), and changes in fuels (for example, increased availablity of electricity, which reduced the use of kerosene). In addition, development of poison control centers has no doubt contributed to the remarkable decline in poisoning mortality in recent decades. The success of this

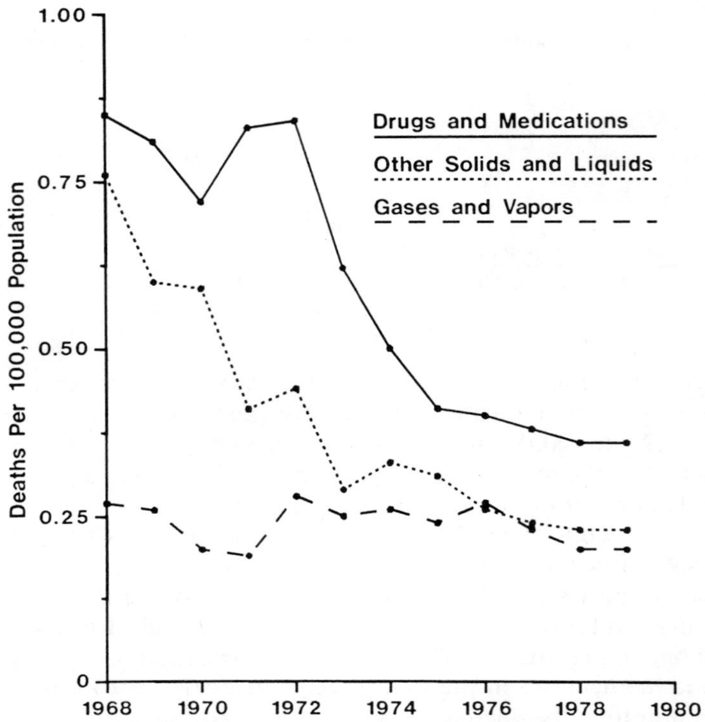

Figure 15-10. Death Rates from Poisoning of Children Ages 0-4 by Year and Category of Poison, 1968-1979

broad approach, which did not depend on changing the behavior of children or parents, illustrates what can be achieved with intensive efforts and the use of appropriate preventive measures.

Notes

1. Alphey, R.S., and S.J. Leach. "Accidental Death in the Home." *Royal Society of Health Journal* 3 (1974): 97-102, 144.

2. Baker, S.P., R.S. Fisher, W.C. Masemore, and I.M. Sopher. "Fatal Unintentional Carbon Monoxide Poisoning in Motor Vehicles." *American Journal of Public Health* 62 (1972): 1463-1467.

3. Barry, P.Z. "Individual Versus Community Orientation in the Prevention of Injuries." *Preventive Medicine* 4 (1975): 47-56.

4. Food and Drug Administration. "Poison Control Case Report

Summary — Calendar Year 1980." Rockville, MD: U.S. Department of Health and Human Services, June 14, 1982.

5. Hassall, C., and W.H. Trethowan. "Suicide in Birmingham." *British Medical Journal* 1 (1972): 717-718.

6. Haupt, B.J., and E. Graves. *Detailed Diagnoses and Surgical Procedures for Patients Discharged from Short-Stay Hospitals: United States, 1979*. DHHS Publication No. PHS 82-1274-1. Washington, DC: U.S. Department of Health and Human Services, 1982.

7. McGuire, F.L., H. Birch, L.A. Gottschalk, J.F. Heiser, and E.C. Dinovo. "A Comparison of Suicide and Nonsuicide Deaths Involving Psychotropic Drugs in Four Major U.S. Cities." *American Journal of Public Health* 66 (1976): 1058-1061.

8. Samkoff, J.S., and S.P. Baker. "Recent Trends in Fatal Poisoning by Opiates in the United States." *American Journal of Public Health* 72 (1982): 1251-1256.

9. Trinkoff, A.M., and S.P. Baker. "Childhood Poisonings Resulting in Hospital Admission." Presented at the Annual Meeting of the American Public Health Association, Dallas, 1983.

10. Walton, W.W. "An Evaluation of the Poison Prevention Packaging Act." *Pediatrics* 69 (1982): 363-370.

16 Introduction to Motor Vehicle Crashes

Chapters 8 through 15 highlighted information on a number of the major causes of injury death. As important as these are, they are overshadowed by the large numbers of deaths resulting from motor vehicle use. Crashes* of motor vehicles are the leading cause of death in the United States for people ages 1-34. From age 5 to 29, *more than one-fifth of deaths from all causes* are caused by motor vehicles (figure 16-1).[17] For people in their late teens and early twenties (ages 16-22), motor vehicle crashes account for more than 40 percent of *all* deaths. They cause more deaths of people ages 1-75 than any other injury-producing event. Motor vehicle crashes are also the leading cause of work-related injury deaths; about one-third of all such deaths involve road vehicles (figure 16-2).

In recent years, motor vehicle crashes on public roads (sometimes referred to as "in traffic") have caused between 45,000 and 53,000 deaths and between 4 and 5 million injuries each year.[20,22] Approximately half a million of these injuries require hospital admission,** involving an average length of stay of 9 days.[21] Clearly, motor vehicle crashes constitute the single most important component of the overall injury problem.

At the same time, motor vehicles are an integral part of our lives. They transport people and goods, provide recreational opportunities, and are used by millions of Americans on their jobs. Although motor vehicles thus provide mobility for much of our society, their widespread use and the speeds at which they travel create the potential (although not the necessity) for injury and death to occupants and other road users.

Most injuries from motor vehicles result when mechanical energy is conveyed to people in amounts or at rates that exceed their injury thresholds. Contrary to the popular belief that the human body is very fragile, with adequate protection it can withstand high forces without

---

*The terms *crash* and *collision* are used interchangeably in this book. Unless otherwise specified, both terms include multiple-vehicle, single-vehicle, motorcycle, bicycle, and pedestrian collisions, as well as other motor vehicle crashes.

**The National Accident Sampling System estimates 420,000 admissions per year in 1979-1980 based on police-reported accidents, which substantially underestimate injuries.

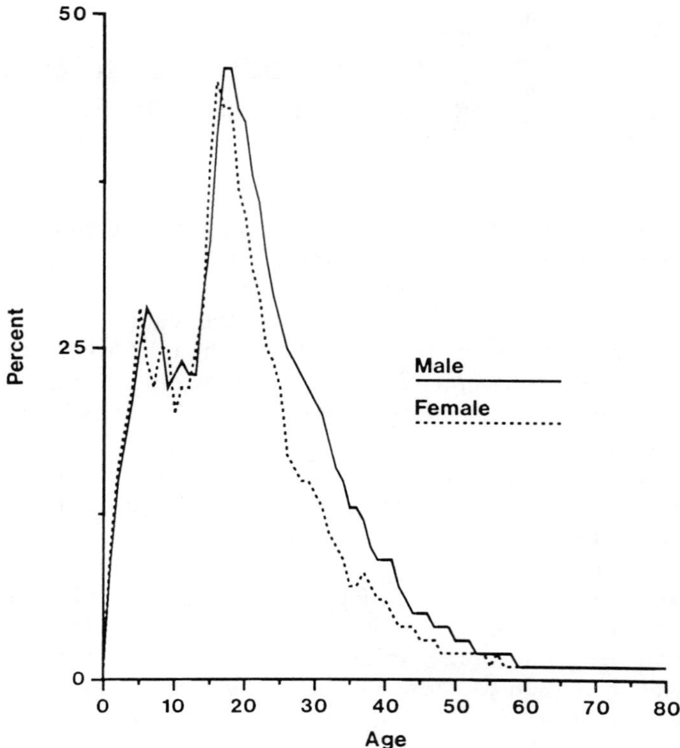

Source: Reprinted with permission from: R.S. Karpf and A.F. Williams, "Teenage Drivers and Motor Vehicle Deaths," *Accident Analysis and Prevention,* 1983. Copyright Pergamon Press, Ltd.

Figure 16-1. Motor Vehicle Deaths as a Percent of Deaths from All Causes by Age and Sex, 1978

injury. In addition to De Haven's work (see Chapter 10), early evidence also was provided by Colonel John Stapp, who withstood deceleration in a rocket sled from 632 to 0 mph in 1.4 seconds without serious injury. This was possible because of the relatively long stopping distance involved, the high resistance of the body to transient forces, and the use of a belt harness system which spread the forces over a large body area.[25]

Understanding motor vehicle crash injuries and possible countermeasures can be aided by a model developed by Haddon,[8-11] which divides the time sequence of a crash into three phases. The *pre-crash phase* includes all of the events that determine whether a crash actually takes place — for example, whether the driver was impaired by alcohol,

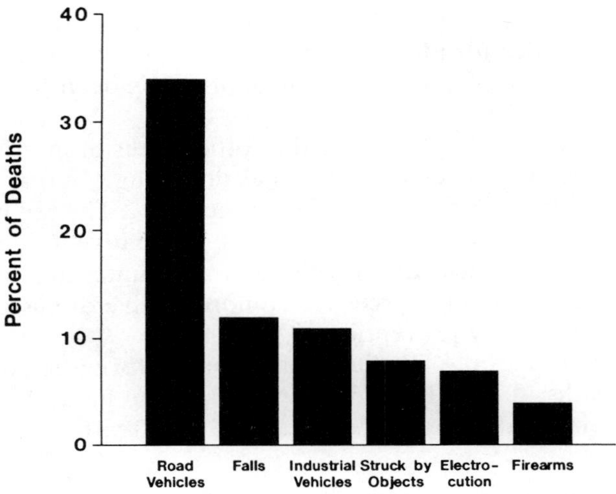

Figure 16-2. Percent of Occupational Injury Deaths by Cause, Workplaces with More Than 10 Employees, Bureau of Labor Statistics, 1980-1981

the vehicle had deficient brakes, or the road lighting was inadequate. The *crash phase* includes all that determines whether injury occurs in the crash and, if so, its type and severity — for example, whether the occupant was wearing a seat belt, how large the car was, and whether the signpost it struck was designed to break away. The *post-crash phase* includes everything that determines the consequences of the injury — for example, how quickly bleeding can be stopped, whether or not a fire occurs after the crash, and how fast the emergency medical system responds.

For decades, most intervention efforts focused on the pre-crash phase, especially efforts to change driving behavior in order to prevent crashes from occurring. Although there is a role for this approach, concentration exclusively on any one factor is inappropriate. Moreover, many efforts to reduce injuries by changing human behavior have had limited success or have failed. In the last 15-20 years, a somewhat more balanced approach has been adopted, one that incorporates many countermeasures aimed at changing events in the crash and post-crash phases, as well as preventing crashes through measures aimed at driver and pedestrian behavior and vehicle and environmental design.

Interacting with each of the three crash phases are three sets of factors: human, vehicle and equipment, and physical and socioeconomic environment. Combining the three crash phases and three groups of factors results in a nine-cell matrix (table 16-1), each cell of which offers opportunities for intervention to reduce motor vehicle crash injuries. A discussion of each cell of the matrix has been provided elsewhere by Haddon.[9-11]

This basic model can be adapted to other types of injuries and has been applied to such diverse problems as drowning,[6] burns,[7] asphyxiation by food,[15] rape,[5] and injuries from machines.[8] The ten basic strategies described in Chapter 7 provide an alternative framework for considering motor vehicle injuries and relevant countermeasures. Readers are referred to other sources for comprehensive discussions of the subject of crash injury prevention.[8-9,11-14,16,23]

Two data sources provide detailed national information on virtually all traffic deaths: the NCHS mortality file and the Fatal Accident Reporting System (FARS) of the National Highway Traffic Safety Admin-

Table 16–1
Examples of Factors Related to the Likelihood of Injury

	Human	*Vehicle*	*Physical and Social Environment*
Pre-Crash	Driver vision Alcohol intoxication Experience and judgement Amount of travel	Brakes, tires Center of gravity Jackknife tendency Speed of travel Ease of control Load characteristics	Laws related to drunk driving Visibility of hazards Road curvature and gradient Surface coeffient of friction Divided highways, one-way streets Intersections, access control Signalization Speed limits
Crash	Seat belt use Osteoporosis	Speed capability Vehicle size Automatic restraints Placement and hardness and sharpness of contact surfaces Load containment	Speed limits Recovery areas Guard rails Characteristics of fixed objects Median barriers Roadside embankments
Post-Crash	Age Physical condition	Fuel system integrity	Emergency communication systems Distance to and quality of emergency medical services Rehabilitation programs

istration (NHTSA). These sources agree closely as to the total number of deaths (see Appendix). In this book we have used NCHS data for all analyses by race, place of residence, or income level, because FARS data do not indicate race and generally specify place of residence only for drivers. In other respects, FARS records provide greater detail and therefore are used in most of the other analyses of motor vehicle traffic deaths.

Except where otherwise noted, the information presented in this section pertains to deaths or injuries categorized as "traffic-related." In addition to the 50,000 or so such deaths each year, NCHS mortality data include 1,200 people killed by road vehicles in nontraffic situations — for example, in driveways, private roads, and worksites. Pedestrians, the largest component of non-traffic deaths, number about 500 annually; more than one-third are children younger than 5 years.

In contrast to deaths, nonfatal injuries are not as clearly defined or easily enumerated. The best national estimates of the incidence of nonfatal injuries are based on samples, such as NCHS's National Health Interview Survey (NHIS) or NHTSA's National Accident Sampling System (NASS). NHIS provides only limited information on motor vehicle crash injuries, which are a subset of a continuing national sample of health conditions. NASS, a relatively recent data collection system, is more detailed. The 1981 file contains data from a stratified sample of police-reported crashes in 30 geographic areas. This system is designed to provide a nationally representative sample of all such events. In addition, estimates of the incidence of specific categories of motor vehicle-related injuries have been obtained from several population-based regional studies (table 16-2).

Hospital-based research reveals significant underreporting of nonfatal injuries by most official statistics. A major study of injuries in northeastern Ohio, for example, found that the number of people injured in traffic collisions and treated in emergency rooms was 43 percent greater than the total number of injured people known from police reports.[3] Since police reports include many injured people who did not receive emergency room treatment, the actual discrepancy is probably even greater.

Injuries related to motor vehicles but not involving crashes are generally identifiable only from surveys, medical records, or death certificates rather than from police reports. Examples include carbon monoxide poisoning (see Chapter 15), scalds and chemical burns from radiators and batteries, flame burns from ignited upholstery or other fires in cars, broken fingers from being caught in doors, strangulation of children by electrically powered windows, and injuries in sudden stops.[1,7,18]

Table 16–2
Estimates of the Incidence of Motor Vehicle Injuries from Population-Based Regional Studies

Type of Injury Studied	*Population and Year of Injury*	*Motor Vehicle Injuries Per 100,000 Study Population Per Year*	*Total Number Projected to 1980 U.S. Population*	*Percent of Injuries Studied Caused by Motor Vehicles*
Injury requiring emergency room treatment[a] (Barancik, et al., 1983)	5 counties in Northeastern Ohio, 1977	2,071 injuries	4,690,000	10
Facial injury treated in emergency room[a] (Karlson, 1982)	Dane County, Wisconsin, June 1978-May 1979	278 facial injuries including:	630,000	20
		(169 facial lacerations)	(383,000)	20
		(28 facial fxs)	(63,000)	26
Brain injury diagnosed by a physician[b] (Kraus, et al., 1984)	San Diego County, California, 1981	79 brain injuries	179,000	44
Acute spinal cord injuries[b] (SCI) (Kraus, et al., 1975)	18 counties in N. Carolina, 1970–71	3 spinal cord injuries	6,800	56
Burns, including scalds, resulting in hospitalization (Feck and Baptiste, 1979)	New York state, excluding New York City, 1974-1975	1.6 burns	3,700	6

[a]Also includes hospital admissions and deaths.
[b]All cases were admitted to hospitals and/or died.

This chapter describes motor vehicle death rates and compares fatalities in major types of crashes. Analyses by per capita income and place of residence are presented mainly in this chapter. Analyses by age, sex, and state are presented here and in greater detail in Chapters 17 through 20. The latter chapters add detailed analyses on the circumstances of crashes, based on data from NASS and FARS.

Age and Sex

Motor vehicle death rates vary tremendously by age and sex, with peaks in the late teenage years and early twenties (figure 16-3). After that, death rates decline, then increase again beginning at about age 65.

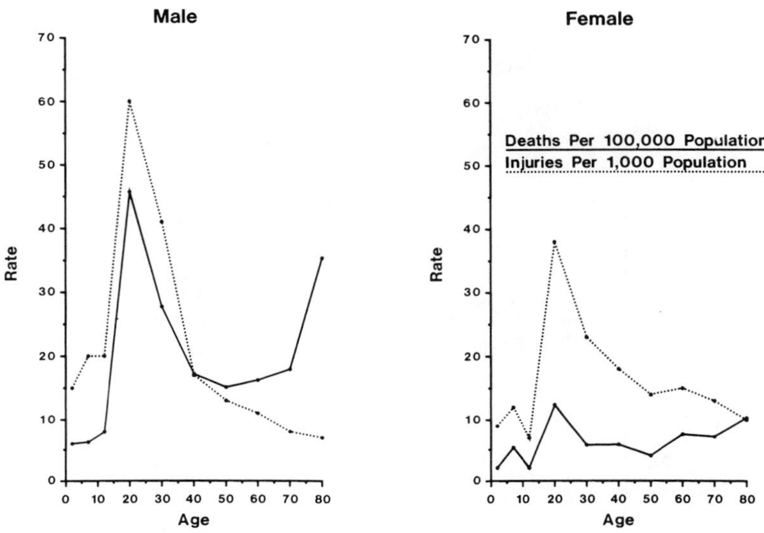

Figure 16-3. Motor Vehicle Crash Injury and Death Rates by Age and Sex, Northeastern Ohio, Emergency Room Visits in 1977 and Deaths in 1976-1978

Males are much more frequently involved than females, especially males in their twenties. The ratio of male to female death rates is 2.8:1 for all ages combined, and almost 4:1 for ages 20-29. The only age for which there is no sex difference in death rates is during the first year of life, when virtually all deaths are to vehicle occupants. The drop in occupant death rates after the first year of life (figure 4-5) is not evident in figure 16-3 because it includes pedestrians and all other motor vehicle fatalities.

As in the case of fatality rates, the rates for motor vehicle crash injuries treated in emergency rooms are highest for ages 15-24 (figure 16-3). The male-female differences, on the other hand, are not as pronounced for injuries as for deaths. Injury rates are higher for males than for females between the ages of 1 and 35. In addition, after about age 15 injuries to males tend to be more severe as well as more frequent than injuries to females. Prior to age 16, males have a slightly higher ratio of deaths to injuries than females. Then the ratio for males jumps sharply, and is 2-3 times as high as the female death:injury ratio among adults (figure 16-4).

The higher ratio of deaths to injuries among older people reflects their greater susceptibility to complications when injured and their

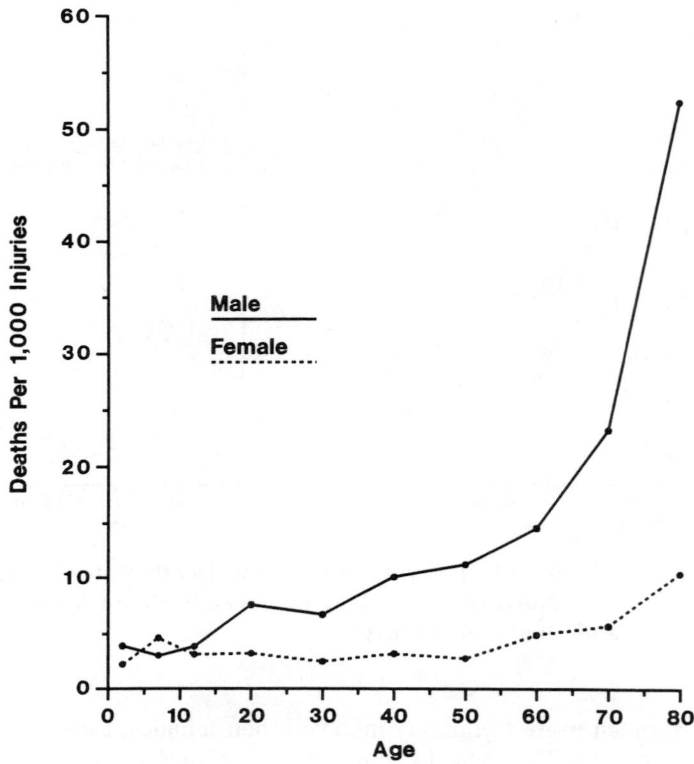

Source: Reprinted with permission from: D. Fife, J.I. Barancik, and B.F. Chatterjee, "Northeastern Ohio Trauma Study II: Injury Rates by Age, Sex, and Cause," *American Journal of Public Health,* 1984. Copyright, American Public Health Association.

Figure 16-4. Deaths Per 1,000 Motor Vehicle Crash Injuries by Age and Sex, Northeastern Ohio, Emergency Room Visits in 1977 and Deaths in 1976-1978

substantially poorer prognosis. This effect is greatest for the least severe injuries. Minor injuries that are rarely fatal in younger people result in significant mortality at ages 70 and older, whereas for the most severe injuries age plays a less important role in survival. Figure 16-5 illustrates this effect, using an overall measure of injury severity, the Injury Severity Score.[2]

A common and misleading oversimplification is to talk about motor vehicle crashes as if all were similar events. Many types of motor vehicle crashes occur — car-to-car, single-car, pedestrian, motorcycle, truck, etc. — and generally the people involved in different kinds of crashes have different characteristics.

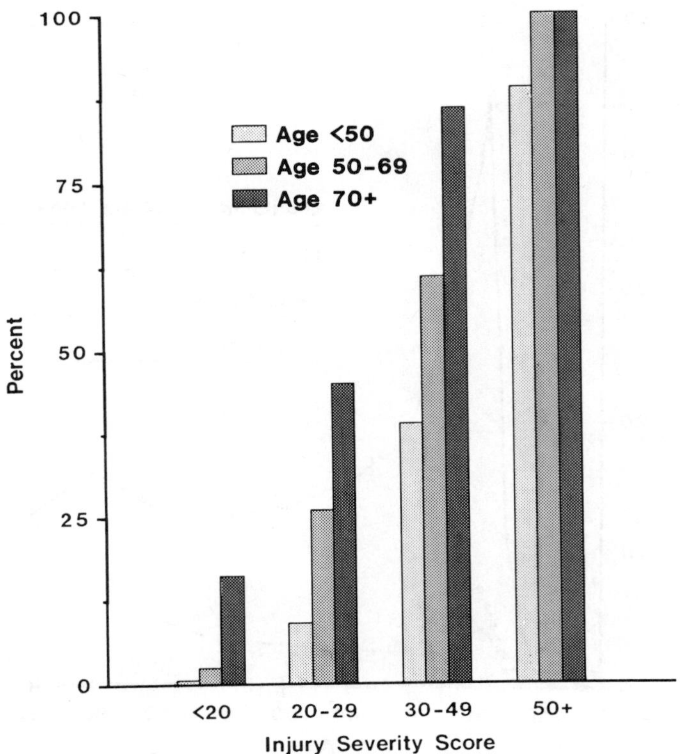

Figure 16-5. Percent of Patients Hospitalized for Motor Vehicle Crash Injuries Who Died by Injury Severity Score and Age, Eight Hospitals in Baltimore, 1968-1969

Death rates for the various types of crashes show distinctive age patterns (figure 16-6). (The rates by single year of age are shown in figures 4-3, 4-4, and 4-5.) Bicyclist death rates are highest at ages 11-15, occupant rates at ages 18-20, and motorcyclist rates at ages 18-22. Pedestrian death rates are highest after age 70, with somewhat lower peaks at ages 6 and 18. The relative importance of each category of motor vehicle fatality varies with age (figure 16-7). Pedestrians account for the majority of all motor vehicle-related deaths in the 5-9-year-old age group,* whereas for all other ages motor vehicle occupants are the largest category. Bicyclist deaths are prominent between the ages of 5

* When analyzed by specific year of age, pedestrian deaths outnumber occupant deaths for children ages 4-8 years.

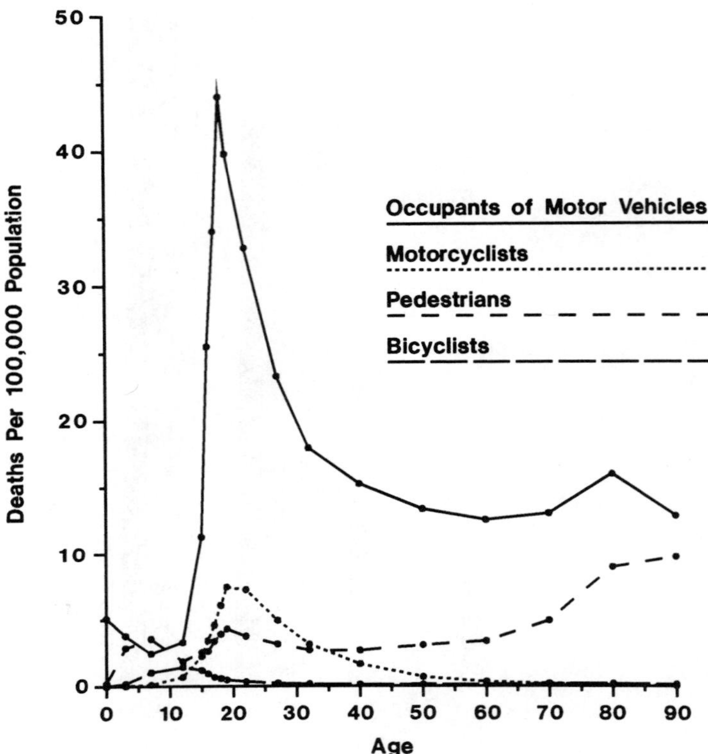

Figure 16-6. Death Rates from Motor Vehicle Crashes by Age and Type of Fatality, 1979-1981

and 14, when they account for about one-sixth of all motor vehicle-related deaths. Among ages 15-34, motorcyclists account for more than one-tenth of such deaths.

Race and Per Capita Income

Death rates from motor vehicle crashes vary tremendously by race and per capita income. Native Americans have the highest death rates from all types of motor vehicle crashes combined — 51 per 100,000, compared to 24 for whites, 19 for blacks, and 9 for Asians. In addition, age patterns vary among racial groups (figure 16-8). Death rates peak for whites at ages 15-24 and for Native Americans and blacks at ages 20-24. After age 30, rates for blacks do not change very much, while

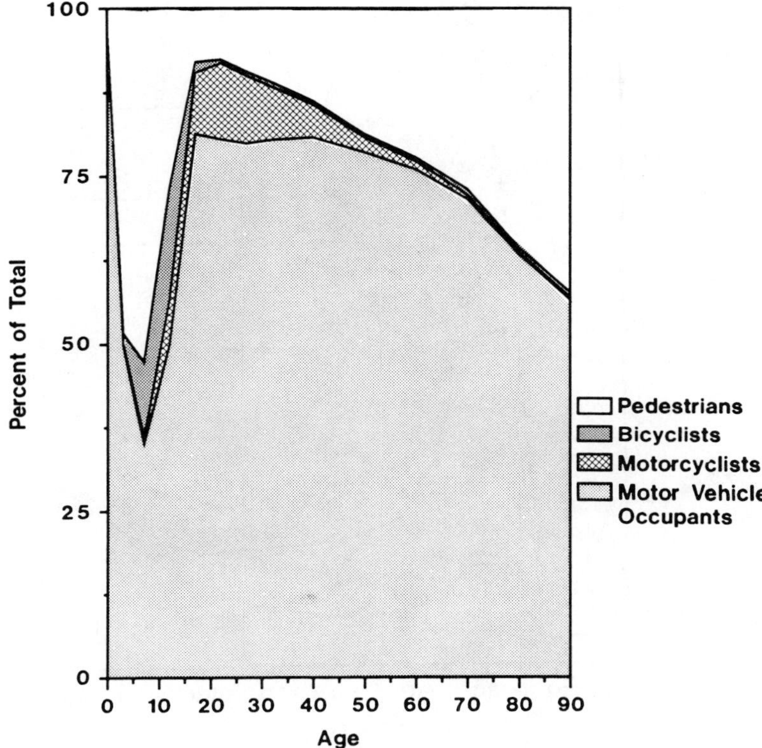

Figure 16-7. Percent of Motor Vehicle Deaths by Age and Type of Fatality, 1979-1981

death rates among Native Americans decline. Rates among whites and Asians drop and then increase.

Separate analyses of the major categories of fatalities show that whites have the highest death rates from motorcycle crashes. Native Americans have the highest rates as occupants and pedestrians. Asians have the lowest rates in all categories (figure 16-9).

The factors underlying these differences need further exploration. While racial differences in injury rates have sometimes been attributed to different patterns of alcohol use, additional factors play a role. Native Americans, for example, may be disproportionately likely to walk on roads without pedestrian areas or to ride in open pickup trucks.[24]

When analyses for whites and blacks are further separated by age and sex as well as by type of fatality, it is clear that the teenage increases in occupant and motorcyclist death rates are not as steep for blacks as

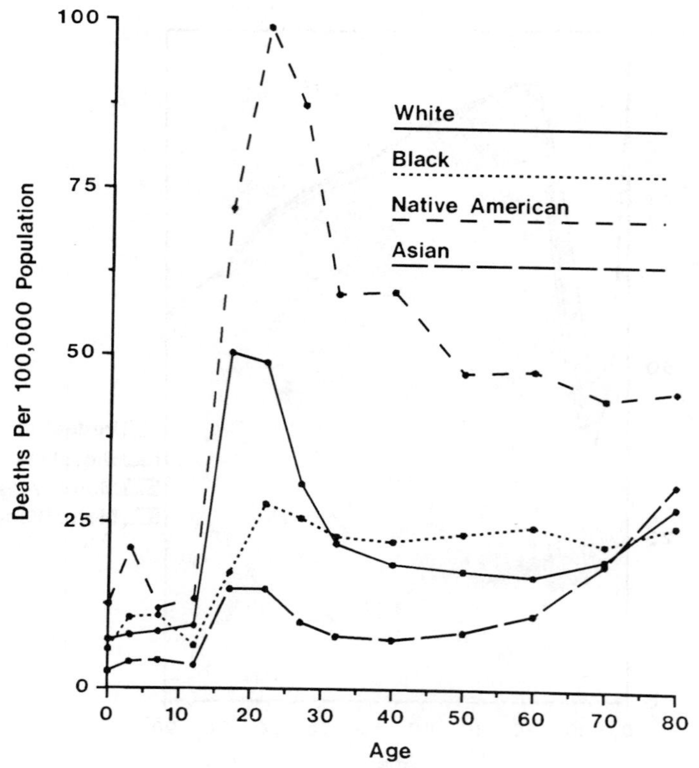

Figure 16-8. Death Rates from Motor Vehicle Crashes by Age and Race, 1977-1979

for whites (figure 16-10). In contrast, bicyclist death rates are virtually the same for black and white males during the high-risk ages.

From about age 30 to 75, the occupant death rate for black males exceeds that for white males, while at other ages it is higher for white males. For females the rate for whites is slightly higher at all ages. Pedestrian death rates are substantially higher for blacks ages 1-9 and 25 or older.

Motor vehicle death rates vary inversely with the per capita income of the area of residence (figure 16-11). For each race, the death rate in counties where the annual per capita income is less than $3,000 is more than double the rate in counties where the average income is $6,000 or more. Most of this difference is attributable to variations in

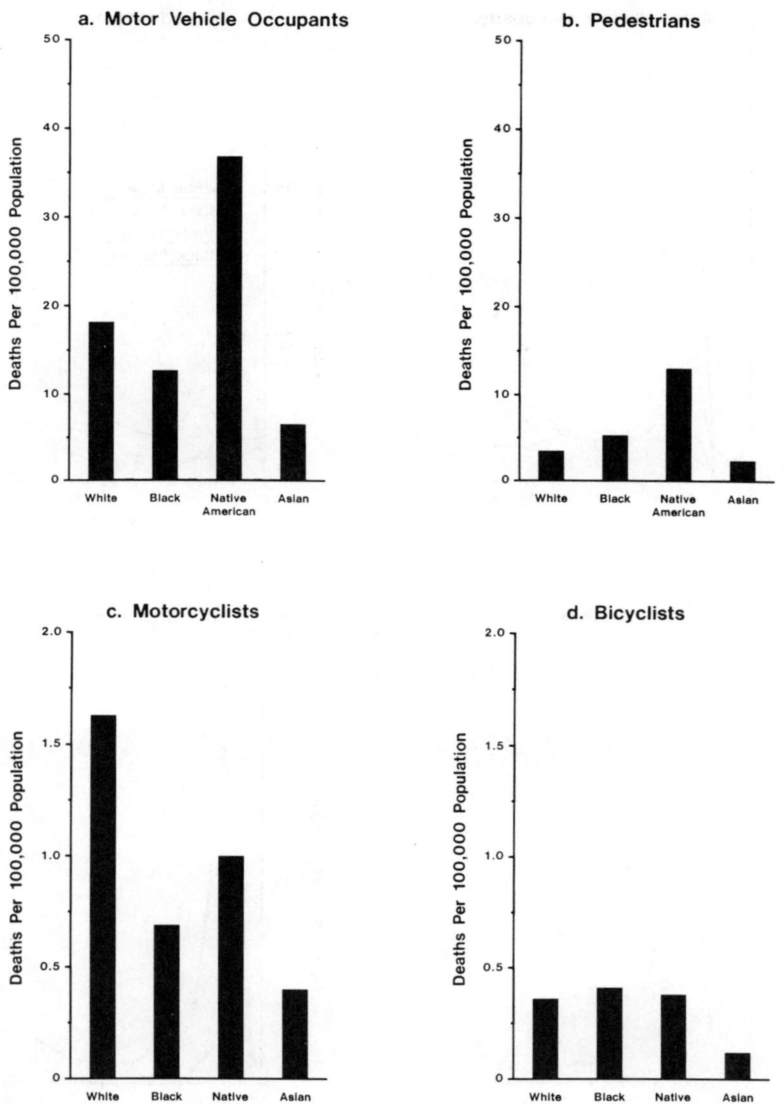

Note: Vertical scales differ

Figure 16-9. Death Rates from Motor Vehicle Crashes by Race and Type of Fatality, 1977-1979

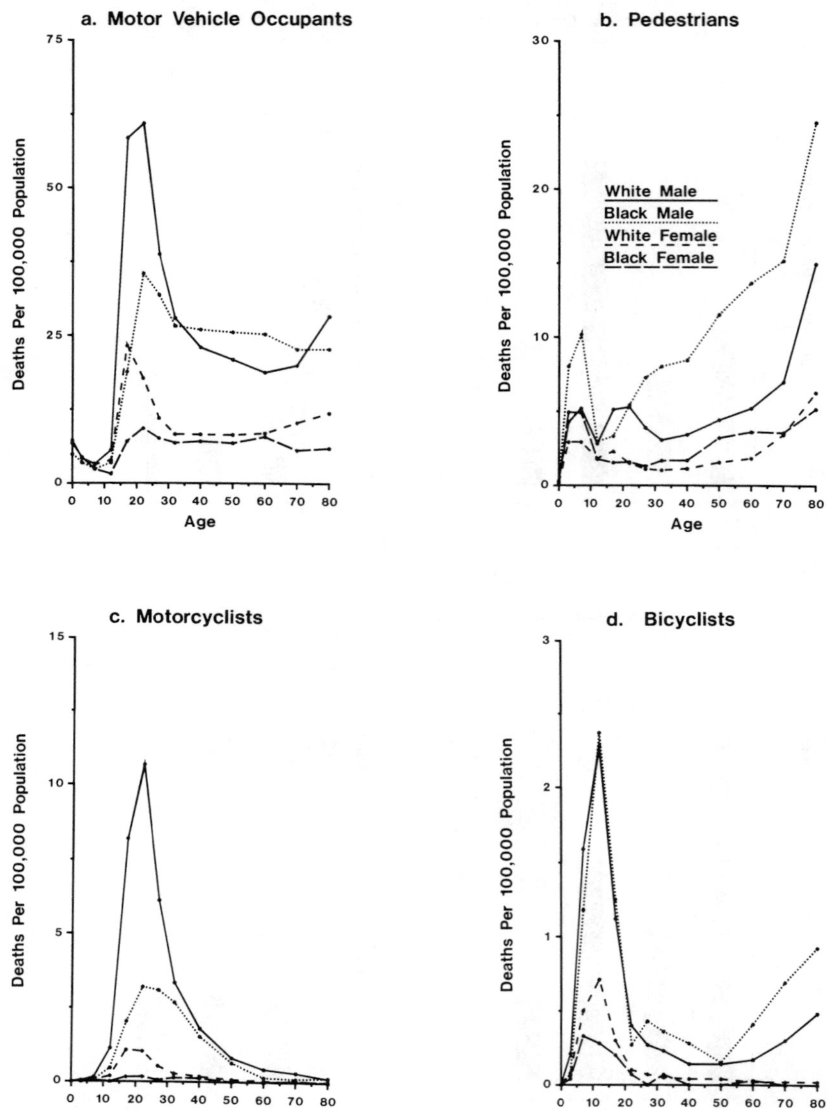

Note: Vertical scales differ

Figure 16-10. Death Rates from Motor Vehicle Crashes by Age, Race, Sex, and Type of Fatality, 1977-1979

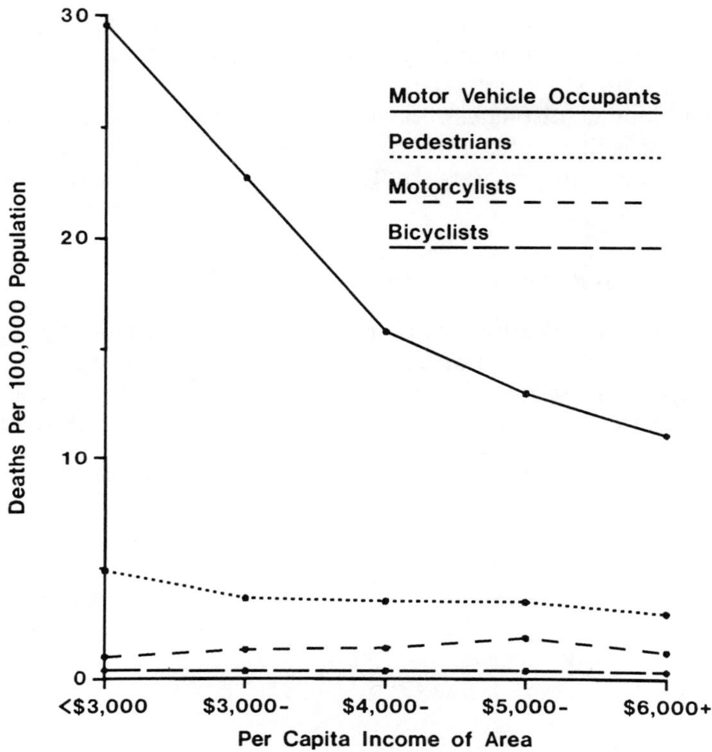

Figure 16-11. Death Rates from Motor Vehicle Crashes by Per Capita Income of Area of Residence and Type of Fatality, 1977-1979

the occupant death rate, which is almost three times as high in low-income areas. The other major categories of motor vehicle deaths show little or no relationship to per capita income.

The higher occupant death rates in lower-income areas are not explained by differences in the amount of motor vehicle travel, since the Nationwide Personal Transportation Study (NPTS) found that the amount of travel per person more than doubles as per capita income increases from $4,000 to $20,000.[4] It is likely that poorer roads in many low-income areas, older vehicles, different driving practices, and poorer emergency and medical care all contribute to the higher death rates. One observational study found that adult drivers in high-income areas use seat belts at three times the rate of adult drivers in low-income areas. This difference is even greater among teenage drivers.[26]

The relationships between occupant death rates and per capita income are similar for blacks and whites (figure 16-12). In higher-income areas, there is little difference between blacks and whites in pedestrian death rates, as was previously noted for all unintentional injuries combined (figure 3-10).

Urban/Rural and Geographic Differences

Motor vehicle death rates are more than twice as high among residents of rural areas as in cities of a million or more, increasing from 14 per 100,000 population in the largest cities to 37 in the most rural areas. As in the case of differences by income of area, these differences pri-

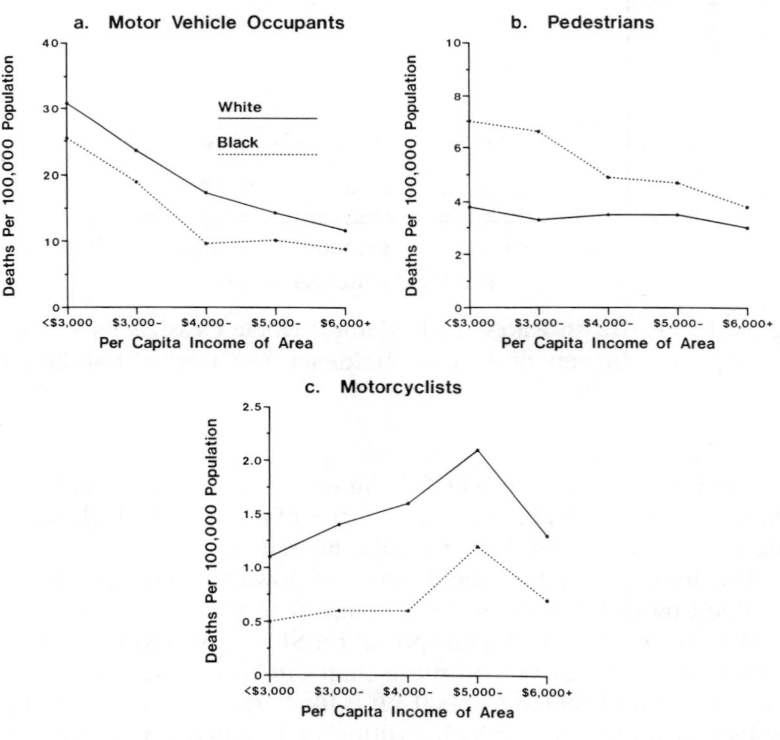

Figure 16-12. Death Rates from Motor Vehicle Crashes by Per Capita Income of Area of Residence, Race, and Type of Fatality, 1977-1979

marily reflect the major contribution of occupant deaths. Among whites, occupant death rates in the most rural areas are three times the rates in the largest cities, and for blacks there is a fivefold difference (figure 16-13). Pedestrian death rates are highest in large cities for whites, but

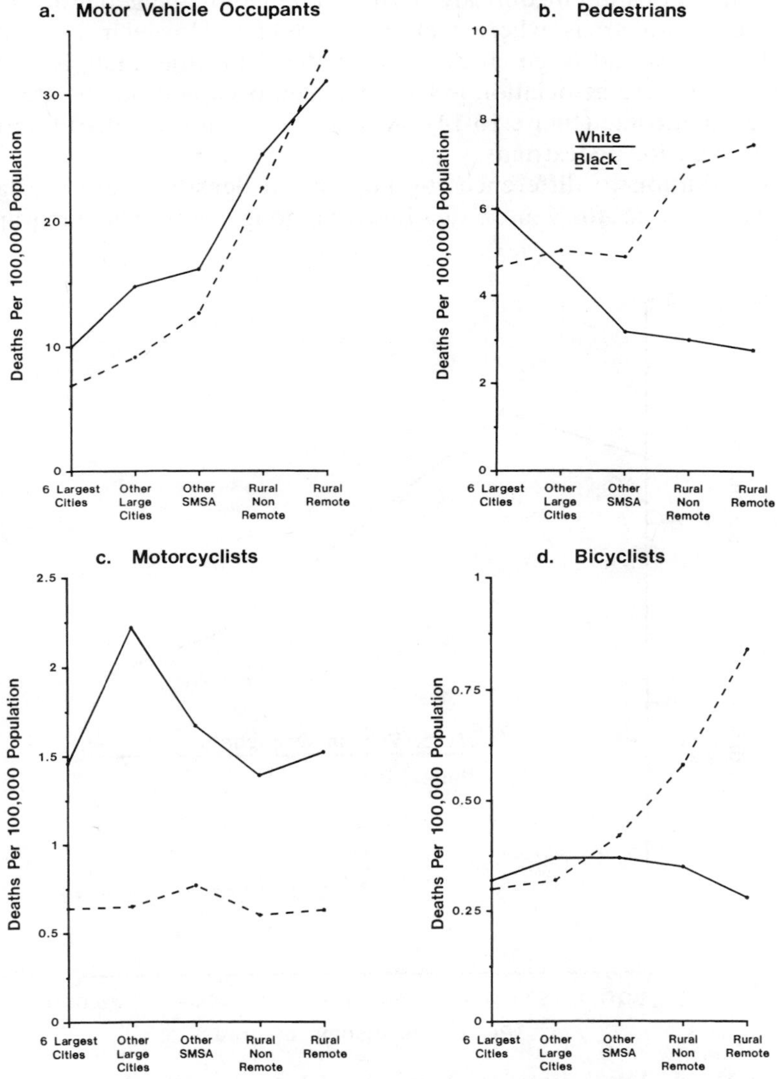

Figure 16-13. Death Rates from Motor Vehicle Crashes by Place of Residence, Race, and Type of Fatality, 1977-1979

the reverse is true for blacks. For motorcyclists, rates are highest for whites who live in large cities (excluding the six largest cities), whereas bicyclist death rates are highest among black residents of very rural areas.

The previously noted relationships between motor vehicle death rates and per capita income are partly explained by the generally lower income in rural areas, where death rates are high. However, even when rural counties and large cities are excluded from the analysis, a pronounced inverse association is seen between occupant death rates and per capita income (figure 16-14). A weaker (but also inverse) relationship is seen for pedestrians.

In addition to differences by population density, there are large differences in motor vehicle death rates among states. The geographic

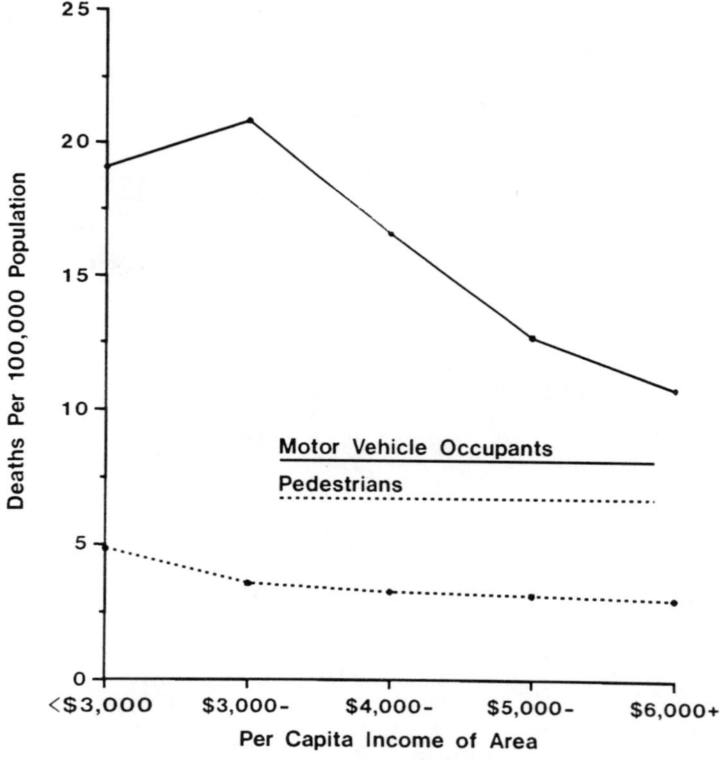

Figure 16-14. Death Rates for Motor Vehicle Occupants and Pedestrians by Per Capita Income of Area of Residence, Non-Urban Parts of SMSA Counties, 1977-1979

patterns in these rates differ among the four major categories of motor vehicle-related deaths (figure 16-15). Occupant death rates are generally lowest in the Northeast and highest in western and southern states. Pedestrian death rates are generally highest in the Southeast

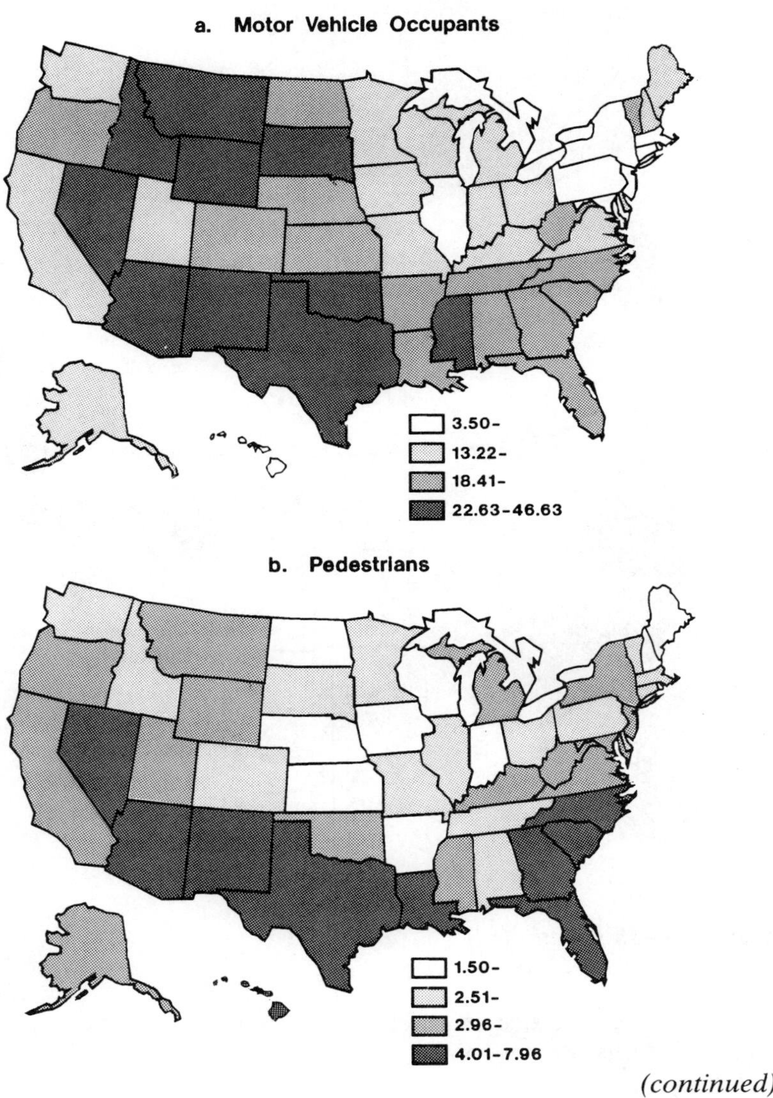

(continued)

Figure 16-15. Death Rates from Motor Vehicle Crashes by State, Per 100,000 Population, 1979-1981

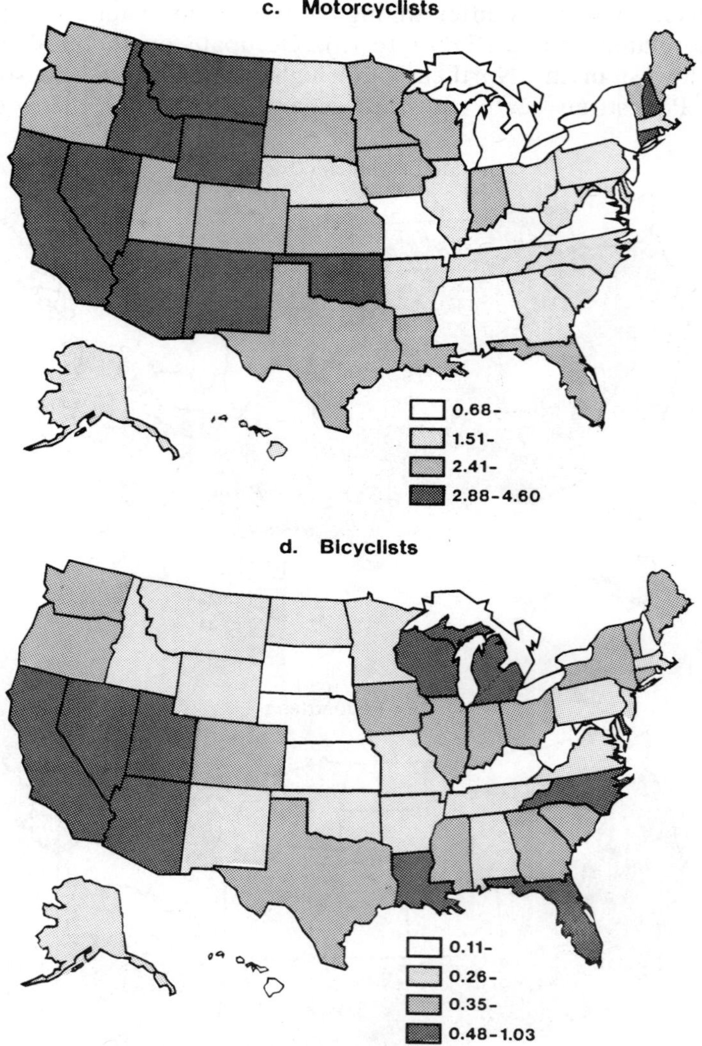

Figure 16–15 *(continued)*

and Southwest, and motorcyclist death rates are highest in western states. Bicyclist deaths, on the other hand, do not show clear regional patterns.*

---

*Figure 16-15, based on FARS data for the state in which the crash occurred, differs from death rates in the Appendix, based on NCHS data for the place of residence of the deceased.

In general, geographic patterns for rates calculated for resident deaths per 100,000 population are similar to those for deaths per 100 million vehicle miles traveled in each state, indicating that variations in the amount of travel do not substantially account for the geographic variations shown in figure 16-15.

Historical Trends

During the past 50 years, the overall motor vehicle death rate per 100,000 population has not shown the major changes that are apparent for many other causes of death (figure 4-16). Rates for some of the categories of motor vehicle deaths, however, have changed dramatically (figure 16-16). The pedestrian death rate, for example, decreased by more than half between 1930 and 1960. The motorcyclist death rate increased fivefold from 1960 to 1980.

In general, the total number of motor vehicle deaths varies with the amount of travel, as illustrated in 1974 when travel decreased somewhat as a result of gasoline shortages (figure 16-17). In this case, substantial decreases in average travel speeds also occurred as a result of the adoption of 55 mph speed limits. Studies have shown that the speed limits were responsible for about half of the reduction in deaths occurring after 1973.[19]

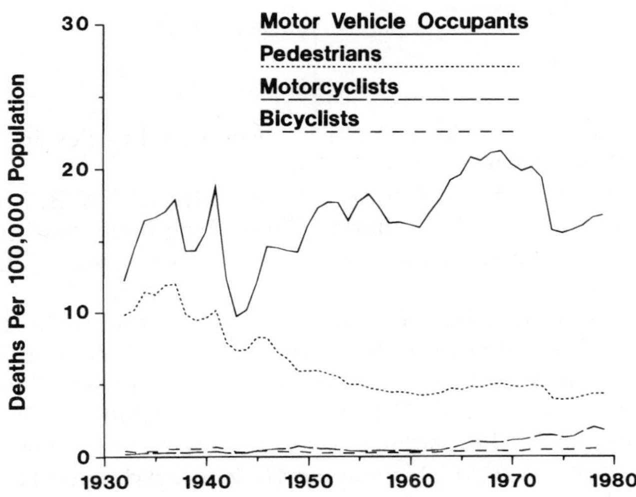

Figure 16-16. Death Rates from Motor Vehicles Crashes by Year and Type of Fatality, 1932-1979

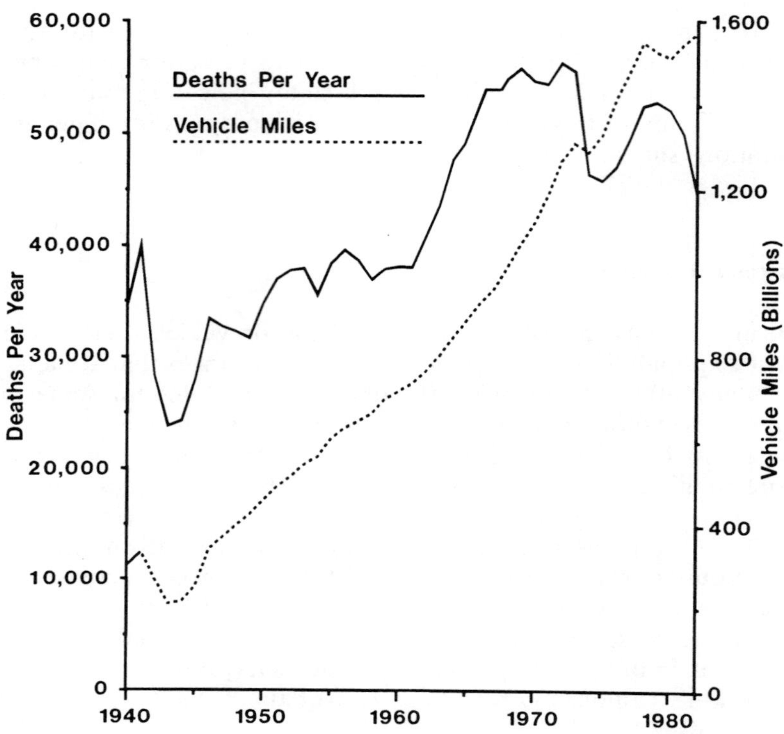

Figure 16-17. Vehicle Miles of Travel and Number of Deaths from Motor Vehicle Injuries, 1940-1982

Notes

1. Agran, P.F. "Motor Vehicle Occupant Injuries in Noncrash Events." *Pediatrics* 67 (1981): 838-840.

2. Baker, S.P., B. O'Neill, W. Haddon, Jr., and W.B. Long. "The Injury Severity Score: A Method for Describing Patients with Multiple Injuries and Evaluating Emergency Care." *The Journal of Trauma* 14 (1974): 187-196.

3. Barancik, J.I., B.F. Chatterjee, Y.C. Greene, E.M. Michenzi, and D. Fife. "Northeastern Ohio Trauma Study: I. Magnitude of the Problem." *American Journal of Public Health* 73 (1983): 746-751.

4. Carsten, O., and K. Weber. "Child and Adult Travel Exposure and Fatality Risk." *Proceedings of the Twenty-Fifth Conference of the American Association for Automotive Medicine*. Arlington Heights, IL: American Association for Automotive Medicine, 1981.

5. Dietz, P.E. *Social Factors in Rapist Behavior*. Philadelphia: University of Pennsylvania School of Medicine, Center for Studies in Social-Legal Psychiatry. Unpublished manuscript, 1977. (Portions of this manuscript appear in Dietz, P.E., "Social Factors in Rapist Behavior," *Clinical Aspects of the Rapist*, edited by R. Rada, New York: Grune and Stratton 1978.

6. Dietz, P.E., and S.P. Baker. "Drowning-Epidemiology and Prevention." *American Journal of Public Health* 64 (1974): 303-312.

7. Feck, G., M.S. Baptiste, and C.L. Tate, Jr. *An Epidemiologic Study of Burn Injuries and Strategies for Prevention*. Atlanta: U.S. Department of Health and Human Services, Public Health Service, Centers for Disease Control, 1978.

8. Haddon, W., Jr. "Advances in the Epidemiology of Injuries as a Basis for Public Policy." *Public Health Reports* 95 (1980): 411-421.

9. Haddon, W., Jr. "Approaches to Prevention of Injuries." *Proceedings of the American Medical Association Conference on Prevention of Disabling Injuries*. Chicago: American Medical Association, 1983.

10. Haddon, W., Jr. "The Changing Approach to the Epidemiology, Prevention, and Amelioration of Trauma: The Transition to Approaches Etiologically Rather than Descriptively Based." *American Journal of Public Health* 58 (1968): 1431-1438.

11. Haddon, W., Jr. "Options for the Prevention of Motor Vehicle Crash Injury." *Proceedings of the Conference on the Prevention of Motor Vehicle Crash Injury*. Beersheba, Israel: Ben-Gurion University of the Negev, January 10, 1979. Reprinted in *Israel Journal of Medical Sciences* 16 (1980): 45-68.

12. Haddon, W., Jr. "Reducing the Damage of Motor-Vehicle Use." *Technology Review* 77 (1975): 1-9.

13. Haddon, W., Jr., and S.P. Baker. "Injury Control." In *Preventive and Community Medicine*, edited by D. Clark and B. MacMahon. Boston: Little, Brown and Company, 1981, pp. 109-140.

14. Haddon, W., Jr., E.A. Suchman, and D. Klein. *Accident Research: Methods and Approaches*. New York: Harper and Row, 1964.

15. Harris, C.S., S.P. Baker, G.A. Smith, and R.M. Harris. "Childhood Asphyxiation by Food: A National Analysis and Overview," *Journal of the American Medical Association,* in press.

16. Insurance Institute for Highway Safety. *Policy Options for Reducing the Motor Vehicle Crash Injury Cost Burden*. Washington, DC: Insurance Institute for Highway Safety, 1981.

17. Karpf, R.S., and A.F. Williams. "Teenage Drivers and Motor Vehicle Deaths." *Accident Analysis and Prevention* 15 (1983): 55-63.

18. Kraus, J.F. "The Epidemiology of Suffocation Deaths in Infants and Children, California, 1960-1981," submitted for publication.

19. Mela, D.F. "Review of Information on the Safety Effects of the 55 MPH Speed Limit in the U.S." Technical Report DOT HS-802-383. Washington, DC: National Highway Traffic Safety Administration, 1977.

20. National Center for Health Statistics. "Persons Injured by Class of Accident and Whether Activity Restricting, 1981." Unpublished data from the National Health Interview Survey, 1982.

21. National Highway Traffic Safety Administration. *Report on Traffic Accidents and Injuries for 1979-1980*. Washington, DC: U.S. Department of Transportation, February 1982.

22. National Safety Council. *Accident Facts — 1982 Edition*. Chicago: National Safety Council, 1982.

23. Robertson, L.S. *Injuries: Causes, Control Strategies, and Public Policy*. Lexington, MA: Lexington Books, 1983.

24. Simpson, S.G., R. Reid, S.P. Baker, and S.P. Teret. "Injuries Among the Hopi Indians, A Population-Based Survey." *Journal of the American Medical Association* 249 (1983): 1873-1876.

25. Stapp, J.P. "Effects of Mechanical Force on Living Tissues. I. Abrupt Deceleration and Windblast." *Journal of Aviation Medicine* 26 (1955): 268-287.

26. Williams, A.F., J.K. Wells, and A.K. Lund. "Voluntary Seat Belt Use Among High School Students." *Accident Analysis and Prevention* 15 (1983): 161-165.

17 Motor Vehicle Occupants

Injuries to passenger vehicle occupants are the predominant cause of motor vehicle crash deaths. In recent years almost 70 percent of all traffic-related deaths were to people injured as occupants of passenger vehicles.* Among 15-19-year-old males, one out of every three deaths from *all* causes results from injuries as a motor vehicle occupant.

Preventing or reducing the severity of occupant injury in crashes can be achieved by spreading crash forces over a wide area of the body, by increasing the distance in which the body is decelerated (that is, by making that deceleration less abrupt), and by reducing the overall change in velocity in the crash. It is essential also to design the occupant compartment to maintain its integrity in crashes, keeping occupants inside and preventing intrusion by outside objects.[9]

One way to decrease the abruptness of deceleration is with occupant restraints such as vehicle seat belts. Lap/shoulder belts, when worn, reduce the chances of occupant death in a crash by about 50 percent.[22] The actual effectiveness of this kind of restraint, however, is severely limited by the fact that only a very small minority — about 1 in 10 — of passenger car occupants uses belts.[19] Furthermore, among many high-risk groups, such as teenagers and people in low-income areas, usage is almost nonexistent.[31]

In some countries and jurisdictions outside the United States, non-use of seat belts is now illegal. The results of this approach have varied. In jurisdictions that have aggressively enforced such laws, daytime belt use levels of between 70 and 80 percent have been achieved in urban areas. Unfortunately, people who are at greatest risk of crash involvement continue to be overrepresented among the nonusers.[30] In jurisdictions where such laws are not enforced, belt use levels typically are only slightly higher than they were before the laws.

In addition to trying to increase the use of existing seat belt systems, there is need for automatic (or "passive") restraints that require no action on the part of the motor vehicle occupant in order to be effective. Two basic design approaches for such restraints, automatic seat belts and air bags, have been developed and tested on production automo-

*Passenger vehicles are defined here as cars, light trucks, vans, and on/off road vehicles such as CJ Jeeps. Occupants include drivers and passengers.

biles and used extensively in cars driven in the United States and Canada.[11-12]

Automatic seat belts position themselves around outboard front-seat occupants after they have entered the car. The air bag is an automatic crash protection cushion. The basic components of an air bag system are one or more crash sensors, inflators, and nylon bags. The sensors determine when a frontal crash is of sufficient violence that the air bag should be activated. The inflators, when triggered by the crash sensors, produce harmless nitrogen gas that inflates bags stored out of sight in the center of the steering wheel and in the passenger side of the instrument panel. In a crash, the bags are inflated in a fraction of a second to provide a relatively soft, energy-absorbing cushion between the occupants and the hard structures in front of them. Lap belts are provided with the air bags for people who choose to use them. In this way, air bags offer improved protection for everyone: for the belt user, an air bag plus a lap belt is a more effective restraint system than a lap/shoulder belt; for the non-belt user, an air bag provides greatly improved protection compared to no restraint system.

Special problems for occupant restraint are posed by infants who cannot sit up unassisted, for whom neither seat belts nor air bags provide sufficient protection. This is not true for young children who can sit up. Despite many claims to the contrary, young children can be protected by seat belts or air bags.[29] Infants should be transported in one of the various infant restraint systems available. Typically, this is a rearward facing seat, held in place by the seat belt, in which the infant is belted in a semi-reclining position. However, infant and child restraints have the same problem as seat belts: lack of sufficient use. An additional problem is incorrect use, especially failure to correctly attach the child restraint to the car or to secure the child properly. Unlike laws for adults, laws that require restraints for children appear to be acceptable politically and have now been enacted in most states. Their effect on child deaths and injuries remains to be determined.

Age and Sex

Very large age and sex differences exist in the death and injury rates for passenger vehicle occupants, with young males having especially high rates. Some of these differences are due to variations in the amount of travel and the consequent exposure to risk. Data from the Nationwide Personal Transportation Study show the great variation in exposure, expressed as person-miles traveled (figure 17-1).

The greater amount of travel by males contributes to their high

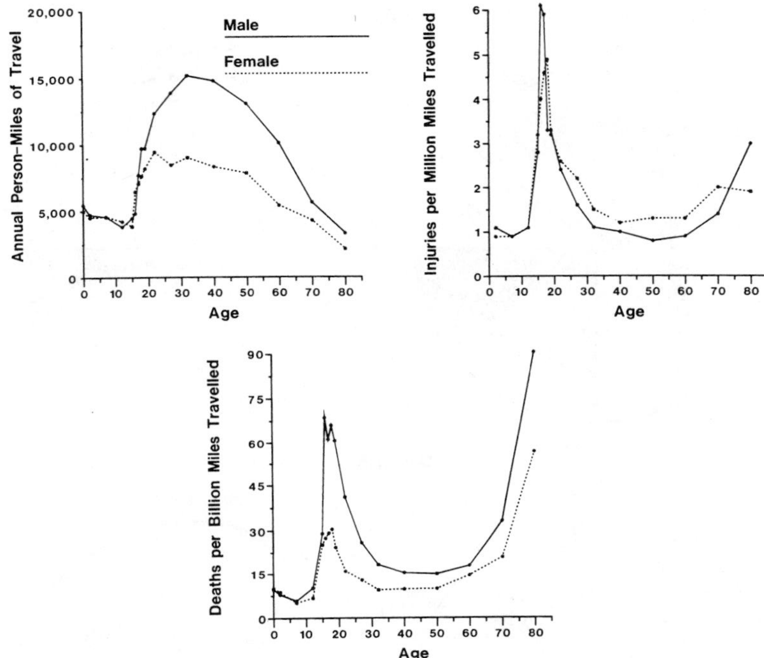

Figure 17-1. Amount of Travel (1977) and Occupant Injury and Death Rates Per Person-Mile of Travel by Age and Sex, 1979-1981

death and injury rates. However, even when variations in the amount of travel are taken into consideration by calculating rates per person-mile of travel, the death rates for males are still substantially higher than those for females after about age 10. For both sexes, the peaks for ages 16-19 remain prominent (figure 17-1).

The higher death rates for males probably reflect differences in speed, alcohol use, and other variables related to serious crashes and high fatality rates. Compared to crashes of female drivers, fatal crashes involving male drivers are more likely to be single-vehicle crashes or nighttime crashes, which typically are very severe (figure 17-2). As drivers, males account for about 70 percent of miles driven and 70 percent of drivers in crashes, but 82 percent of the drivers in fatal crashes. Thus, the amount of travel appears to explain more of the sex difference in crash rates than in death rates.

Exposure is a factor that can be manipulated in order to reduce

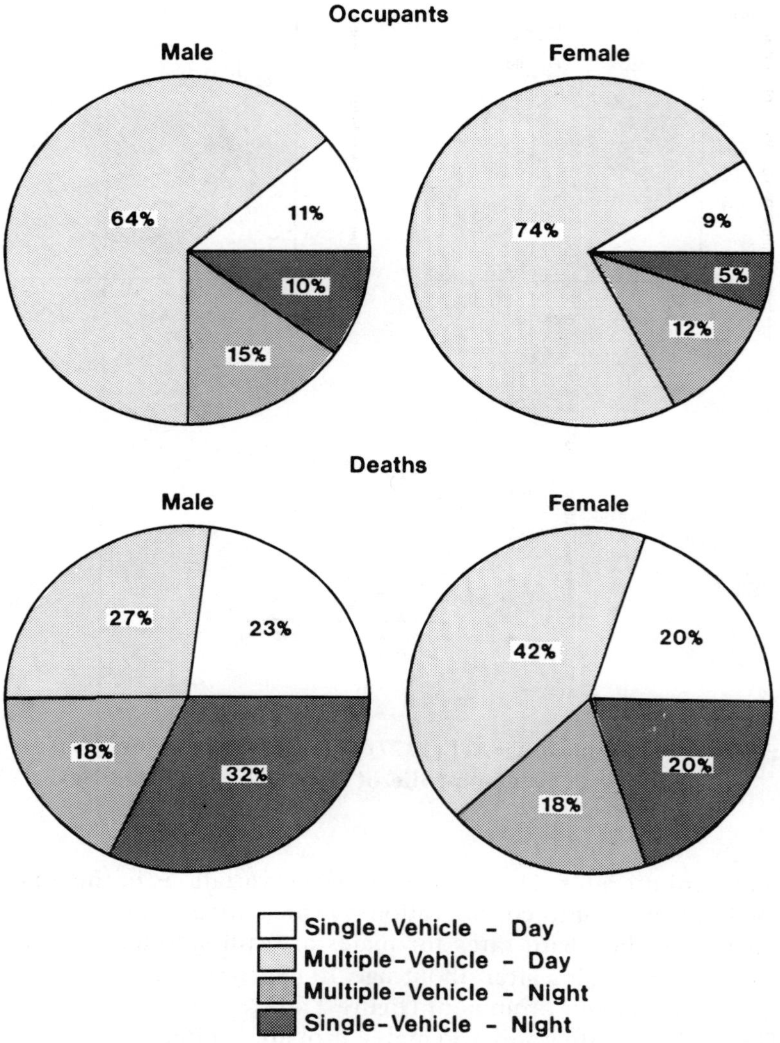

Figure 17-2. Percent of Occupants Involved in Crashes and Deaths in Crashes by Sex, Time of Day, and Number of Vehicles, 1979-1981

injuries and deaths. Some states have curfew laws that prohibit driving by young people during certain nighttime hours. Such laws have substantially reduced crashes of 16 year olds.[20] Conversely, the very availability of high school driver education courses influences many teenagers to drive sooner than they would otherwise, thereby increasing the amount of driving by this very high-risk group. In some communities, large reductions in teenage crashes have followed decreases in licensure and driving by 16 year olds when high school driver education courses were discontinued.[24]

Fatal crash involvement rates per 10,000 licensed drivers for both multiple- and single-vehicle crashes are highest for 18-year-old drivers and lowest for drivers ages 35-64 (figure 17-3). The involvement rate of drivers 70 years and older increases for multiple-vehicle crashes at intersections. This finding suggests age-related changes in the ability to perceive, gauge the speed of, and respond to the movements of other vehicles. Despite such changes, the fatal crash involvement rate of drivers 70 years and older (3.1 per 10,000 licensed drivers) is slightly lower than the average involvement rate (3.6) for drivers of all ages

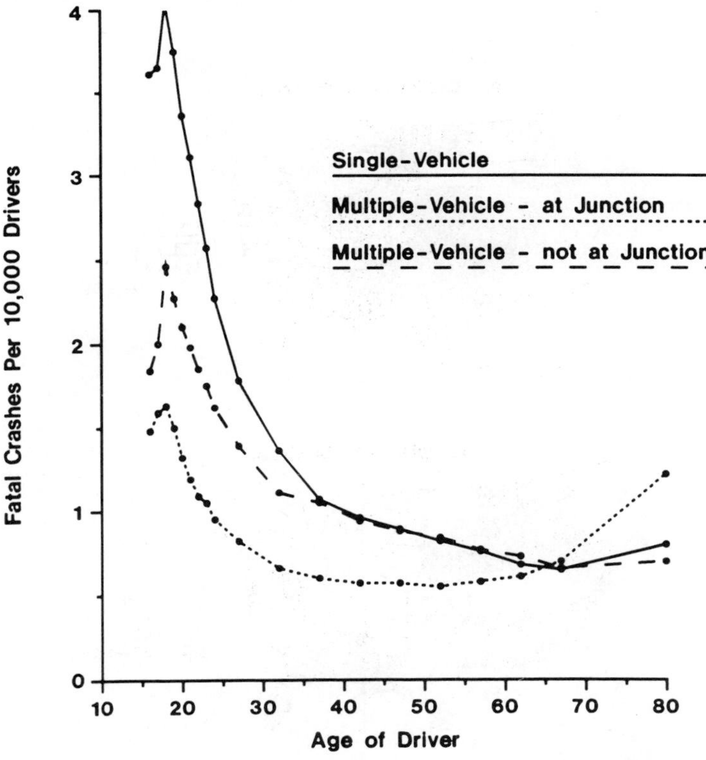

Figure 17-3. Fatal Crash Involvement Rate by Age of Driver and Type of Crash Per 10,000 Licensed Drivers, 1979-1981

combined. The higher death rates among elderly drivers compared to middle-aged drivers probably reflect their lower injury thresholds and greater likelihood of complications following injury as well as increases in some types of crashes.

Geographic Differences

Occupant death rates in all types of crashes combined are highest in the southern and western parts of the United States (figure 16-15a), but the patterns vary for different types of crashes. For example, death rates from collisions with trains, which kill about 800 motor vehicle occupants annually, are highest in the central part of the United States (figure 17-4). Most of these states have especially large numbers of rail-highway crossings on the same level (referred to as "at grade") with no protection other than warning or stop signs. In northeastern states

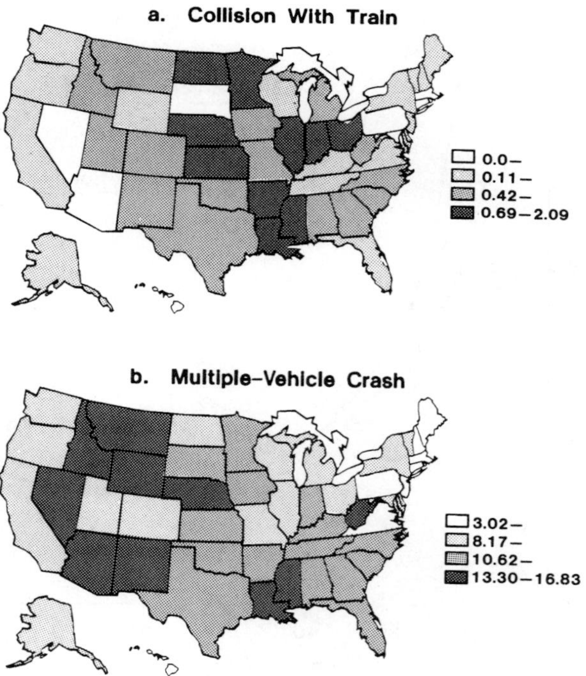

Figure 17-4. Death Rates from Motor Vehicle Crashes by State and Type of Crash, Per Billion Vehicle Miles, 1979-1981

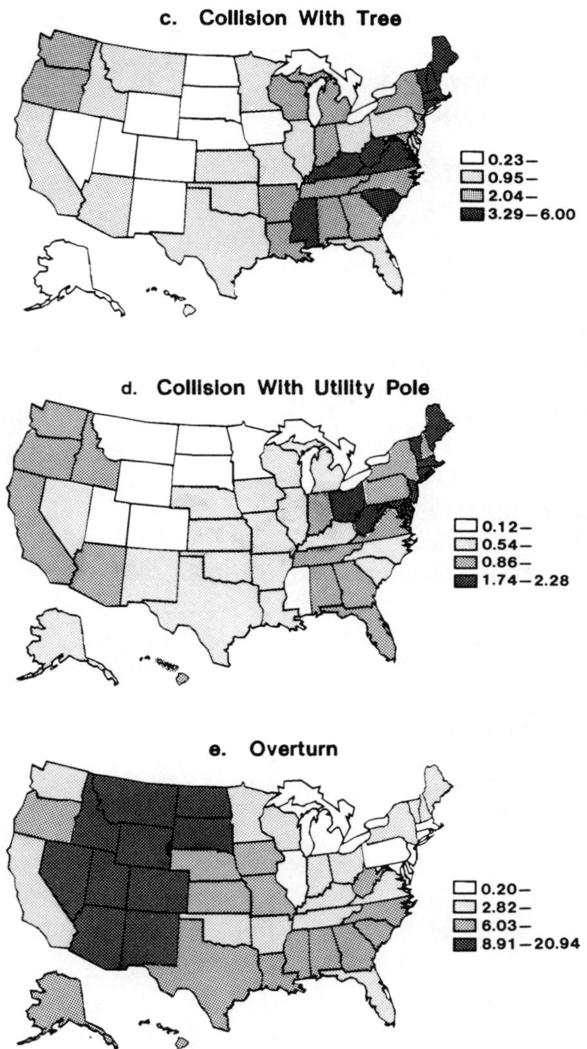

Figure 17–4 *(continued)*

such as New York and Pennsylvania where death rates from collisions with trains are generally low, the trains pass over or under highways at one-third or more of all crossings, and one-third to one-half of the at-grade crossings are protected by gates, flashing lights, or other active warning devices.[7] Because of the tremendous forces involved and the high death rates, collisions between trains and motor vehicles should be prevented wherever possible with failure-proof measures such as elimination of rail-highway intersections at grade, rather than relying on motor vehicle drivers' perceptions of risk.

Death rates for occupants in multiple-vehicle crashes, excluding collisions with trains, are lowest in the northeastern, north central, and Pacific coast states. They are highest in the mountain states (figure 17-4b).

Collisions with trees, which claim about 3,600 lives each year, are associated with high death rates in the eastern third of the country (figure 17-4c). Collisions with utility poles, which result in 1,800 deaths annually, also have high rates in eastern states, especially the Northeast (figure 17-4d). These differences reflect the greater numbers of trees in the East and also suggest that utility poles generally may be closer to the road. It is possible to identify trees, poles, and other structures that are in especially hazardous locations (for example, sites that combine a downhill gradient with a curve in the road of more than six degrees) and to remove, reposition, or shield such fixed objects in ways that protect vehicle occupants.[33] Placing utility poles farther from lanes of travel and burying electrical and telephone lines also reduce or eliminate the risk of collision with poles. In addition, breakaway poles that yield on impact reduce injuries when crashes occur.

About 8,000 occupants are killed each year in vehicles that overturn. Death rates for such "rollover" crashes, which are highest in the mountain states (figure 17-4e), are related not only to the gradient and curvature of roads, but also to the absence of recovery areas and guardrails where vehicles leaving the roadway can roll down an embankment.[32]

Season, Day, and Time

Passenger vehicle occupant fatalities are most common in the summer months and least common in the winter (figure 17-5). This seasonal pattern holds true for all regions of the country including the southern states, but it is most extreme in Alaska.

Time of day is also an important factor in the incidence of injuries and deaths (figure 17-6). More than one-third (37 percent) of passenger vehicle occupant fatalities occur in crashes between 10:00 P.M. and 3:59 A.M., even though only 17 percent of crashes occur during these hours. Less than 40 percent of deaths occur in daytime crashes (6:00 A.M. to 5:59 P.M.), even though more than 60 percent of crashes reported to the police and three-fourths of all passenger miles traveled are during the day.[6]

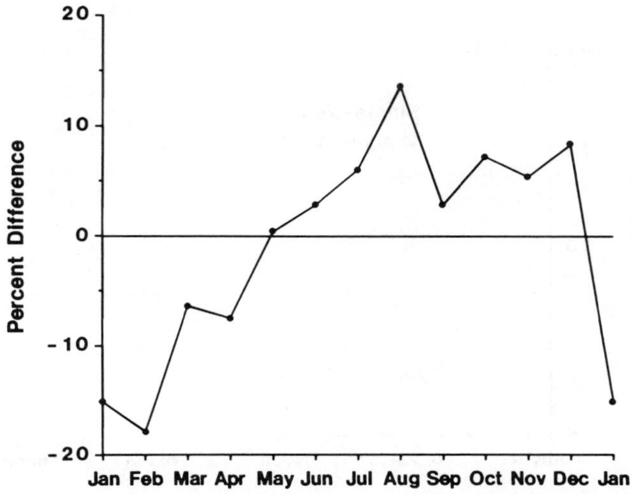

Figure 17-5. Percent Difference from the Average Number of Occupant Deaths by Month, 1979-1981

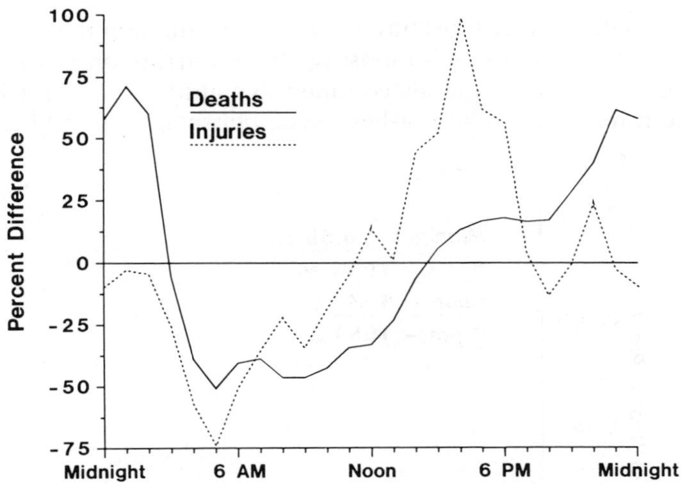

Figure 17-6. Percent Difference from the Average Number of Occupant Deaths and Injuries by Time of Crash, 1979-1981

A larger proportion of multiple-vehicle than of single-vehicle crashes occur during the daytime (figure 17-7). There is a pronounced peak in deaths from multiple-vehicle crashes at about 5:00 P.M. Single-vehicle crashes exhibit a dramatic peak from 1:00 to 2:59 A.M.

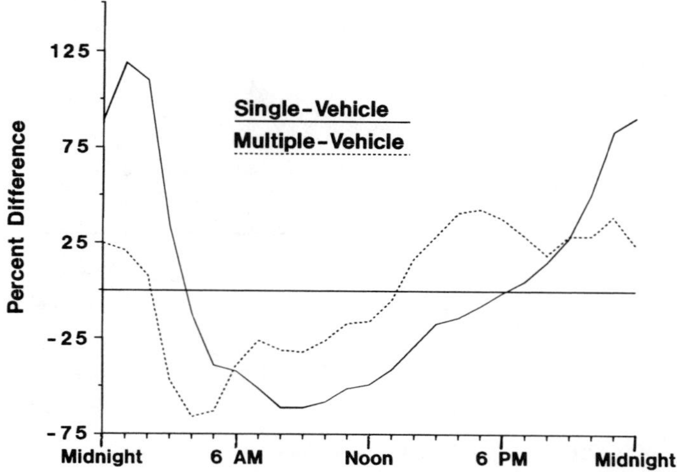

Figure 17-7. Percent Difference from the Average Number of Single- and Multiple-Vehicle Fatal Crashes by Time of Crash, 1979-1981

Although there is substantial variation in the number of occupant deaths by day of week, with most deaths occurring on weekends, the day-to-day variation is mainly confined to nighttime crashes (figure 17-8). One-third of all fatal crashes occur between 6:00 P.M. and 5:59

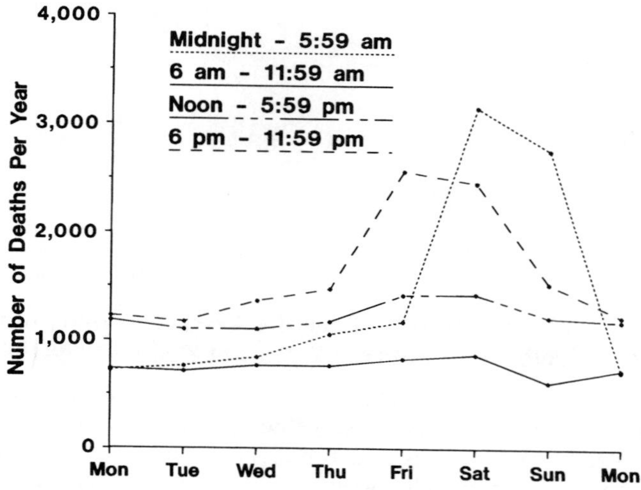

Figure 17-8. Average Number of Motor Vehicle Occupant Deaths Per Year by Time and Day of Crash, 1979-1981

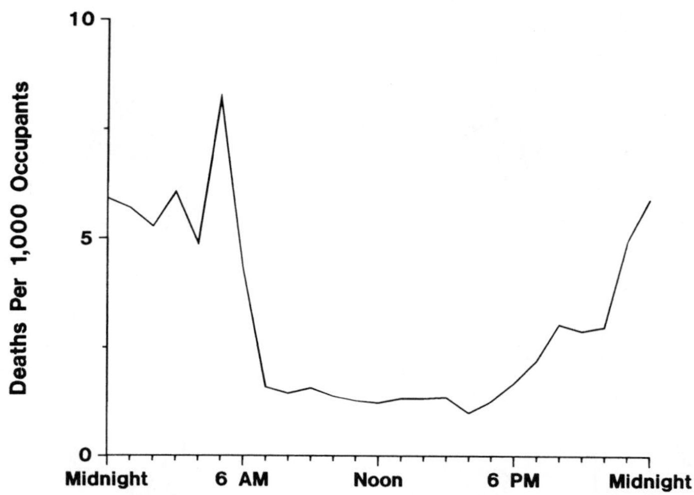

Figure 17-9. Deaths Per 1,000 Occupants in Crashes by Time of Crash, 1979-1981

A.M. on Friday and Saturday nights. The occupant death rate per person-mile of travel is highest on Fridays and Saturdays and lowest on Tuesdays and Wednesdays.

Seasonal and temporal variations in the incidence of crashes are influenced not only by hours of daylight and corresponding visibility, but also by amounts of travel, which are greater in the daytime and during the summer. Alcohol-impaired driving, which is more common at night and is a more important factor in single-vehicle crashes than in multiple-vehicle crashes, contributes significantly to the greater severity of nighttime crashes. The number of deaths per 1,000 occupants in crashes is about four times as great between midnight and 5:59 A.M. as it is during the daytime (figure 17-9).

Types of Crashes

Single-vehicle crashes are associated with higher death rates than multiple-vehicle crashes (figure 17-10). This is true of daytime as well as nighttime crashes.

More than half of all occupants of passenger cars in towaway crashes*

*In general, much better information is available for towaway crashes, and they are more likely to be reported to the police. Some analyses in this book are restricted to towaway crashes, which represent a subset of all crashes and overlap with the subset of fatal crashes.

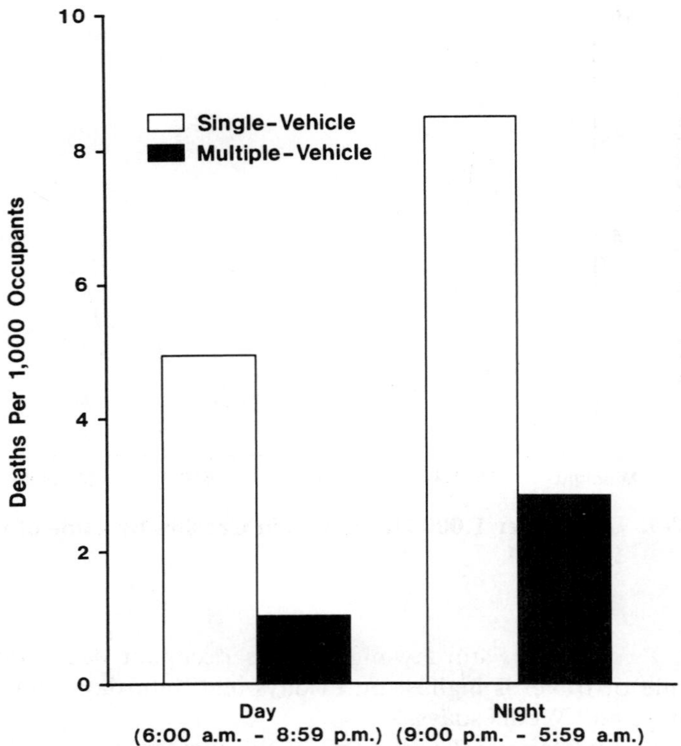

Figure 17-10. Deaths Per 1,000 Motor Vehicle Occupants in Daytime and Nighttime Single- and Multiple-Vehicle Crashes, 1979-1981

(i.e., those where one or more vehicles are towed from the scene) and fatal crashes are in direct-frontal and front-corner impacts (figure 17-11). The largest number are in direct-frontal impacts, which account for 41 percent of the occupants in towaway crashes and 44 percent of the fatalities. Rear impacts, which are common in minor, non-towaway crashes, account for only 2 percent of the fatalities. The prominence of frontal impacts in serious crashes makes it especially important to provide automatic crash protection that is effective in these kinds of impacts. Better protection is also needed in side impacts, the second largest component of fatal crashes.

About one-tenth of all occupants in towaway crashes are in vehicles that overturn. Called rollovers, these crashes have high death rates — more than twice the rate for non-rollovers (figure 17-12). This is partly because a much larger proportion of occupants (8 percent) are ejected

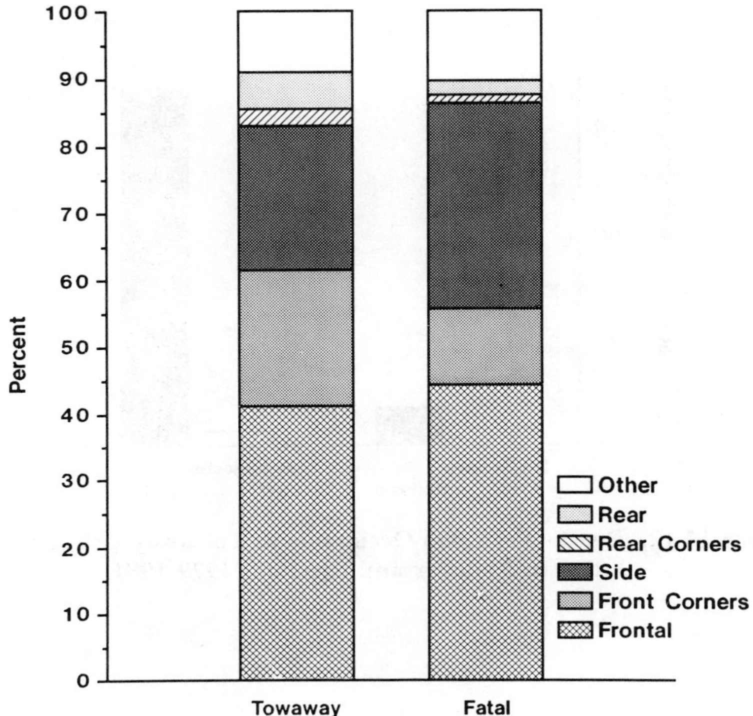

Figure 17-11. Percent Distribution of Passenger Car Occupants in Towaway and Fatal Crashes by Direction of Impact, 1979-1981

from their vehicles in rollovers, compared to only 0.4 percent ejected from vehicles that do not roll over. Ejection is associated with a 25-fold increase in the risk of death: 259 deaths per 1,000 people ejected compared to about 10 per 1,000 among those not ejected. The ability of a vehicle to keep occupants inside when it crashes (whether or not the vehicle overturns) is a major determinant of the likelihood of severe injury or death.

Vehicle Type and Size

Motor vehicle occupant deaths are almost evenly divided between single- and multiple-vehicle crashes. Another major split in the single-vehicle category involves impacts with fixed objects and rollovers. The

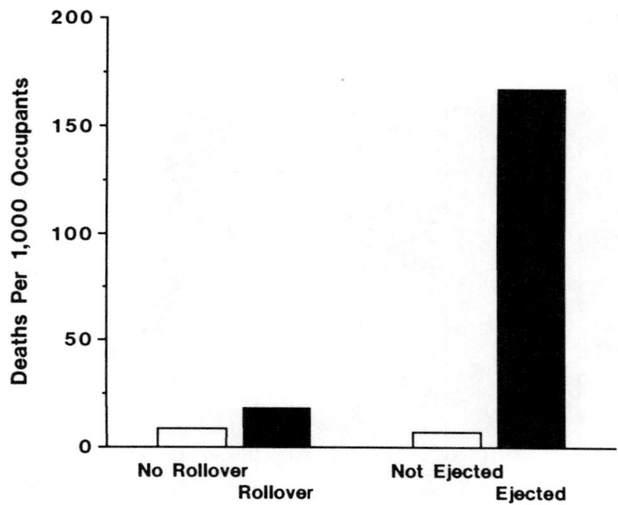

Figure 17-12. Deaths Per 1,000 Occupants in Towaway Crashes in Relation to Rollover and Ejection, 1979-1981

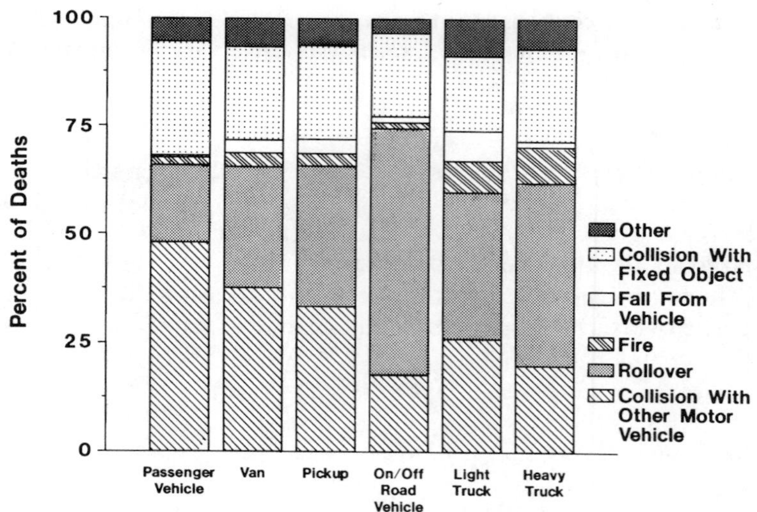

Figure 17-13. Percent Distribution of Occupant Deaths by Most Harmful Event and Type of Vehicle, 1979-1981

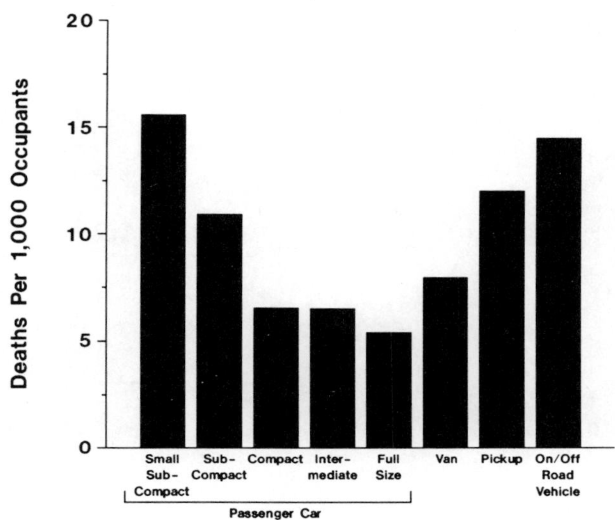

Figure 17-14. Deaths Per 1,000 Occupants in Towaway Crashes by Size of Car or Type of Vehicle, 1979-1981

mix of crash types varies with the type and size of the vehicle (figure 17-13); in general, as the size of the vehicle decreases, the proportion of deaths due to multiple-vehicle crashes increases. This reflects the fact that occupants of smaller vehicles in two-vehicle collisions are at a major disadvantage because of the greater forces inflicted on the smaller vehicle by the larger one. The proportion of deaths involving rollover or overturn also varies tremendously with vehicle type. Rollovers are involved in 17 percent of occupant deaths in passenger cars and 41 percent in heavy trucks. Other research has shown that certain small on/off road vehicles have especially high rates of overturn in crashes.[21,27]

The circumstances surrounding fatalities vary with vehicle type. Fatal falls from vehicles, for example, are relatively rare for most vehicle types, but account for about 180 occupant deaths annually in pickup trucks.

The relative frequency of each type of crash has important implications for prevention. Carrying passengers in the open beds of pickup trucks could be made illegal. To reduce the high incidence of rollover, small vehicles designed for on/off road use could be designed with lower centers of gravity and wider and longer wheelbases.

Vehicle size is a major determinant of the severity of occupant injuries in a crash.[13] The death rate per 1,000 occupants in passenger

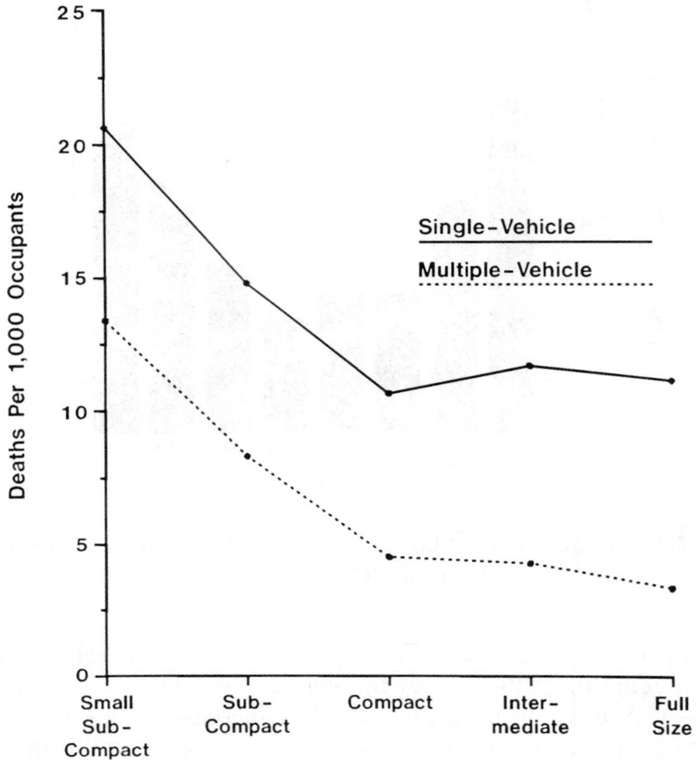

Figure 17-15. Deaths Per 1,000 Occupants in Towaway Crashes by Size of Car and Type of Crash, 1979-1981

cars involved in towaway crashes ranges from a low of about 5 deaths per 1,000 in full sized-cars (with wheelbases greater than 120 inches) to a high of about 15 in the smallest cars, small subcompacts with wheelbases less than or equal to 96 inches (figure 17-14). The most pronounced increases in death rates occur in cars smaller than compacts. Among vans, pickup trucks, and on/off road vehicles, the last group has the highest death rate and vans have the lowest.

The relationship between car size and occupant death rates holds for both single- and multiple-vehicle crashes (figure 17-15). This fact refutes claims that the greater risk of injury and death to small-car occupants is primarily due to collisions with larger vehicles and that if all cars were small the risk would be substantially reduced. Clearly,

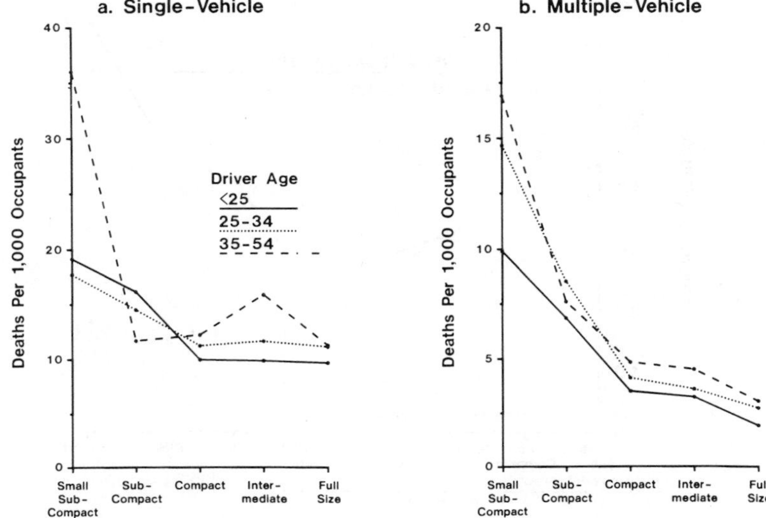

Figure 17-16. Deaths Per 1,000 Occupants in Towaway Crashes by Size of Car, Type of Crash, and Driver Age, 1979-1981

single-vehicle crashes account for a large number of small-car occupant deaths, and these would remain even if all cars were small. Furthermore, in collisions between vehicles of the *same* size, occupant death and injury rates are higher in smaller cars.[5]

The high death rates in small cars are not strongly influenced by driver age. Because young drivers are more likely to drive small cars as well as more likely to be involved in crashes, there is a notion that the high death rates in small cars reflect age differences among drivers. However, regardless of driver age, death rates per 1,000 occupants in crashes show similar relationships to car size (figure 17-16).

The proportions of crashes involving rollover or ejection vary considerably by size and type of vehicle. For single-vehicle crashes, two-thirds of the deaths in on/off road vehicles involve rollovers, compared to one-fourth of the deaths in full-sized passenger cars (figure 17-17). Among small cars and pickup trucks, the corresponding proportion is about 45 percent. Similar variations and patterns may be noted for the proportion of fatally injured occupants who were ejected from their vehicles during a crash, with on/off road vehicles having the highest percentage of occupants ejected and full-sized cars having the lowest (figure 17-18).

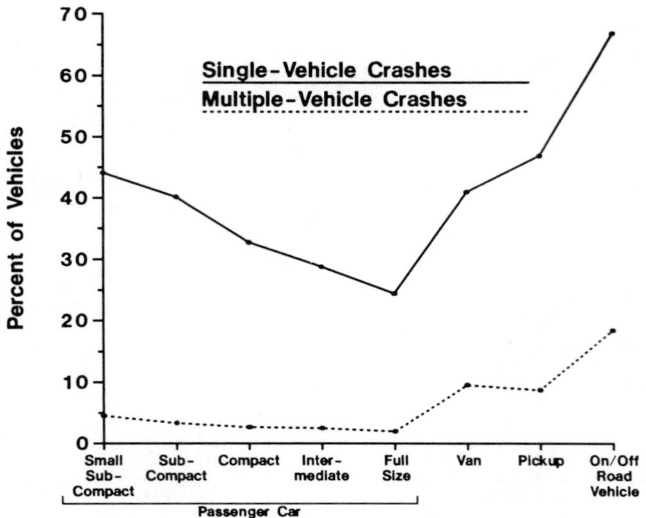

Figure 17-17. Percent of Fatally Injured Occupants Whose Vehicles Overturned, by Size of Car or Type of Vehicle and Type of Crash, 1979-1981

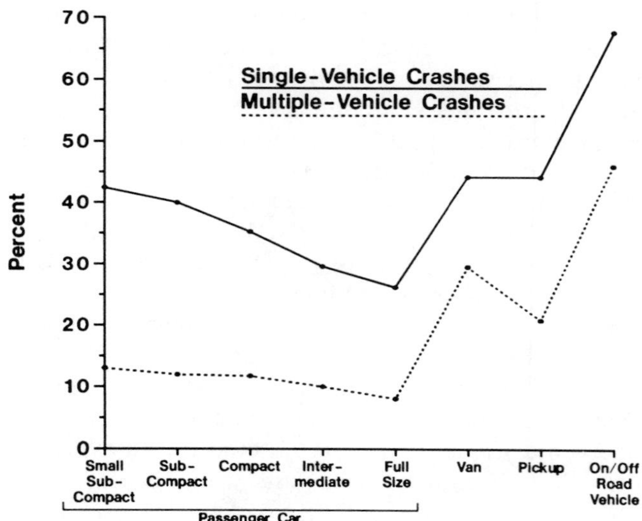

Figure 17-18. Percent of Fatally Injured Occupants Who Were Ejected by Size of Car or Type of Vehicle and Type of Crash, 1979-1981

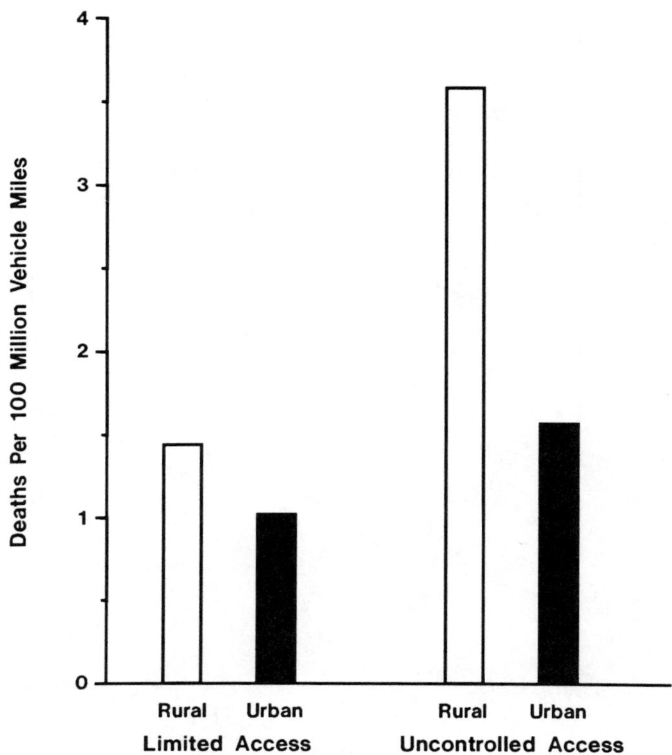

Figure 17-19. Occupant Deaths per 100 Million Vehicle Miles by Type of Road and Urban/Rural Classification, 1981

Type of Road and Speed Limit

Death rates on various types of road depend on the amount and type of travel, which influence both the incidence and severity of crashes. When adjustments are made for the amount of travel by calculating rates per 100 million miles, the lowest death rate is for interstate highways (1.2, compared to 2.5 for all roads). Rural roads have higher death rates per 100 million miles than urban roads. This is true for interstates and other limited-access roads and, to an even greater extent, for roads where access is not controlled (figure 17-19).

Interstate highways have relatively low crash rates because they are usually designed with gentler grades and curves and with wider recovery areas. In addition, access control and separation of opposing lanes of traffic greatly reduce the potential for frontal and side impacts. The

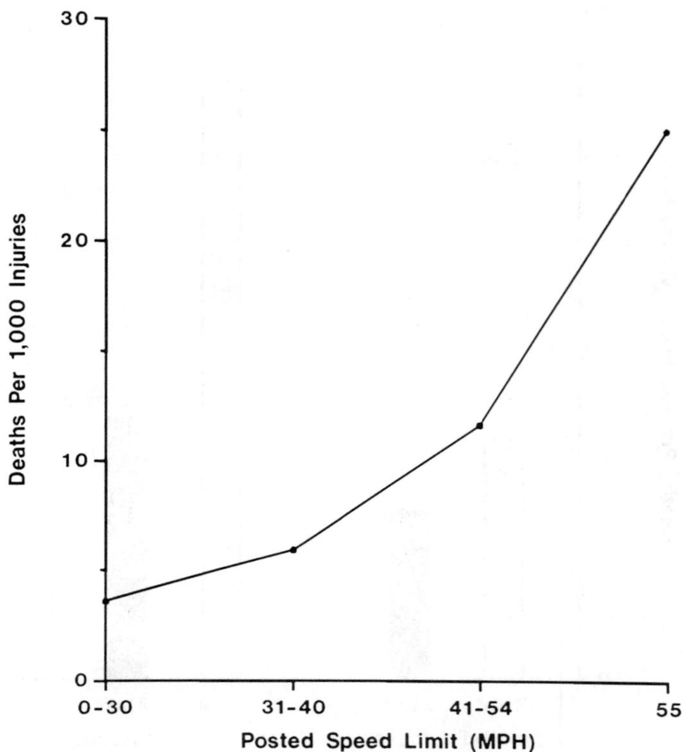

Figure 17-20. Motor Vehicle Occupant Deaths Per 1,000 Injuries by Posted Speed Limit, 1979-1981

prevalence of alcohol-impaired driving may also be relatively low on interstate highways. When crashes do occur, the consequences are often severe because the average speed of travel (and therefore the typical impact speed) is greater than on most other roads.

The ratio of occupant deaths to injuries increases dramatically with the posted speed limit, from less than 4 deaths per 1,000 injuries where the limit is 30 mph or less, to 25 per 1,000 where the limit is 55 mph (figure 17-20).

Alcohol

Alcohol-impaired driving is one of the leading factors in passenger-vehicle crashes that result in serious and fatal injuries. Approximately half of all crashes with fatalities involve drivers who have consumed

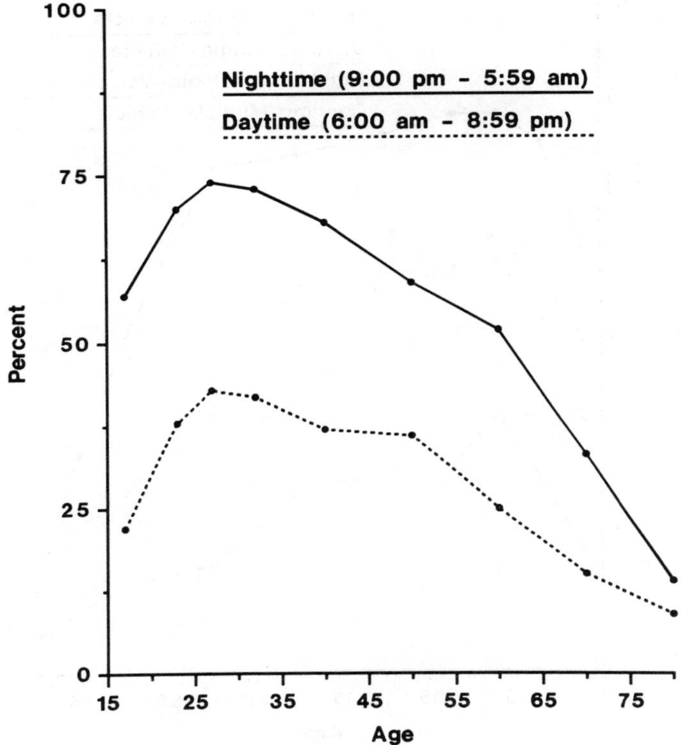

Figure 17-21. Percent of Fatally Injured Passenger Vehicle Drivers with Blood Alcohol Concentrations At or Above 0.10 Percent by Age and Time of Crash, 1979-1981

enough alcohol to be considered legally intoxicated.* Research studies have shown that half or more of the fatally injured drivers in single-vehicle crashes or "at fault" drivers in multiple-vehicle crashes had illegal BACs. In contrast, fatally injured drivers who were not "at fault" and drivers not involved in crashes are much less likely to be intoxicated.[3,8,14-15,28] A classic study by McCarroll and Haddon found that 50 percent of the drivers killed in single-vehicle crashes had BACs of 0.10 percent or higher, compared to 3 percent of a comparison group of drivers who did not crash but who were matched on the basis of day,

*In most jurisdictions, a blood alcohol concentration (BAC) of 0.10 percent by weight or higher in a driver is considered either presumptive evidence of intoxication or an offense in its own right.

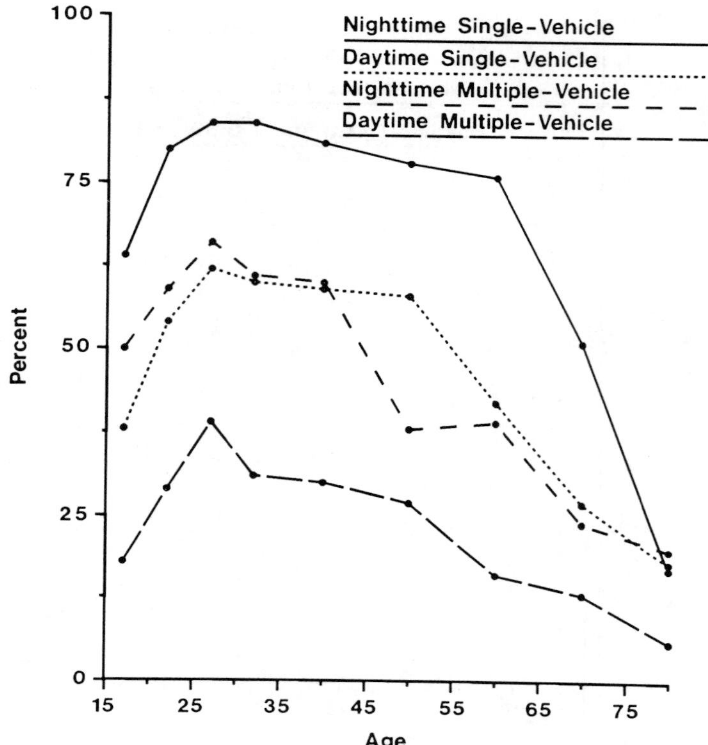

Figure 17-22. Percent of Fatally Injured Passenger Vehicle Drivers with Blood Alcohol Concentrations At or Above 0.10 Percent by Age, Time of Crash, and Type of Crash, 1979-1981

time, site, and direction of travel.[15] Studies in other jurisdictions have yielded comparable results, but national data on the incidence of alcohol impairment among drivers in fatal crashes are incomplete because fewer than 60 percent of all fatally injured drivers, and only 20 percent of surviving drivers involved in fatal crashes, are tested for alcohol.[18]

Alcohol impairs driving skills measurably at BACs of 0.05 percent (half of the legal limit in most states) and at lower BACs for some drivers, including many teenagers and elderly people.[4] The impairment effect increases substantially with higher BACs.

Generally, the more violent the crash the greater the likelihood that alcohol is a factor. Alcohol is a contributing factor in about 20 percent of all crashes resulting in an injury to a driver or passenger, about 50 percent of all fatal crashes, and approximately 60 percent of all single-vehicle fatal crashes.[10]

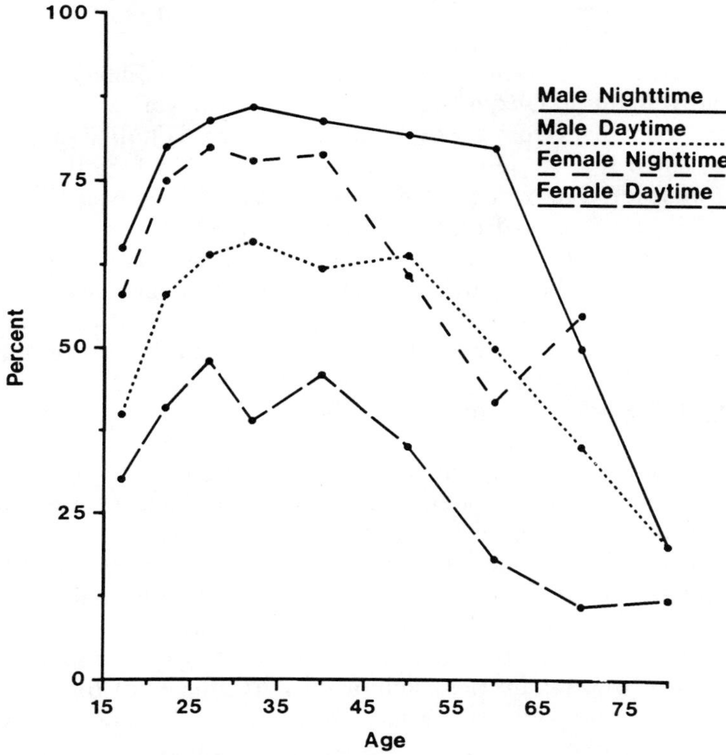

Figure 17-23. Percent of Fatally Injured Passenger Vehicle Drivers in Single-Vehicle Crashes with Blood Alcohol Concentrations At or Above 0.10 Percent by Age, Sex, and Time of Crash, 1979-1981

The likelihood of fatally injured drivers* having illegal BACs varies by driver age and time of day of the crash (figure 17-21). Alcohol involvement is most common in nighttime crashes (9:00 P.M. to 5:59 A.M.) and among drivers ages 20-49.

Alcohol involvement varies by type of crash (figure 17-22). Except in the case of elderly drivers, among whom alcohol involvement is uncommon, drivers killed in nighttime single-vehicle crashes are much

---

*Information on the BACs of nonfatally injured drivers involved in crashes resulting in death to others and/or serious injury are not routinely obtained in any jurisdiction. Consequently, statistics on alcohol involvement tend to be confined to fatally injured drivers whose BACs are measured as part of an autopsy. FARS data from 13 states where more than 80 percent of the fatally injured drivers are tested for alcohol were used for the alcohol analyses in this book.

more likely to have illegal BACs than drivers killed in nighttime multiple-vehicle crashes. In the 20-64 age group, over 75 percent of the drivers killed in nighttime single-vehicle crashes have illegal BACs.

Involvement in alcohol-related crashes also varies by sex, with crashes of male drivers more often involving alcohol than those of females (figure 17-23). In single-vehicle crashes in which the driver is killed, male drivers in nighttime crashes have the highest alcohol involvement and female drivers in daytime crashes the lowest. There is little sex difference in alcohol involvement among drivers less than 45 years old who are killed in single-vehicle nighttime crashes.

The very frequent and longstanding involvement of alcohol in serious and fatal motor vehicle crashes illustrates the difficulty of reducing deaths and injuries by changing human behavior. The major contribution of alcohol to motor vehicle deaths and injuries, both in the United States and in virtually all other industrial societies, has led to programs, laws, and enforcement activities intended to deter people from driving while intoxicated and thereby to reduce the incidence of such crashes. Only in some Scandinavian countries with major programs spanning decades — including types of police enforcement that would not be possible in the United States because of constitutional guarantees against unreasonable search and seizure — is there evidence that these efforts have somewhat reduced the incidence of alcohol-impaired driving. Even in these countries, significant percentages of the fatally injured and hospitalized drivers have high BACs. It appears that it is principally the behavior of adult social drinkers that has been affected by the legislation. Elsewhere the evidence indicates that programs intended to change alcohol-related driving behavior have produced either no effect or at best only short term reductions in alcohol-related deaths and injuries.[8,25,26]

Occupants of Large Trucks

Large trucks have high rates of involvement in fatal crashes, which usually involve the deaths of road users other than the truck occupants. This is principally because of the very large differences in mass between trucks and other road vehicles. However, even though truck operators involved in crashes are less likely to be fatally injured than the other road users they collide with, the amount of travel by many truck operators places them at a high risk of death and injury. In fact, truck operators have one of the highest occupational death rates. In view of this, there is need for trucks designed to provide better occupant protection in crashes.[2]

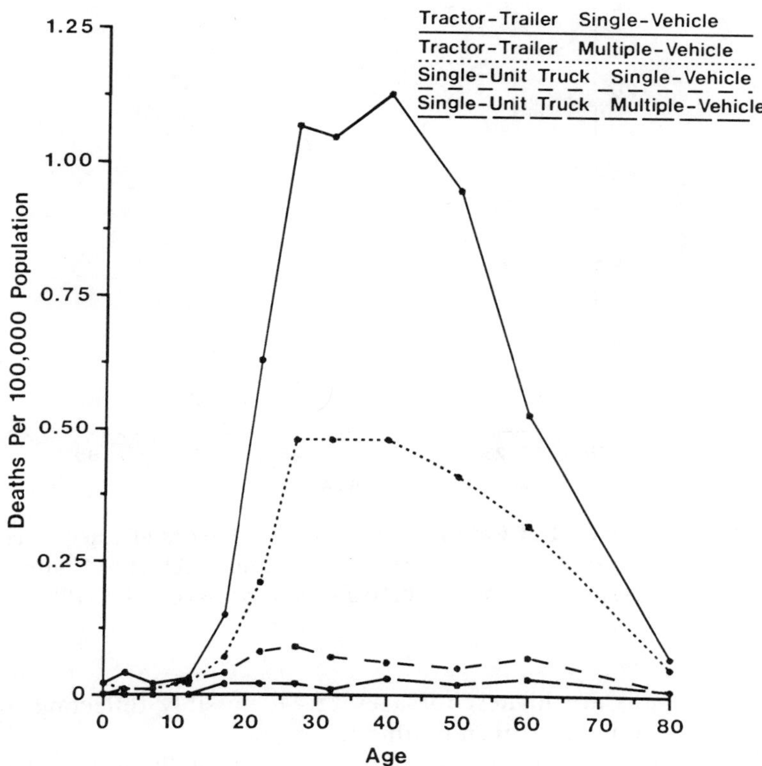

Figure 17-24. Large Single-Unit Truck and Tractor-Trailer Occupant Death Rates Per 100,000 Population by Type of Crash and Age, for Males, 1979-1981

Large truck occupant death rates are influenced by many factors, especially the amount and type of exposure, which varies tremendously among different truck types and configurations. Ideally, deaths per licensed truck driver would provide a useful basis for comparing the occupational risks associated with different truck types, but information on licensed drivers by truck type is not readily available. To present some relevant information, truck occupant death rates per 100,000 population have been computed. For all age groups except children, there are many more deaths of tractor-trailer occupants than occupants of other large trucks (figure 17-24). The death rate is much higher for single-vehicle than for multiple-vehicle crashes. Unlike passenger car occupant death rates, which peak in the teenage years, tractor-trailer

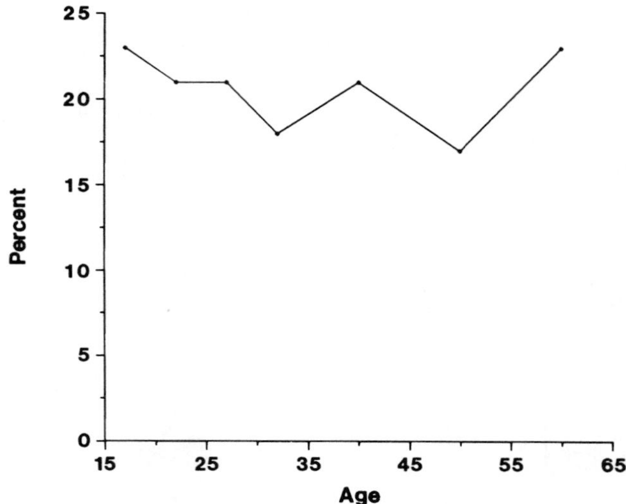

Figure 17-25. Percent of Fatally Injured Male Drivers of Large Trucks in Single-Vehicle Crashes with Blood Alcohol Concentrations At or Above 0.10 Percent by Age, 1977-1981

occupant deaths are highest for ages 25-44, possibly reflecting more tractor-trailer mileage driven by this age group.

Although alcohol is less commonly found in fatally injured drivers of large trucks than in fatally injured drivers of passenger cars, it is nevertheless a serious problem.[1] Approximately one in five drivers of large trucks who are fatally injured in single-vehicle crashes have illegal blood alcohol concentrations. There is little variation in this proportion with driver age (figure 17-25). In the vast majority of multiple-vehicle fatal crashes involving large trucks, the truck operator is not killed. Consequently, there is no systematic alcohol testing of such drivers. The results for the operators of large trucks killed in single-vehicle crashes, however, suggest that a significant proportion of truck drivers in multiple-vehicle fatal crashes may also have illegal BACs.

Historical Trends

During recent decades, motor vehicle occupant death rates have reflected not only improvements in roads but also changes in vehicles, patterns of use, speed limits, and the economy. Since the mid-1960s, a declining trend has occurred in occupant death rates based on vehicle miles traveled (figure 17-26), in part because of federal standards for

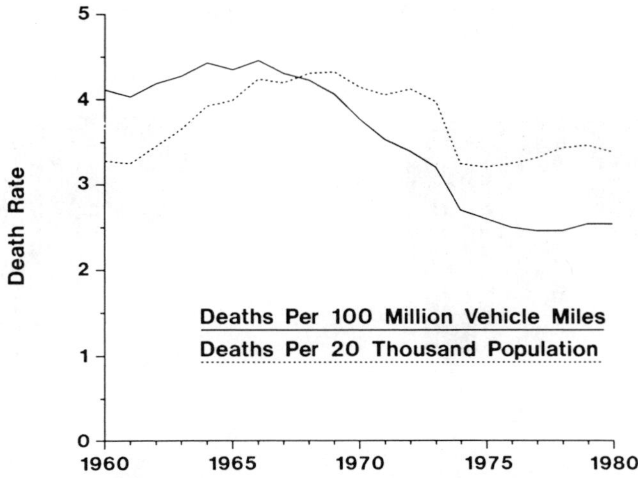

Figure 17-26. Motor Vehicle Occupant Deaths Per 100 Million Vehicle Miles of Travel, and Per 20,000 Population by Year, 1960-1980

state and local highway safety programs and federal motor vehicle safety standards, which began in 1967-1968. Federal standards for vehicles require virtually all new passenger cars sold in the United States to be designed to meet performance requirements to reduce the likelihood of crashes (e.g., standards for brakes), of injuries when crashes occur (e.g., standards for windshields and restraint systems), and of post-crash injuries (e.g., standards to make fuel systems less likely to leak and start post-crash fires). Research studies have documented the substantial reductions in deaths and injuries in cars designed to meet the requirements of these standards.[17,23]

Gasoline shortages and the subsequent nationwide institution of 55 mph speed limits in 1974 caused a dramatic decline in highway deaths. Although this was partly due to a decrease in driving, there were also fewer deaths per 100 million miles of travel, largely because of reduced travel speeds and more uniform speeds; that is, fewer vehicles were traveling at speeds much faster or slower than the average.[16]

The percent changes in occupant death rates calculated from 1968-1979 trendlines show an overall reduction of 26 percent during this period. The smallest reduction in death rates occurred among 15-19 year olds, while the greatest reductions occurred among children younger than 1 year (a 40 percent reduction, not shown) and adults 55 or older (figure 17-27). Females in their twenties showed substantially less decrease than males, so their death rates, although still lower, are now somewhat closer to male rates.

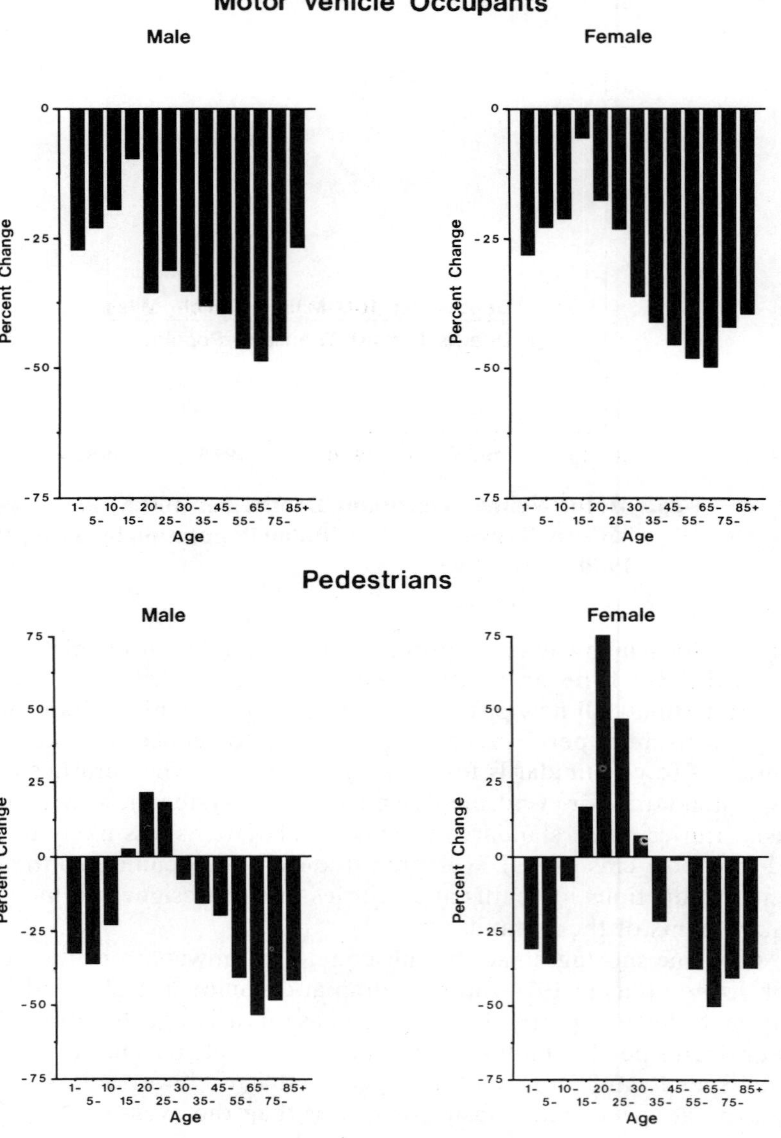

Figure 17-27. Percent Change in Death Rates for Motor Vehicle Occupants and Pedestrians by Age and Sex, Based on 1968-1979 Trend

Notes

1. Baker, S.P. "Alcohol in Fatal Tractor Trailer Crashes." *Proceedings of the Nineteenth Conference of the American Association for Automotive Medicine*. Arlington Heights, IL: American Association for Automotive Medicine, 1975.

2. Baker, S.P., J.S. Samkoff, R.S. Fisher, and C.B. Van Buren. "Fatal Occupational Injuries." *Journal of the American Medical Association* 248 (1982): 692-697.

3. Baker, S.P., and W.U. Spitz. "Age Effects and Autopsy Evidence of Disease in Fatally Injured Drivers." *Journal of the American Medical Association* 214 (1970): 1079-1088.

4. Borkenstein, R.F., R.F. Crowther, R.O. Shumute, W.B. Ziel, R. Zylman, and A. Dale. "The Role of the Drinking Driver in Traffic Accidents (Grand Rapids Study)." *Blutalkohol* 2 (1974) Supp. 4.

5. Campbell, B.J., and D.W. Reinfurt. *Relationship Between Driver Crash Injury and Passenger Car Weight*. Chapel Hill, NC: University of North Carolina, Highway Safety Research Center, 1973.

6. Carsten, O., and K. Weber. "Child and Adult Travel Exposure and Fatality Risk." *Proceedings of the Twenty-Fifth Conference of the American Association for Automotive Medicine*. Arlington Heights, IL: American Association for Automotive Medicine, 1981.

7. Federal Railroad Administration, Office of Safety. *Rail-Highway Crossing Accident/Incident and Inventory Bulletin, No. 4 Calendar Year 1981*. Washington, DC: U.S. Department of Transportation, June 1982.

8. Haddon, W., Jr. *Automobile Injuries Related to Drug Abuse: An Introduction to Some of the Basic Considerations in Prevention and Research*. Washington, DC: Insurance Institute for Highway Safety, 1984.

9. Haddon, W., Jr., and S.P. Baker. "Injury Control." *Preventive and Community Medicine*, edited by D. Clark and B. MacMahon. Boston: Little, Brown and Company, 1981, pp. 109-140.

10. Haddon, W., Jr., and M. Blumenthal. "Foreword." In *Deterring the Drinking Driver: Legal Policy and Social Control* by H.L. Ross. Lexington, MA: Lexington Books, 1981.

11. Insurance Institute for Highway Safety. "Air Bags: A Special Issue." *The Highway Loss Reduction Status Report* 14 (August 21, 1979): 1-19.

12. Insurance Institute for Highway Safety. "The Human Costs of Air Bag Delay: 39,000 Lives Might Have Been Saved." *The Highway Loss Reduction Status Report* 14 (September 7, 1979): 1-8.

13. Insurance Institute for Highway Safety. "A Special Issue: Small-

Car Deaths, Injuries Worst; Models Vary Greatly." *The Highway Loss Reduction Status Report* 17 (December 30, 1982): 1-11.

14. Jones, R.K., and K.B. Joscelyn. *Alcohol and Highway Safety 1978: A Review of the State of Knowledge*. Report No. UM-HSRI-78-5. Ann Arbor, MI: University of Michigan Highway Safety Research Institute, 1978.

15. McCarroll, J.R., and W. Haddon, Jr. "A Controlled Study of Fatal Automobile Accidents in New York City." *Journal of Chronic Diseases* 15 (1962): 811-826.

16. Mela, D.F. "Review of Information on the Safety Effects of the 55 MPH Speed Limit in the U.S." Technical Report DOT HS-802-383. Washington, DC: National Highway Traffic Safety Administration, 1977.

17. National Highway Traffic Safety Aministration. *Effectiveness, Benefits, and Costs of Federal Safety Standards for Protection of Passenger Car Occupants*. Washington, DC: U.S. Department of Transportation, 1976.

18. National Highway Traffic Safety Administration. *Fatal Accident Reporting System 1981*. Technical Report DOT HS-806-251. Washington, DC: U.S. Department of Transportation, 1983.

19. O'Neill, B., A.F. Williams, and R.S. Karpf. "Passenger Car Size and Driver Seat Belt Use." *American Journal of Public Health* 73 (1983): 588-590.

20. Preusser, D.F., A.F. Williams, P.L. Zador, and R.D. Blomberg. "The Effect of Curfew Laws on Motor Vehicle Crashes." *Law and Policy Quarterly*, in press.

21. Reinfurt, D.W., L.K. Li, C.L. Popkin, B. O'Neill, P.F. Burchman, and J.K. Wells. *A Comparison of the Crash Experience of Utility Vehicles, Pickup Trucks and Passenger Cars*. Chapel Hill, NC: University of North Carolina, Highway Safety Research Center, September 1981.

22. Reinfurt, D.W., C.Z. Silva, and A.F. Seila. *A Statistical Analysis of Seatbelt Effectiveness in 1973-1975 Model Cars Involved in Towaway Crashes*. Technical Report DOT HS-5-01255. Chapel Hill, NC: University of North Carolina, Highway Safety Research Center, May 1976.

23. Robertson, L.S. "Automobile Safety Regulations and Death Reductions in the United States." *American Journal of Public Health* 71 (1981): 818-822.

24. Robertson, L.S. "Crash Involvement of Teenaged Drivers When Driver Education is Eliminated from High School." *American Journal of Public Health* 70 (1980): 599-603.

25. Robertson, L.S. *Injuries: Causes, Control Strategies, and Public Policy*. Lexington, MA: Lexington Books, 1983.

26. Ross, H.L. *Deterring the Drinking Driver: Legal Policy and Social Control*. Lexington, MA: Lexington Books, 1982.

27. Smith, S.R. "Analysis of Fatal Rollover Accidents in Utility Vehicles." Washington, DC: National Highway Traffic Safety Administration, February 1982.

28. U.S. Congress, House of Representatives, Committee on Public Works. *1968 Alcohol and Highway Safety Report: A Study Transmitted by the Secretary of the Department of Transportation to the Congress, in Accordance with Requirements of Section 204 of the Highway Safety Act of 1966, Public Law 89-564*. 90th Congress, 2nd sess., 1968.

29. Williams, A.F. "Restraint Use Legislation: Its Prospects for Increasing the Protection of Children in Cars." *Accident Analysis and Prevention* 11 (1979): 255-260.

30. Williams, A.F., and B. O'Neill. *Seat Belt Laws: Implications for Occupant Protection*. SAE Technical Paper No. 790683. Warrendale, PA: Society of Automotive Engineers, 1979.

31. Williams, A.F., J.K. Wells, and A.K. Lund. "Voluntary Seat Belt Use Among High School Students." *Accident Analysis and Prevention* 15 (1983): 161-165.

32. Wright, P.H., J.W. Hall, and P.L. Zador. "Low-Cost Countermeasures for Ameliorating Run-Off-Road Crashes." Washington, DC: Insurance Institute for Highway Safety, August 1982.

33. Wright, P.H., and L.S. Robertson. "Priorities for Roadside Hazard Modification: A Study of 300 Fatal Roadside Object Crashes." *Proceedings of the Twentieth Conference of the American Association for Automotive Medicine*. Arlington Heights, IL: American Association for Automotive Medicine, 1976, pp. 114-127.

18 Pedestrians

Pedestrian deaths represent the second largest category of motor vehicle deaths. In 1981, about 8,000 people were killed as pedestrians, comprising about one-sixth of all traffic-related deaths, half of the traffic deaths for ages 1-9, and one-third for ages 70 or older. Among all categories of people injured by motor vehicles, pedestrians have the highest ratio of deaths to injuries: the number of deaths per 1,000 police-reported injuries is about 52 for pedestrians, compared to 27 for motorcyclists and 12 for motor vehicle occupants. These differences, while important, should not be taken as indicative of the relative risks of various means of travel since they do not reflect exposure.

Age and Sex

Unlike motor vehicle occupant deaths, the highest pedestrian death rates are for the elderly, with lower peaks seen for children and teenagers (figure 16-6). Pedestrian injury rates are highest for children in the 5-14-year-old age group. As with other causes of injury, the high pedestrian death rates for the elderly reflect high fatality rates among those injured. In addition, when adjustment is made for exposure, elderly pedestrians are more likely to be injured than younger adults.[4,8]

Seventy percent of the pedestrians killed are males. After age 18, the male:female ratio of death rates is about 3:1. Among children, the sex difference is apparent beginning in the second year of life.

One-fifth of all collisions that are fatal to adult pedestrians occur at intersections, compared to one-eighth in the case of children younger than 5 years.[5] Among children, 82 percent who are killed as pedestrians are in the roadway but not at an intersection.

Urban/Rural and Geographic Differences

Pedestrian collisions are predominantly an urban phenomenon. Five out of six injuries to pedestrians and two out of three deaths occur in urban areas. However, for pedestrian collisions in rural areas the ratio of deaths to injuries is higher, about 120 per 1,000 compared to 40 per

1,000 in urban areas, reflecting the generally higher impact speeds in rural areas. For all residents of large cities combined, the death rate is higher than for other SMSA residents and people in rural counties. For blacks, however, the reverse is true (figure 16-13). Among the states, death rates range from about 2 per 100,000 in several midwestern states to 8 in New Mexico (figure 16-15).

Season, Day, and Time

The number of pedestrian deaths per month increases throughout the year to a peak in December (figure 18-1). Saturday is the peak day for fatalities, but injury rates are highest on weekdays. Two-thirds of all pedestrian fatalities occur between 6:00 P.M. and 5:59 A.M., with the

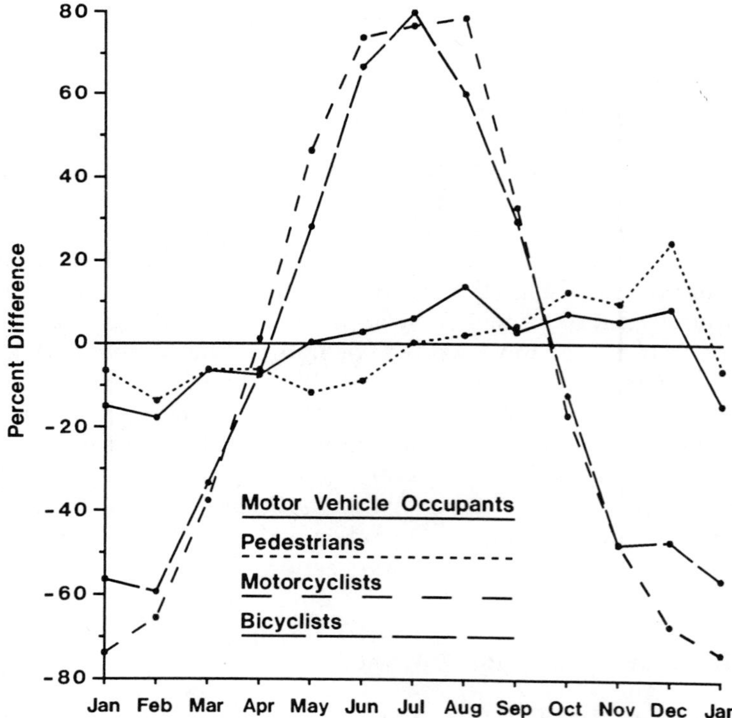

Figure 18-1. Percent Difference from the Average Number of Deaths of Motor Vehicle Occupants, Pedestrians, Motorcyclists, and Bicyclists by Month, 1979-1981

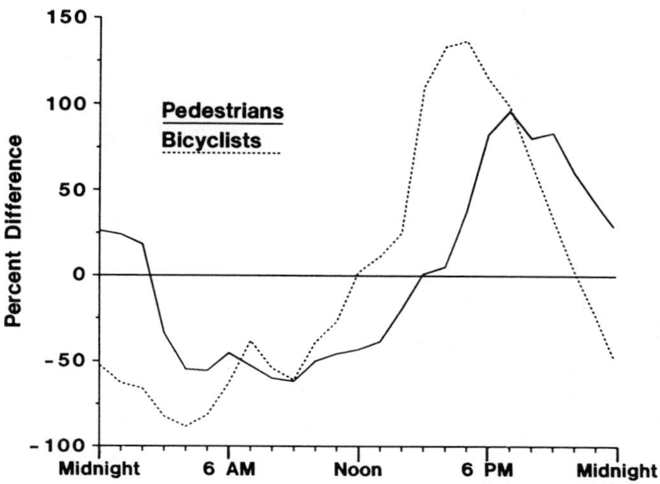

Figure 18-2. Percent Difference from the Average Number of Pedestrian and Bicyclist Deaths by Time of Day, 1979-1981

highest incidence at 6:00-9:59 P.M. (figure 18-2). Nonfatal injuries, on the other hand, more closely reflect the periods of greatest pedestrian activity, predominantly the daytime, with the highest incidence at about 4:00 P.M.

The peak hour for pedestrian fatalities changes with the seasonal variation in the hour of dusk (figure 18-3). Each month the peak hour occurs about an hour after the average time of sunset. Between December and June, the peak varies by about two hours, local standard time (three hours, when daylight saving time is considered). Pedestrian conspicuousness, street lighting, other visibility factors, and associated variations in weather probably play important roles.

Alcohol

As with passenger vehicle occupant deaths, alcohol intoxication plays a major role in adult pedestrian fatalities.[3,4,9] Blood alcohol concentrations of 0.10 percent or greater are found in almost half of all fatally injured adult pedestrians. Moreover, if all drivers involved in pedestrian fatalities were tested for alcohol, its contribution to pedestrian deaths would undoubtedly prove even greater.[3] Unlike the alcohol involvement of fatally injured drivers, which declines after age 40, the percentage of fatally injured pedestrians with high BACs remains above

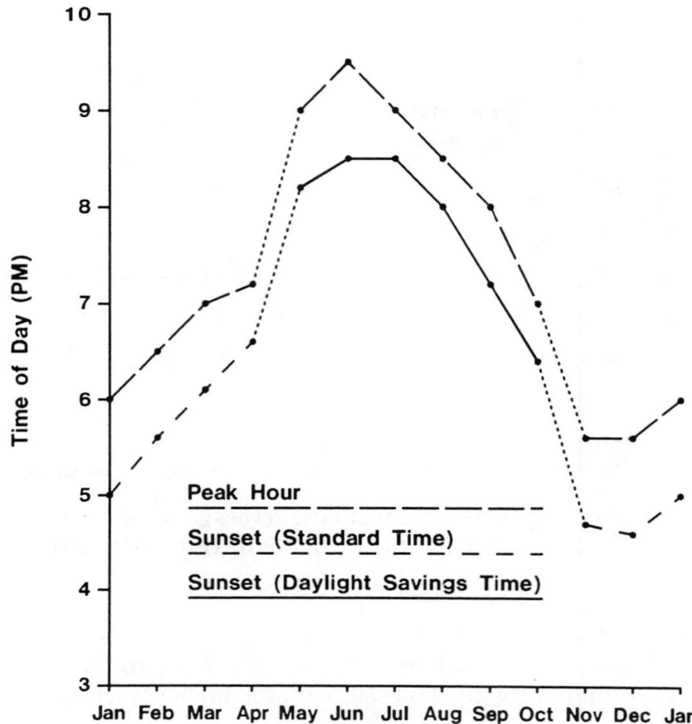

Figure 18-3. Peak Hour of Pedestrian Fatalities and Time of Sunset by Month, 1978-1980

50 throughout ages 20-64 (figure 18-4). Pedestrians in this age range, who are more likely to be intoxicated than elderly pedestrians, are greatly overrepresented among nighttime fatalities.

About half of all pedestrian fatalities occur on weekends, between 4:00 P.M. Friday and midnight Sunday. Only one-fourth of nonfatal pedestrian injuries occur during the same period, reflecting the fact that alcohol is less commonly involved in nonfatal injuries.

Vehicle Factors

Vehicle size and design are major factors in pedestrian injuries. In Great Britain, the death rate among pedestrians struck by various types of vehicles was found to range from 4 per 1,000 for bicycles to 106 per 1,000 for heavy trucks. Of people struck by cars, 31 per 1,000 were

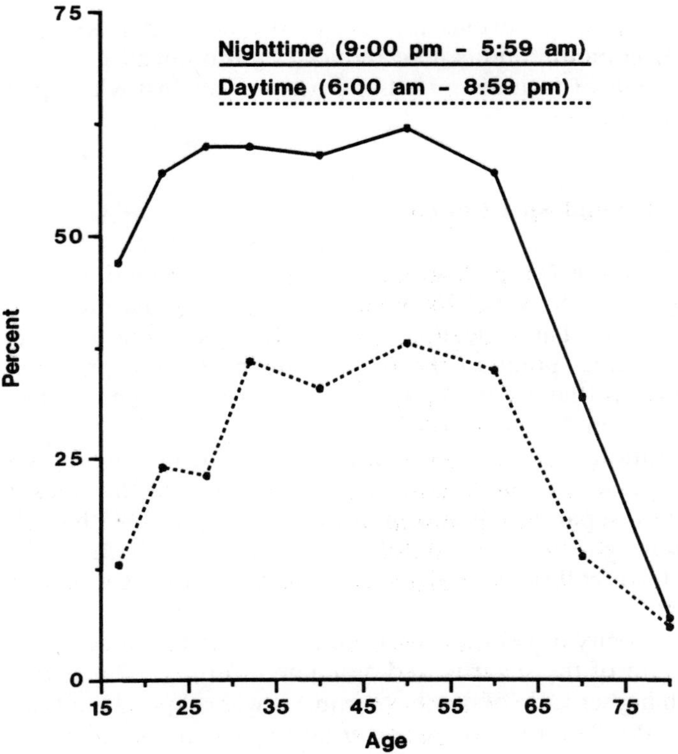

Figure 18-4. Percent of Fatally Injured Pedestrians with Blood Alcohol Concentrations At or Above 0.10 Percent by Age and Time of Day, 1979-1981

killed.[1] In Maryland, the number of pedestrians killed per 10,000 vehicles was twice as high among cars with wheelbases greater than 120 inches compared to those with wheelbases less than 111 inches.[7]

Impacts with pedestrians usually involve the front structures of vehicles. Other circumstances include children running into the sides of cars and pedestrians being struck by mirrors or other protruding structures or run over by the rear wheels of trucks or buses. The dynamics of the collision depend on many factors, including the vehicle's shape, speed at impact, braking action, contact point, and the height of the pedestrian relative to the bumper and the front of the hood. A pedestrian may be run over (especially common when the vehicle is a truck or the pedestrian is a child) but, more often, sustains the most serious injuries as a result of being thrown onto the hood, windshield, or top of the car. Serious injuries to the head, pelvis, and legs are especially common and can be reduced by modifications in the design and materials of frontal and other structures against which pedestrians may be thrown.[1-2]

Road Design and Speed Limit

Each year about 600 pedestrians are struck and killed while on crosswalks, and an additional 200 while on sidewalks and median strips or traffic islands.[5] These deaths, representing about one-tenth of all pedestrian deaths, point to the inadequate protection provided by pedestrian areas that are on the same level as roadways but not physically separated from vehicle traffic.

Separation of pedestrians from motor traffic is sometimes achieved with overpasses and underpasses and/or barriers at the sides of roads. More often, separation is absent or merely temporal, with traffic lights. Permitting right turns at red lights has resulted in significant increases in pedestrian collisions at signalized intersections, especially in urban areas.[6,10]

The velocity of vehicles involved in pedestrian impacts is the major determinant of the severity and outcome of injury. This is reflected in the much higher ratio of deaths to injuries where speed limits are higher (figure 18-5). The ratio of deaths to injuries is about ten times as high where the speed limit is 55 mph as on roads where it is 30 mph or less. In addition, vehicle travel speeds influence the likelihood that a pedestrian will be struck.

Historical Trends

Pedestrian death rates declined by more than half between 1935 and 1955. The trend roughly paralleled occupant death rates from the early 1930s until after World War II (figure 16-16). Subsequently, as motor vehicle ownership and use increased, pedestrian death rates continued to decline for another decade, possibly because fewer people walked to their destinations. The reductions in vehicle mileage, changes in travel patterns, and reduced travel speeds subsequent to the 1974 gas shortage substantially reduced pedestrian as well as occupant deaths. While the overall trend from 1968 to 1979 was downward, the death rates increased for ages 15-29 (figure 17-27). As with death rates from many other causes, the increases were greatest among females in this age range.

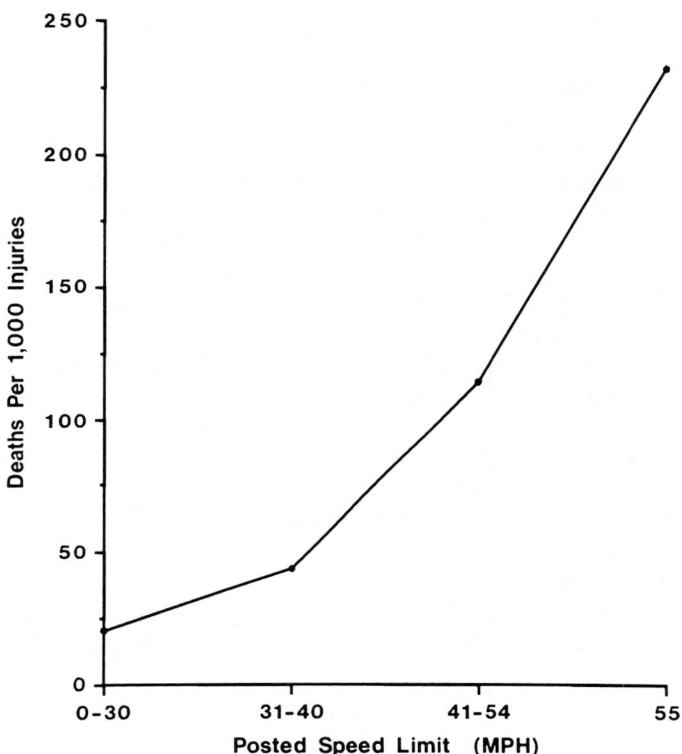

Figure 18-5. Pedestrian Deaths Per 1,000 Injuries by Posted Speed Limit, 1979-1981

Notes

1. Ashton, S.J. "Vehicle Design and Pedestrian Injuries." In *Pedestrian Accidents*, edited by A.J. Chapman, F.M. Wade, and H.C. Foot. New York: John Wiley and Sons Ltd., 1982.

2. Ashton, S.J., J.B. Pedder, and G.M. Mackay. "Pedestrian Leg Injuries, the Bumper and Other Front Structures." Presented at the International Research Committee on the Biokinetics of Impacts, 3rd International Conference on Impact Trauma. Berlin: September 7-9, 1977.

3. Baker, S.P., L.S. Robertson, and B. O'Neill. "Fatal Pedestrian Collisions." *American Journal of Public Health* 64 (1974): 319-325.

4. Haddon, W., Jr., P. Valien, J.R. McCarroll, and C.J. Umberger. "A Controlled Investigation of the Characteristics of Adult Pe-

destrians Fatally Injured by Motor Vehicles in Manhattan." *Journal of Chronic Diseases* 14 (1961): 655-678.

5. National Highway Traffic Safety Administration. *Fatal Accident Reporting System 1981*. Technical Report DOT HS-806-251. Washington, DC: U.S. Department of Transportation, 1983.

6. Preusser, D.F., W.A. Leaf, K.B. DeBartolo, and R.D. Blomberg. "The Effect of Right-Turn-On-Red on Pedestrian and Bicyclist Accidents." Technical Report DOT HS-806-182. Washington, DC: National Highway Traffic Safety Administration, October 1981.

7. Robertson, L.S., and S.P. Baker. "Motor Vehicle Sizes in 1440 Fatal Crashes." *Accident Analysis and Prevention* 8 (1976): 167-175.

8. Smeed, R.J. "Pedestrian Accidents." *Proceedings of the International Conference on Pedestrian Safety, Vol. 2.* Haifa, Israel: Technion, 1976.

9. U.S. Congress, House of Representatives, Committee on Public Works. *1968 Alcohol and Highway Safety Report: A Study Transmitted by the Secretary of the Department of Transportation to the Congress, in Accordance with Requirements of Section 204 of the Highway Safety Act of 1966, Public Law 89-564*. 90th Congress, 2nd sess., 1968.

10. Zador, P.L. "Right-Turn-On-Red Laws and Motor Vehicle Crashes." *Accident Analysis and Prevention* 14 (1982): 219-234.

19 Motorcyclists

Motorcyclist deaths, numbering almost 5,000 in 1981, comprise one-tenth of all traffic deaths. For ages 15-34, one out of every 6 or 7 motor vehicle fatalities is a motorcycle driver or passenger. Analyses of FARS and NASS data indicate that for every death, there are 37 injuries reported to the police. In addition, many injuries are not reported to the police.[3] This is especially likely when no other motor vehicle is involved.

Motorcyclists generally travel at speeds similar to or greater than passenger vehicle occupants but lack the stability and protection of an enclosed vehicle. It is therefore not surprising that the death rate per 100 million person-miles of travel is more than 15 times the rate for cars (table 8-1). The ratio of deaths to reported injuries (about 27 per 1,000) is twice as great for motorcyclists as for occupants of passenger vehicles.

Age and Sex

About 55 percent of all motorcyclist deaths occur in the 15-24-year-old age group and more than 80 percent among ages 15-34. Death rates are highest for ages 18-24 (figures 4-4 and 19-1). The death rate is about ten times as high for males as for females (figure 4-4). Males killed as motorcycle operators outnumber by about 15:1 those killed as passengers. For females, the difference is in the opposite direction; female passengers outnumber operators by about 5:1.

The best population-based data on nonfatal injuries are from California. These show a very sharp peak in incidence at age 18.[3] FARS and NASS data indicate that injuries tend to be more severe among somewhat older motorcyclists. For ages 20-44, there are about 30 to 35 deaths per 1,000 reported injuries, compared to about 20 per 1,000 for younger motorcyclists.

Geographic Differences and Helmet Laws

Differences among states in motorcyclist death rates are determined to a large extent by two factors: amount of motorcycle travel and helmet

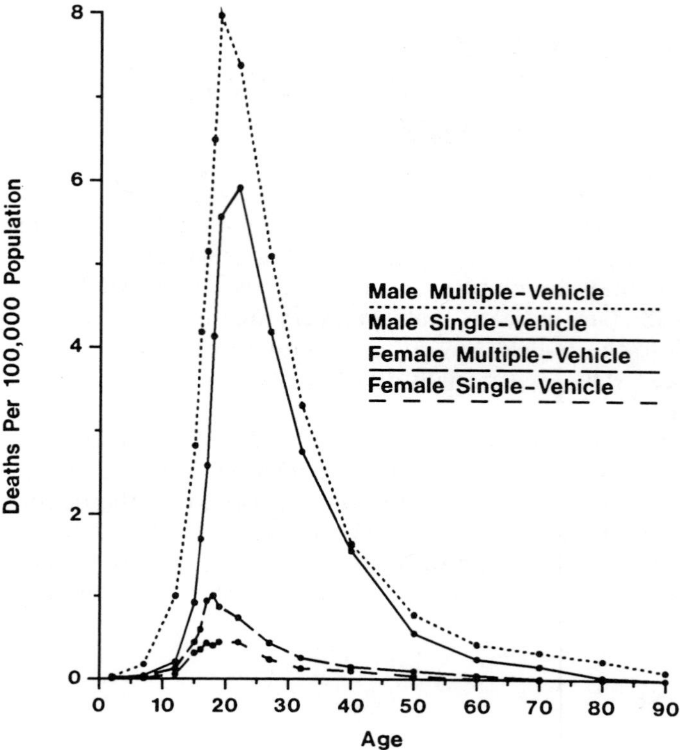

Figure 19-1. Motorcyclist Death Rates by Age, Sex, and Type of Crash, 1979-1981

use. Laws requiring helmet use have been shown by a variety of studies to reduce motorcyclist deaths by about 30 percent. States that revoked their helmet laws after a 1976 change in federal requirements experienced a substantial drop in helmet use and an increase of about 40 percent in deaths.[6] The elevated national death rate continues to reflect the repeal or weakening of helmet laws enacted in about half of the states in the wake of the 1976 federal legislation (figure 19-2).

Season, Day, and Time

Because motorcycles expose their riders to the weather, motorcycle use is seasonal and the pattern of deaths reflects this. The number of motorcyclist deaths per month ranges from a low of about 100 in January to a monthly average of 700 in June, July, and August. This seasonal

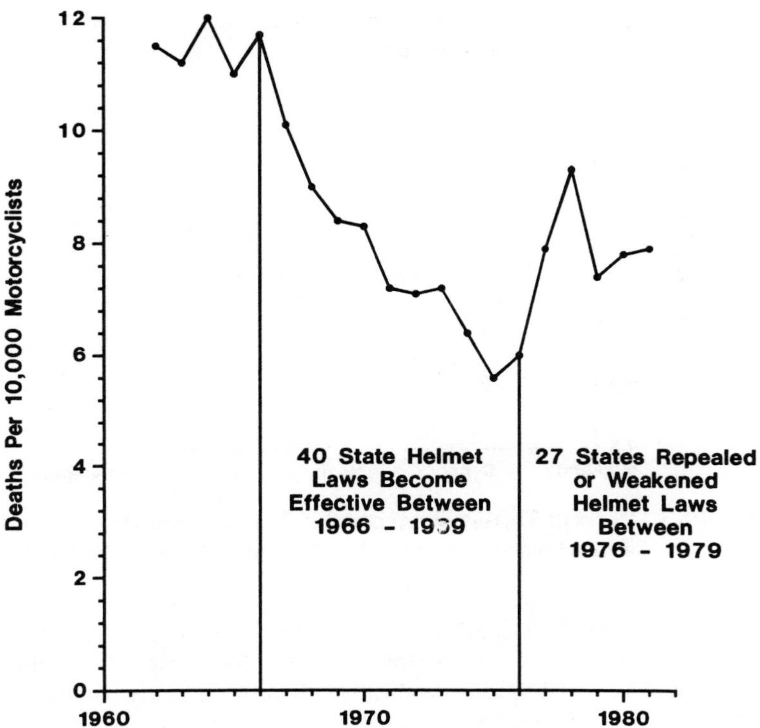

Figure 19-2. Motorcyclist Deaths Per 10,000 Motorcycles by Year, 1962-1981

pattern differs from the pattern for car occupants and pedestrians and more closely resembles that for bicyclists, where use is also seasonal (figure 18-1).

As with other motor vehicle fatalities, most motorcyclist deaths occur on weekends and during the evening or night. The peak hours begin at about 4:00 P.M., earlier than the peak for passenger vehicle occupant deaths, and extend to about 2:00 A.M. (figure 19-3). The peak time for nonfatal motorcyclist injuries is 3:00 P.M. to 6:59 P.M., when more than one-third of all injuries occur.

Types of Crashes

Collisions with other motor vehicles cause 55 percent of motorcyclist deaths. Motorcycle characteristics related to the likelihood of crashes and injuries include speed capability (injury rates are higher for more

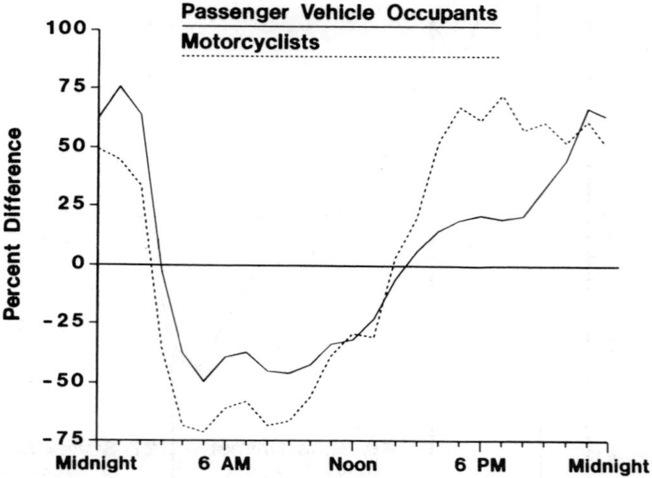

Figure 19-3. Percent Difference from the Average Number of Occupant and Motorcyclist Deaths by Time of Day, 1979-1981

powerful motorcycles), stability, and visibility, which can be improved with light-colored paint, reflectors, and daylight use of headlights.[2-4] The characteristics of vehicle and other structures likely to be impacted by motorcyclists in crashes, such as hardness, degree of curvature or sharpness, and lack of energy attenuation, also play a role in injury causation.

About 8 motorcycle occupant deaths per 10,000 registered motorcycles occur each year.[5] This ratio is three times as high as for passenger vehicles. Assuming that a motorcycle is used for as many years as a car, this means that, on average, each motorcycle manufactured is about three times as likely as a car to have one of its users killed. The potential benefit to be realized from motorcycle modifications that prevent severe or fatal injuries is therefore substantial.

Alcohol

The likelihood of alcohol involvement in fatal motorcycle crashes varies markedly with operator age, type of crash, and time of crash (figure 19-4). Fatally injured motorcycle drivers, like passenger car drivers, are most likely to have illegal BACs if they are killed in nighttime single-vehicle crashes. About 80 percent of the drivers ages 25-29 killed in such crashes have illegal BACs. Research in Maryland indicated that for the majority of motorcyclists who were found at post mortem to

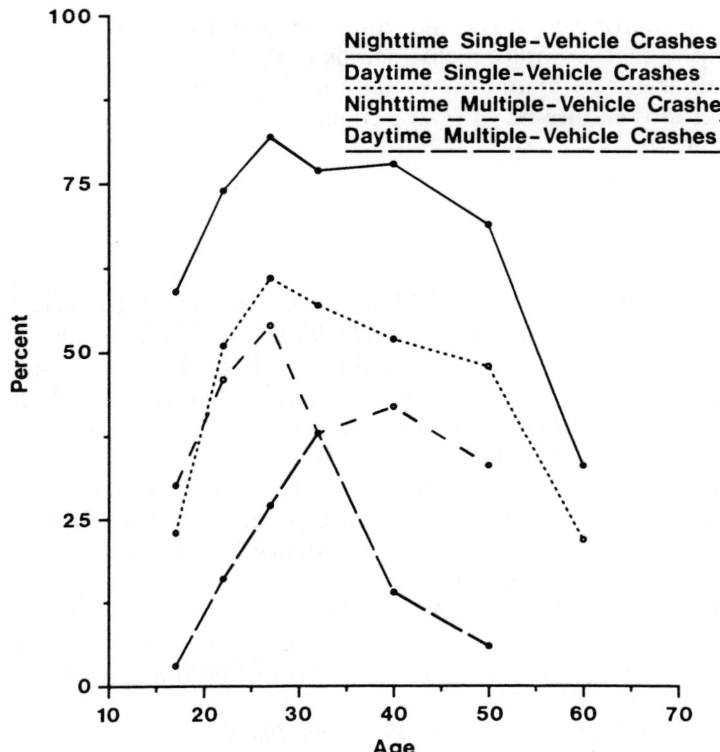

Figure 19-4. Percent of Fatally Injured Motorcycle Drivers with Blood Alcohol Concentrations At or Above 0.10 Percent by Age, Time of Day, and Type of Crash, 1979-1981

have illegally high BACs, the police reports did not indicate that the motorcyclists had been drinking.[1]

Historical Trends

Most causes of death, from diseases as well as injuries, have decreased in recent years. No major cause of death has experienced an increase approaching that for motorcyclist mortality. Trendline calculations for 1968-1979 indicate an increase of 158 percent for all ages combined in motorcyclist death rates. This increase occurred while deaths from unintentional injuries as a whole decreased by 23 percent. Contributing to the exceptional increase in motorcyclist deaths are increases in the amount of motorcycle travel and the decrease in helmet use. The relative importance of motorcyclist deaths in the high-risk 15-24-year-old age group (figure 4-4) and the increasing size of the problem in almost all age groups should be of major concern to health professionals and policy makers.

Notes

1. Baker, S.P., and R.S. Fisher. "Alcohol and Motorcycle Fatalities." *American Journal of Public Health* 67 (1977): 246-249.

2. Hurt, H.H., J.U. Ouelett, and D.R. Thom. *Motorcycle Accident Cause Factors and Identification of Countermeasures, Final Report.* Technical Report DOT HS-5-01160. Washington, DC: National Highway Traffic Safety Administration, 1981.

3. Kraus, J.F., R.S. Riggins, and C.E. Franti. "Some Epidemiologic Features of Motorcycle Collision Injuries: I. Introduction, Methods and Factors Associated with Incidence." *American Journal of Epidemiology* 102 (1975): 74-98.

4. Kraus, J.F., R.S. Riggins, and C.E. Franti. "Some Epidemiologic Features of Motorcycle Collision Injuries: II. Factors Associated with Severity of Injuries." *American Journal of Epidemiology* 102 (1975): 99-109.

5. National Safety Council. *Accident Facts — 1982 Edition.* Chicago: National Safety Council, 1982.

6. Watson, G.S., P.L. Zador, and A. Wilks. "The Repeal of Helmet Use Laws and Increased Motorcycle Mortality in the United States, 1975-1978." *American Journal of Public Health* 70 (1980): 579-585.

20 Bicyclists

Almost 1,000 bicyclists were killed in 1981, comprising 2 percent of all traffic deaths. Two-thirds of all bicyclist deaths occur in the 5-14-year-old age group. At this age, injuries to bicyclists cause about 15 percent of all traffic deaths and are a major cause of injury death. About 90 percent of all bicyclist deaths involve collisions with motor vehicles. Nonfatal injuries, on the other hand, generally result from falls from bicycles, which are rarely reported.[2]

Age and Sex

The death rate rises rapidly beginning at about age 4 and is highest for 13-year-old males. The male:female ratio increases at age 5 and for all ages combined is about 4:1 (figures 4-5 and 3-4) .

Geographic Differences

Regional differences in bicyclist death rates are less pronounced than for other deaths related to motor vehicles (figure 16-15). Similarly, variation by degree of urbanization and per capita income of the area of residence shows no pronounced patterns. This lack of effect is probably because the majority of fatally injured bicyclists are children. The possibility that childhood injury death rates from some causes may show less variation by region, urbanization, and income group than adult death rates deserves exploration. Further research is also needed on injuries to adult bicyclists, a growing problem.

Season, Day, and Time

The seasonal distribution of bicyclist deaths is similar to that of motorcyclist deaths (figure 18-1). Two-thirds occur during the five-month period from May through September.

Unlike motorcyclist deaths, the peak time of day is from 3:00 P.M. to 7:59 P.M. This peak begins during "after school" hours and is substantially earlier than for pedestrians (figure 18-2). The importance of visibility is suggested by the fact that among injury-producing collisions between bicyclists and motor vehicles during twilight or darkness, 28 percent involve a motor vehicle striking a bicycle from the rear or

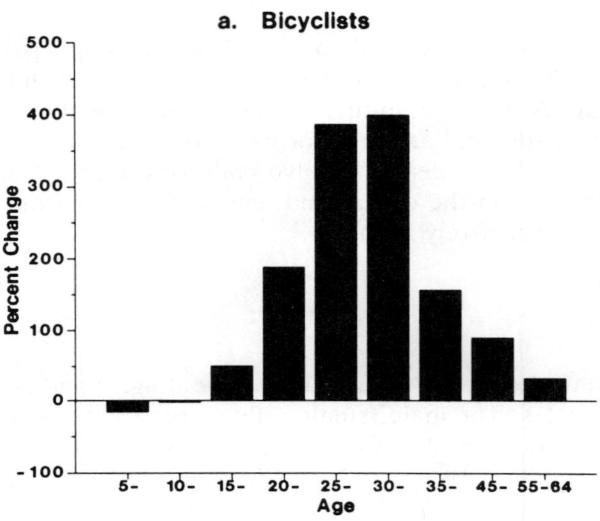

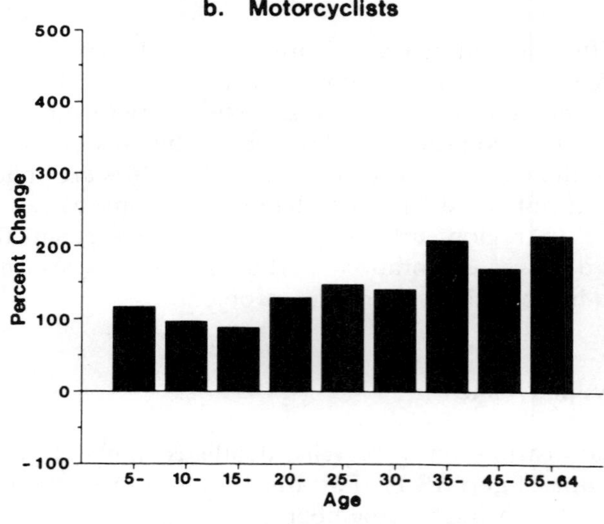

Figure 20-1. Percent Change in Bicyclist and Motorcyclist Death Rates by Age, Based on 1968-1979 Trend

making a left turn in front of an oncoming bicycle.[3] About one-third of all bicyclist deaths occur between 6:00 P.M. Friday and midnight Sunday. Because half of the fatally injured bicyclists are children, who are less likely than adults to use alcohol, this "weekend effect" is less pronounced than for other types of motor vehicle deaths.

Historical Trends

Changes in bicyclist death rates calculated from 1968-1979 trendlines show only a 4 percent increase overall but large increases for some age groups. The greatest increase occurred in the 25-34-year-old age group, which experienced a fourfold increase (figure 20-1). For these ages, the increase in death rates from bicycle-related injuries far surpassed the increase from any other type of motor vehicle crash in any age group. Even the motorcyclist death rate, which increased by about 160 percent during the same period for all ages combined, did not show as dramatic a change for any single age group.

Few bicyclists wear helmets. A review of bicyclist deaths in Dade County, Florida, indicated that the head or neck is the most seriously injured part of the body in 5 out of 6 fatally injured bicyclists. Typically, bicyclists who die with serious head injuries do not have other life-threatening or potentially disabling injuries. Thus, if bicyclists used helmets, many fatalities and serious head injuries would not occur.[1]

Notes

1. Fife, D., J. Davis, L. Tate, J.K. Wells, D. Mohan, and A.F. Williams. "Fatal Injuries to Bicyclists: The Experience of Dade County, Florida." *The Journal of Trauma* 23 (1983): 745-755.

2. Waller, J.A. "Bicycle Ownership, Use and Injury Patterns Among Elementary School Children." *Pediatrics* 47 (1971): 1042-1050.

3. Williams, A.F. "Factors in the Initiation of Bicycle-Motor Vehicle Collisions." *American Journal of Diseases of Children* 130 (1976): 370-377.

21 Conclusion

Injuries impose a greater burden on modern societies than any disease. Unlike other major health problems, a variety of effective preventive measures are available, well within the state of the art, and inexpensive in relation to their potential benefits. Unfortunately, these measures typically are not applied. More often, efforts to reduce the injury problem have utilized unproductive approaches. The results of neglect and misdirected efforts are reflected in the death rates portrayed in the preceding chapters.

Analyses in this book identify population subgroups at high risk of injury and death. A comprehensive discussion of ways to reduce injuries and of related public policies is presented elsewhere by Robertson.[14] Many new questions raised by the analyses, however, can be answered only by additional research requiring better data or the enhancement of existing sources of data. A major information gain would result, for example, if the causes of injury were determined and coded for a statistical sample of hospitalized patients. It would then be possible to study the morbidity and incidence of serious injuries in relation to various causes, as we have done with mortality data in this book. At present, data on people hospitalized for injuries include the nature of the injury itself but seldom its cause. As a result, the potential value of NCHS's Hospital Discharge Survey and of many statewide hospital-based data systems for developing and evaluating countermeasures is not realized. Further gains would result from including relevant questions on injury causation in the National Health Interview Survey. The most recent attempt to identify products other than motor vehicles was in 1975, and more than a decade has elapsed since questions were included on the incidence of gunshot wounds.[2,11]

Data for fatal injuries, while far better than those for nonfatal injuries, also leave much to be desired. For instance, the place of injury (home, nursing home, school, etc.) is not recorded on most death certificates, nor are the circumstances of falls (on one level, on stairs, from a ladder, etc.). Similarly, ICD codes for describing the specific type of firearm that caused an injury generally are not used. In many states death certificates indicate whether a fatal injury occurred at work, but this information is not uniformly available or compiled by NCHS.

Until some of these gaps in hospital and death certificate data are filled, we remain overly dependent on sources of information such as work injury data furnished by employers, which are widely regarded as being underreported and do not provide the detail needed for setting priorities and planning interventions.[13] Similarly, police data greatly underestimate the incidence of injuries from assaults and motor vehicle crashes. Such incidence data are almost nonexistent for other injuries.[2,4]

Far more serious than the gaps in our information base is the discrepancy between what is already known about the etiology and prevention of injuries and the application of that knowledge. More than four decades ago, Hugh De Haven, in his classic study of falls from heights, noted that the "structural environment is the dominant cause of injury" and that fatal injuries in aircraft and automobiles "are often sustained under moderate and controllable circumstances."[6] Despite some progress in making automobiles more crashworthy, the statement is still true. Protection against serious injury in crashes at impact speeds below 50 mph not only is theoretically possible but was incorporated several years ago in prototype cars that were also lightweight and fuel efficient, and that would have been reasonable in cost if mass produced.[10] These lifesaving features, however, have not been incorporated into cars produced for the public. In addition, most roads today are not designed to provide state-of-the-art protection against foreseeable events.[12] Nor have available knowledge and technology been adequately applied in the designs of trucks, aircraft, boats, tractors, cranes, forklifts, and other products associated with high injury rates.

The literature on injuries has given an inordinate amount of attention to the behavior of the people involved. Little emphasis has been placed on the relationships between high-risk groups and effective means of protecting people. Failure to use automotive seat belts, for example, has been shown to be especially common among those at greatest risk of being involved in crashes, such as teenagers, intoxicated drivers, people traveling at night, drivers who follow other cars too closely or ignore red traffic lights, and people in low-income areas. Thus, the people least apt to change their behavior are often the ones most at risk.[*3,7,15] If injuries among the people at greatest risk are to be reduced, this must be taken into account in planning effective approaches. Virtually all available evidence indicates that for injuries as for diseases, the most effective way to protect high-risk groups as well as the rest of the population is with measures — such as pasteurization and household fuses — that do not require individual motivation and frequent effort.[1,5,8-9,14]

---

*This does not necessarily imply unreasonable behavior, as illustrated by children unaware of hazards, farmers hurrying to harvest a crop before it rains, truck drivers paid by the mile rather than by the hours worked, and many others.

Some of the facts in this book document the success of measures that have protected the public against injury. Nonpoisonous domestic fuels and stringent elevator regulations, for example, have virtually eliminated hazards that once caused hundreds of deaths each year. Most of the analyses, however, reveal the need to apply equally effective countermeasures to the hazards that still are prevalent. In doing so, particular attention should be given to protecting groups whose activities, age, income, location, and other characteristics render them especially liable to serious injury. If that task is now easier, this book will have met its objective.

Notes

1. Baker, S.P. "Childhood Injuries: The Community Approach to Prevention." *Journal of Public Health Policy* 2 (1981): 235-246.

2. Baker, S.P. "Medical Data and Injuries." *American Journal of Public Health* 73 (1983): 733-734.

3. Baker, S.P., and P.E. Dietz. "The Epidemiology and Prevention of Injuries." In *The Management of Trauma*, edited by G.D. Zuidema, R.B. Rutherford, and W.F. Ballinger, II. Philadelphia: W.B. Saunders Company, 1979.

4. Barancik, J.I., B.F. Chatterjee, Y.C. Greene, E.M. Michenzi, and D. Fife. "Northeastern Ohio Trauma Study: I. Magnitude of the Problem." *American Journal of Public Health* 73 (1983): 746-751.

5. Barry, P.Z. "Individual Versus Community Orientation in the Prevention of Injuries." *Preventive Medicine* 4 (1975): 47-56.

6. De Haven, H. "Mechanical Analysis of Survival in Falls from Heights of Fifty to One Hundred and Fifty Feet." *War Medicine* 2 (1942): 539-546.

7. Deutsch, D., S. Sameth, and J. Akinyemi. "Seat Belt Usage and Risk-Taking Behavior at Two Major Traffic Intersections." *Proceedings of the Twenty-Fourth Conference of the American Association for Automotive Medicine*. Arlington Heights, IL: American Association for Automotive Medicine, 1980.

8. Haddon, W., Jr. "Advances in the Epidemiology of Injuries as a Basis for Public Policy." *Public Health Reports* 95 (1980): 411-421.

9. Haddon, W., Jr. "Strategy in Preventive Medicine: Passive vs. Active Approaches to Reducing Human Wastage." *Journal of Trauma* 14 (1974): 353-354.

10. Haddon W., Jr. "The Safety of the Automobile — An International Perspective." Presented at the Nordic Seminar on the Safety of the Automobile, Linkoping, Sweden, June 14, 1983.

11. Jagger, J., and S.P. Baker. "National Health Statistics and

Injury Prevention." *Proceedings of the 1983 Public Health Conference on Records and Statistics*. Bethesda, MD: August 1983.

12. Kelley, A.B. "Our Booby-Trapped Highways." *World* 2 (March 13, 1973): 30-32.

13. Kronebusch, K. "Occupational Injury Data: Are We Collecting What We Need for Prevention and Evaluation?" *Proceedings of the 1983 Public Health Conference on Records and Statistics*. Bethesda, MD: August 1983.

14. Robertson, L.S. *Injuries: Causes, Control Strategies, and Public Policy*. Lexington, MA: Lexington Books, 1983.

15. Williams, A.F., and B. O'Neill. *Seat Belt Laws: Implications for Occupant Protection*. SAE Technical Paper No. 790683. Warrendale, PA: Society of Automotive Engineers, 1979.

Appendix

Computational Methods

Death rates, unless otherwise indicated, are calculated per year and for the entire United States. They are not adjusted for age, race, or other population characteristics.

Sex ratios were calculated by dividing the unadjusted death rate for males by the unadjusted death rate for females.

Age-specific rates, plotted at age 90, are for persons 85 and older. Where the last rate plotted is at age 80, it represents age group 75–84. Where the last group plotted is 75, it is for ages 65 and over.

Maps divide the 50 states and Washington, D.C., into four strata: the 10 areas with the lowest rates, the 16 next lowest, the 15 next to the highest, and the 10 with the highest rates.

Percent change in death rates over the period 1968 through 1979 is calculated from regression estimates of the rates for 1968 and 1979. These regression estimates are calculated from NCHS mortality figures for each year and from 1970 and 1980 census data.

Urban/rural analyses divide the population into five subgroups: residents of cities of 1 million or more; residents of cities of 250,000 to 1 million; other SMSA residents; residents of "rural remote" counties that are not adjacent to an SMSA and contain no town as large as 2,500; and other non-SMSA residents called "rural non-remote."

Per capita income for the area of residence is usually for the county of residence. For counties that include cities of 250,000 or more, the per capita income was calculated separately for city and non-city residents.

Sources of Data and Basis for Computations

Except where otherwise indicated, rates in figures were based on the following data:

Type of Figure	*Source of Numerator*	*Source of Denominator*
Death rates per 100,000 population for 1977-1979*	Underlying cause of death, U.S. residents, 1977-1979[1]	U.S. resident population, 1980 census[2]
Death rates by year for 1968-1979	Underlying cause of death, U.S. residents, for each year[3]	Straight-line estimates from 1970 and 1980 census[4]
Death rates by year for 1930-1979	1930-1977 underlying cause of death, U.S. residents, for each year[5]; 1978-1979 from mortality tapes[1]	U.S. resident population estimates for each year as of July 2 (Census Bureau)
Death rates per 100,000 population 1979-1981 (motor vehicle-related)	Deaths in U.S. from motor vehicle crashes on public roads in 1979-1981, from FARS[6]	U.S. resident population, 1980[2]
Deaths per 1,000 injuries or per 1,000 occupants in crashes, 1979-1981	Deaths in U.S. from motor vehicle crashes on public roads in 1979-1981, from FARS[6]	Estimates of injured persons or occupants in 1979-1981 from NASS[7]
Death rates per million vehicle miles, 1979-1981	Deaths in U.S. from motor vehicle crashes on public roads in 1979-1981, from FARS[6]	Estimates of vehicle miles of travel in 1979-1981 from publication "Highway Statistics,"[8] FHWA

1. *Mortality Detail Tapes, 1979 (1977, 1978),* National Center for Health Statistics.
2. *Census of Population and Housing 1980:* Summary Tape File C1, Bureau of the Census.
3. *Mortality Detail Tapes, 1968-1979,* National Center for Health Statistics Series P-25, April 1979.
4. *Census of Population and Housing 1980;* 1970 Census figures from Current Population Reports.
5. *Vital Statistics of the United States.* Annual volumes, National Center for Health Statistics.
6. *Fatal Accident Reporting System (FARS) 1981 (1979, 1980),* National Highway Traffic Safety Administration.
7. *National Accident Sampling System (NASS) 1981 (1979, 1980),* National Highway Traffic Safety Administration.
8. *Highway Statistics 1981 (1979, 1980),* Federal Highway Administration.

---

*All rates calculated for deaths from machinery, collission with object or person, and caught or crushed, are based on 1979 data alone.

Number of Motor Vehicle-Related Deaths in 1979, FARS vs. NCHS

	Occupants		*Motorcyclists*		*Pedestrians*		*Bicyclists*		*Other/ Unknown*		*Total*	
	FARS	*NCHS*	*FARS*	*NCHS*	*FARS*	*NCHS*	*FARS*	*NCHS*	*FARS*	*NCHS*	*FARS*	*NCHS*
< 1 Year	174	209	0	0	7	7	0	0	2	0	183	216
1-4	521	519	3	1	416	468	23	14	13	0	976	1002
5-9	458	495	24	17	671	709	191	165	13	5	1357	1391
10-14	644	714	135	92	354	380	289	264	15	3	1437	1453
15-19	7026	7541	1168	882	766	786	161	152	17	5	9138	9366
20-24	7155	7724	1520	1126	795	810	63	53	14	7	9547	9720
25-29	4545	4859	884	639	597	609	39	39	13	2	6078	6148
30-34	3071	3245	496	363	440	420	35	34	8	2	4050	4064
35-44	3903	4144	395	285	714	719	28	26	8	3	5048	5177
45-54	3068	3229	149	100	728	789	23	23	14	4	3982	4145
55-64	2765	2903	74	54	755	830	24	26	11	2	3629	3815
65-74	2052	2205	33	26	808	834	29	24	6	2	2928	3091
75-84	1246	1339	5	6	670	753	16	17	0	1	1937	2116
85+	267	280	1	1	207	228	4	5	1	0	480	514
Other	141	14	7	0	168	21	7	0	0	0	323	35
Total	37036	39420	4894	3592	8096	8363	932	842	135	36	51093	52253

For all analyses of NCHS data on traffic deaths, persons of unknown status were included with occupants, which are probably overestimated by about 6 percent. The number of motorcyclist deaths identified by NCHS is about one-third less than the number identified by FARS; the number of bicyclist deaths is about one-tenth less. The number of pedestrian deaths identified by NCHS is 3 percent greater. The totals for the two files differ by only 1 percent. Appendix tables are based on NCHS data.

Table 1
Number of Deaths in 1979 and 1980, 69 Causes, and ICD E-Code for Each Cause

Cause	ICD E-Code (9th Rev.)	1979	1980
Transportation			
1. Motor Vehicle-Train	810	826	739
2. Motor Vehicle Occupant	810-819(.0,.1,.9)	39,420	38,919
3. Motorcyclist	810-819(.2,.3)	3,592	3,841
4. Bicyclist	810-819(.6)	842	861
5. Pedestrian	810-819(.7)	8,363	8,290
6. Motor Vehicle-Traffic (Total)	810-819	52,253	51,930
7. Pedestrian-Nontraffic	822.7	538	551
8. Pedestrian-Train	805.2	399	450
9. Aircraft	840-845	1,764	1,494
Drowning			
10. Boat-Related	830,832	1,194	1,214
11. Non-Boat	910	5,678	6,043
12. Drowning (Total)	830,832,910	6,872	7,257
Poisoning			
13. Opiates	850.0	341	322
14. Barbiturates	851	180	155
15. Tranquilizers	853	106	110
16. Antidepressants	854.0	105	141
17. Alcohol	860	416	385
18. Solids/Liquids (Total)	850-866	3,165	3,089
19. Motor Vehicle Exhaust	868.2	717	611
20. Gas/Vapor (Total)	867-869	1,472	1,242
Falls			
21. Stairs	880	1,315	1,349
22. Ladder/Scaffold	881	371	387
23. Building/Structure	882	653	734
24. Different Level	884	1,145	1,113
25. Same Level	885	454	406
26. Other/Unspecified	883,886-888	9,278	9,305
27. Fall (Total)	880-888	13,216	13,294
Fires and Burns			
28. Housefires	890	4,715	4,509
29. Clothing Ignition	893	289	311
30. Fires/Burns Excl. Scalds	890-899	5,991	5,822
31. Fires/Burns (Total)	890-899,924	6,183	6,016
Other Unintentional			
32. Firearm	922	2,004	1,955
33. Excessive Heat	900	148	1,700
34. Excessive Cold	901	711	707
35. Exposure, Neglect	904	378	415
36. Lightning	907	87	94
37. Natural Disaster	908-909	158	118
38. Aspiration-Food	911	2,093	1,943
39. Aspiration-Nonfood	912	1,150	1,306
40. Suffocation	913	863	872
41. Struck by Falling Object	916	1,163	1,037
42. Collision with Obj or Pers	917	328	318
43. Caught/Crushed	918	165	135
44. Machinery	919	1,629	1,471
45. Cutting/Piercing	920	136	143
46. Explosion	923	345	339
47. Electric Current	925	1,024	1,095
48. Unint Excl. Traffic	800-807,820-949	53,059	53,788
49. Unintentional (Total)	800-949	105,312	105,718
Suicide			
50. Firearm	955	15,558	15,404
51. Poison Solids/Liquids	950	3,344	3,035
52. Motor Vehicle Exhaust	952.0	1,929	1,998
53. Hanging	953	3,525	3,691
54. Drowning	954	583	547
55. Cutting/Piercing	956	416	395
56. Jumping	957	888	872
57. Non-Firearm (Total)	950-954,956-959	11,648	11,465
58. Suicide (Total)	950-959	27,206	26,869
Homicide			
59. Firearm	965	14,502	15,522
60. Cutting/Stabbing	966	4,077	4,354
61. Strangulation	963	849	930
62. Other	960-962,964,967-969	2,774	3,161
63. Non-Firearm (Total)	960-964,966-969	7,700	8,445
64. Homicide (Total)	960-969	22,202	23,967
65. Legal Intervention-Firearm	970	341	311
66. Undetermined-Firearm	985	641	629
67. Undet.-Poison Sol/Liq	980	960	893
68. Undetermined (Total)	980-989	3,860	3,663
69. Injuries (Total)	800-999	158,938	160,551

Table 2
Number of Deaths by Sex, 69 Causes, 1979, and Death Rates per 100,000 Population by Sex and by Race, 69 Causes, 1977-1979

	Deaths			Death Rate			Race			
	Male	Female	Total	Male	Female	Total	White	Black	Native Amer	Asian
Transportation										
1. Motor Vehicle-Train	589	237	826	.59	.22	.40	.43	.30	.38	.07
2. Motor Vehicle Occupant	28539	10881	39420	25.08	9.31	16.97	18.21	12.70	36.59	6.60
3. Motorcyclist	3247	345	3592	2.71	.26	1.45	1.63	.69	1.01	.40
4. Bicyclist	683	159	842	.58	.14	.35	.36	.41	.38	.12
5. Pedestrian	5844	2519	8363	5.11	2.11	3.58	3.41	5.28	12.88	2.33
6. Motor Vehicle-Traffic (Total)	38344	13909	52253	33.51	11.83	22.37	23.64	19.09	50.88	9.46
7. Pedestrian-Nontraffic	354	184	538	.31	.16	.23	.24	.21	.92	.10
8. Pedestrian-Train	345	54	399	.33	.06	.19	.17	.32	1.22	.06
9. Aircraft	1449	315	1764	1.31	.27	.78	.91	.09	.61	.30
Drowning										
10. Boat-Related	1097	97	1194	1.00	.09	.53	.53	.63	1.69	.27
11. Non-Boat	4682	996	5678	4.32	.87	2.56	2.33	4.74	6.78	1.55
12. Drowning (Total)	5779	1093	6872	5.32	.96	3.09	2.86	5.37	8.47	1.82
Poisoning										
13. Opiates	271	70	341	.23	.06	.14	.13	.27	.00	.09
14. Barbiturates	93	87	180	.07	.08	.08	.08	.08	.07	.04
15. Tranquilizers	65	41	106	.04	.03	.04	.04	.04	.05	.01
16. Antidepressants	75	30	105	.02	.05	.04	.04	.04	.05	.00
17. Alcohol	322	94	416	.25	.08	.16	.13	.48	.42	.02
18. Solids/Liquids (Total)	1964	1201	3165	1.75	1.08	1.41	1.38	2.09	1.88	.31
19. Motor Vehicle Exhaust	559	158	717	.54	.15	.34	.35	.37	.47	.16
20. Gas/Vapor (Total)	1096	376	1472	1.08	.36	.71	.71	.88	1.43	.21
Falls										
21. Stairs	768	547	1315	.69	.49	.59	.63	.51	.42	.18
22. Ladder/Scaffold	357	14	371	.35	.02	.18	.20	.10	.12	.09
23. Building/Structure	581	72	653	.51	.07	.29	.27	.45	.38	.17
24. Different Level	763	382	1145	.75	.34	.54	.58	.38	.70	.23
25. Same Level	231	223	454	.21	.21	.21	.24	.08	.14	.05
26. Other/Unspecified	4228	5050	9278	3.94	4.41	4.18	4.61	2.76	2.32	1.02
27. Fall (Total)	6928	6288	13216	6.46	5.53	5.99	6.53	4.29	4.08	1.73
Fires and Burns										
28. Housefires	2867	1848	4715	2.56	1.58	2.06	1.71	5.15	4.39	.33
29. Clothing Ignition	133	156	289	.14	.15	.15	.14	.26	.21	.03
30. Fires/Burns Excl. Scalds	3712	2279	5991	3.44	2.04	2.72	2.33	6.37	5.59	.40
31. Fires/Burns (Total)	3824	2359	6183	3.53	2.12	2.81	2.41	6.54	5.66	.43
Other Unintentional										
32. Firearm	1715	289	2004	1.50	.24	.85	.83	1.25	2.21	.13
33. Excessive Heat	98	50	148	.14	.07	.11	.09	.24	.33	.01
34. Excessive Cold	526	185	711	.44	.15	.29	.23	.71	3.10	.03
35. Exposure, Neglect	235	143	378	.18	.09	.14	.12	.22	1.69	.00
36. Lightning	76	11	87	.08	.01	.04	.05	.05	.07	.00
37. Natural Disaster	90	68	158	.10	.07	.08	.09	.09	.12	.02
38. Aspiration-Food	1238	855	2093	1.09	.72	.90	.93	1.04	1.08	.25
39. Aspiration-Nonfood	686	464	1150	.56	.39	.47	.44	.81	.80	.17
40. Suffocation	680	183	863	.66	.18	.41	.42	.48	.66	.09
41. Struck by Falling Object	1093	70	1163	.99	.06	.51	.53	.51	.56	.10
42. Collision with Obj or Pers	278	50	328	.25	.04	.14	.14	.18	.28	.06
43. Caught/Crushed	148	17	165	.13	.01	.07	.07	.09	.00	.06
44. Machinery	1541	88	1629	1.40	.08	.72	.79	.49	.77	.17
45. Cutting/Piercing	113	23	136	.10	.02	.06	.05	.14	.14	.00
46. Explosion	300	45	345	.30	.04	.17	.17	.21	.07	.04
47. Electric Current	957	67	1024	.91	.05	.47	.52	.29	.38	.08
48. Unint Excl. Traffic	36059	17000	53059	33.10	15.02	23.84	23.95	30.22	40.86	7.88
49. Unintentional (Total)	74403	30909	105312	66.54	26.84	46.21	45.93	49.31	91.73	17.33
Suicide										
50. Firearm	12919	2639	15558	11.84	2.27	6.92	7.70	3.71	8.24	1.71
51. Poison Solids/Liquids	1384	1960	3344	1.31	1.84	1.58	1.77	.69	1.10	.91
52. Motor Vehicle Exhaust	1277	652	1929	1.23	.57	.89	1.05	.10	.16	.16
53. Hanging	2783	742	3525	2.58	.67	1.60	1.73	.93	2.82	2.09
54. Drowning	329	254	583	.28	.23	.25	.26	.30	.09	.12
55. Cutting/Piercing	311	105	416	.27	.09	.18	.19	.10	.19	.30
56. Jumping	587	301	888	.50	.28	.39	.40	.41	.19	.48
57. Non-Firearm (Total)	7337	4311	11648	6.80	3.92	5.32	5.88	2.78	4.81	4.26
58. Suicide (Total)	20256	6950	27206	18.63	6.19	12.24	13.59	6.49	13.05	5.97
Homicide										
59. Firearm	12023	2479	14502	10.14	2.06	6.00	3.79	23.58	7.06	2.53
60. Cutting/Stabbing	3196	881	4077	2.62	.70	1.64	1.01	6.51	3.73	.67
61. Strangulation	274	575	849	.23	.47	.36	.29	.91	.42	.25
62. Other	1795	979	2774	1.50	.79	1.14	.88	3.17	4.11	.64
63. Non-Firearm (Total)	5265	2435	7700	4.34	1.96	3.13	2.19	10.59	8.26	1.55
64. Homicide (Total)	17288	4914	22202	14.49	4.02	9.13	5.98	34.17	15.32	4.09
65. Legal Intervention-Firearm	333	8	341	.25	.00	.13	.08	.46	.23	.02
66. Undetermined-Firearm	509	132	641	.56	.13	.34	.33	.51	.94	.05
67. Undet.-Poison Sol/Liq	537	423	960	.50	.41	.45	.46	.52	.49	.17
68. Undetermined (Total)	2671	1189	3860	2.58	1.10	1.83	1.67	3.40	3.87	.97
69. Injuries (Total)	114975	43970	158945	97.00	38.16	69.51	65.58	93.86	124.21	23.28

Table 3
Number of Deaths of Males by Age, 69 Causes, 1979

Cause	0	1–	5–	10–	15–	20–	25–	30–	35–	45–	55–	65–	75–	85+
Transportation														
1. Motor Vehicle-Train	5	9	9	14	102	102	81	48	63	45	58	35	11	7
2. Motor Vehicle Occupant	114	251	274	436	5462	6042	3796	2506	3039	2302	1979	1369	791	166
3. Motorcyclist	0	0	14	76	785	1019	588	348	253	90	45	25	4	0
4. Bicyclist	0	11	127	215	122	40	32	30	22	18	24	21	16	5
5. Pedestrian	4	288	468	229	568	652	470	321	531	571	594	527	449	151
6. Motor Vehicle-Traffic (Total)	118	550	888	959	6941	7758	4888	3207	3848	2984	2644	1944	1260	322
7. Pedestrian-Nontraffic	1	110	21	6	9	21	24	16	27	36	27	30	21	5
8. Pedestrian-Train	0	0	8	15	40	54	39	33	49	31	33	23	11	7
9. Aircraft	0	6	14	21	56	154	222	213	336	254	132	26	3	0
Drowning														
10. Boat-Related	0	6	26	40	119	152	138	125	162	138	115	57	18	1
11. Non-Boat	38	466	313	353	840	712	446	254	395	258	251	170	97	41
12. Drowning (Total)	38	472	339	393	959	864	584	379	557	396	366	227	115	42
Poisoning														
13. Opiates	0	4	0	0	10	57	84	61	33	13	7	1	1	0
14. Barbiturates	0	0	1	0	8	20	19	10	10	9	7	4	3	0
15. Tranquilizers	0	0	0	0	0	6	15	8	18	9	5	3	0	1
16. Antidepressants	0	1	0	0	0	4	6	5	6	2	4	2	0	0
17. Alcohol	0	1	0	0	13	14	24	29	61	90	62	24	2	0
18. Solids/Liquids (Total)	8	25	9	15	120	328	386	257	256	210	165	106	52	23
19. Motor Vehicle Exhaust	1	2	0	3	61	98	82	62	84	64	46	30	22	4
20. Gas/Vapor (Total)	6	9	7	17	113	175	136	98	155	130	106	73	58	13
Falls														
21. Stairs	2	5	4	1	3	11	17	21	41	95	155	162	165	86
22. Ladder/Scaffold	0	1	1	1	8	14	20	19	39	64	72	65	40	13
23. Building/Structure	0	30	11	8	37	66	73	38	71	62	71	73	32	9
24. Different Level	19	10	10	20	79	82	57	33	54	65	82	71	101	80
25. Same Level	0	0	0	0	2	5	3	4	6	13	26	59	66	47
26. Other/Unspecified	12	21	12	24	58	79	62	75	201	336	445	720	1126	1054
27. Fall (Total)	33	67	38	54	187	257	232	190	412	635	851	1150	1530	1289
Fires and Burns														
28. Housefires	69	382	188	88	113	190	174	141	253	284	361	299	232	91
29. Clothing Ignition	1	1	0	1	2	2	3	1	7	14	16	24	35	26
30. Fires/Burns Excl. Scalds	71	408	201	105	134	242	224	184	330	394	481	434	346	149
31. Fires/Burns (Total)	73	417	201	106	136	248	230	193	339	407	500	446	361	158
Other Unintentional														
32. Firearm	1	42	61	203	321	268	182	128	165	135	105	70	28	6
33. Excessive Heat	2	3	1	2	2	8	6	3	10	13	26	9	5	6
34. Excessive Cold	1	2	2	3	21	24	17	11	59	70	95	101	85	33
35. Exposure, Neglect	1	0	0	1	2	8	11	8	21	27	31	49	43	29
36. Lightning	0	0	3	7	11	3	11	13	17	7	1	2	1	0
37. Natural Disaster	1	2	2	5	7	13	12	5	8	12	14	7	2	0
38. Aspiration-Food	90	63	11	9	29	39	42	47	111	139	189	235	164	69
39. Aspiration-Nonfood	62	38	6	7	14	15	5	16	35	52	89	133	129	85
40. Suffocation	104	46	33	103	73	70	62	43	53	38	26	16	8	5
41. Struck by Falling Object	5	25	13	17	79	147	118	113	158	171	138	71	36	2
42. Collision with Obj or Pers	6	5	8	10	31	41	27	22	30	34	33	18	6	7
43. Caught/Crushed	6	9	3	4	19	19	14	9	18	24	16	4	3	0
44. Machinery	0	24	39	43	121	176	125	114	209	206	252	176	52	4
45. Cutting/Piercing	2	1	9	1	5	12	11	11	17	12	17	8	7	0
46. Explosion	1	5	2	8	26	43	44	31	41	37	37	14	11	0
47. Electric Current	6	13	17	27	127	208	132	106	131	102	62	17	6	3
48. Unint Excl. Traffic	496	1450	908	1177	2780	3533	2926	2276	3591	3727	3950	3743	3325	2084
49. Unintentional (Total)	614	2000	1796	2136	9721	11291	7814	5483	7439	6711	6594	5687	4585	2406
Suicide														
50. Firearm	0	0	0	53	966	1743	1478	1141	1697	1605	1685	1490	877	180
51. Poison Solids/Liquids	0	0	0	1	56	169	250	178	227	211	139	87	49	16
52. Motor Vehicle Exhaust	0	0	0	0	64	149	181	138	196	213	167	106	47	16
53. Hanging	0	0	0	49	255	458	388	259	293	273	288	257	195	63
54. Drowning	0	0	1	0	13	49	49	25	51	39	33	29	22	17
55. Cutting/Piercing	0	0	0	0	8	31	38	26	42	47	61	33	18	6
56. Jumping	0	0	0	0	33	92	85	76	72	62	58	50	39	18
57. Non-Firearm (Total)	0	0	1	50	486	1050	1109	777	983	922	820	598	388	142
58. Suicide (Total)	0	0	1	103	1452	2793	2587	1918	2680	2527	2505	2088	1265	322
Homicide														
59. Firearm	2	20	43	91	1157	2274	2204	1707	2044	1341	724	305	79	12
60. Cutting/Stabbing	3	8	12	15	381	608	545	407	539	331	211	91	25	3
61. Strangulation	12	6	13	8	23	23	30	21	26	40	37	12	12	5
62. Other	87	120	23	31	73	157	173	158	250	268	203	135	81	25
63. Non-Firearm (Total)	102	134	48	54	477	788	748	586	815	639	451	238	118	33
64. Homicide (Total)	104	154	91	145	1634	3062	2952	2293	2859	1980	1175	543	197	45
65. Legal Intervention-Firearm	0	0	0	0	47	80	76	49	38	24	7	8	3	1
66. Undetermined-Firearm	0	1	3	11	74	111	68	52	65	39	43	25	15	1
67. Undet.-Poison Sol/Liq	1	4	0	2	35	95	139	69	76	53	33	23	7	0
68. Undetermined (Total)	36	57	20	47	208	386	370	274	365	341	273	165	81	34
69. Injuries (Total)	754	2211	1908	2431	13062	17613	13799	10021	13385	11588	10559	8494	6133	2808

Table 4
Death Rates per 100,000 Population for Males by Age, 69 Causes, 1977-1979

Cause	0	1–	5–	10–	15–	20–	25–	30–	35–	45–	55–	65–	75–	85+
Transportation														
1. Motor Vehicle-Train	.26	.21	.12	.13	1.10	1.06	.83	.60	.45	.59	.58	.59	.76	.68
2. Motor Vehicle Occupant	6.44	3.95	3.00	5.10	50.37	55.10	36.32	26.58	22.55	20.80	19.01	19.97	27.50	25.73
3. Motorcyclist	.00	.03	.12	.98	6.92	9.13	5.42	3.11	1.69	.77	.40	.29	.13	.24
4. Bicyclist	.00	.17	1.43	2.19	1.08	.36	.28	.23	.15	.15	.19	.34	.50	.49
5. Pedestrian	.28	4.64	5.70	2.70	4.72	5.16	4.33	3.59	3.96	5.08	6.00	7.77	15.79	20.79
6. Motor Vehicle-Traffic (Total)	6.72	8.79	10.29	11.06	63.16	69.78	46.38	33.54	28.38	26.83	25.64	28.37	43.93	47.25
7. Pedestrian-Nontraffic	.17	1.52	.24	.09	.15	.18	.19	.17	.23	.30	.29	.37	.71	.83
8. Pedestrian-Train	.00	.06	.07	.16	.39	.48	.44	.33	.37	.40	.39	.39	.38	1.03
9. Aircraft	.07	.09	.16	.19	.57	1.58	2.46	2.47	2.52	2.25	1.23	.37	.15	.00
Drowning														
10. Boat-Related	.00	.13	.28	.39	1.14	1.55	1.47	1.39	1.25	1.19	1.13	.88	.53	.15
11. Non-Boat	2.03	6.76	4.04	4.29	8.38	6.79	4.47	3.11	3.04	2.45	2.48	2.57	3.21	4.01
12. Drowning (Total)	2.03	6.89	4.33	4.69	9.52	8.34	5.94	4.51	4.30	3.64	3.61	3.44	3.74	4.16
Poisoning														
13. Opiates	.00	.03	.00	.00	.10	.61	.85	.56	.20	.10	.03	.02	.01	.05
14. Barbiturates	.00	.01	.00	.00	.07	.16	.16	.12	.06	.09	.07	.08	.06	.00
15. Tranquilizers	.00	.01	.00	.00	.02	.08	.09	.06	.08	.05	.04	.03	.01	.05
16. Antidepressants	.04	.03	.01	.00	.02	.03	.04	.03	.04	.02	.03	.01	.00	.00
17. Alcohol	.00	.01	.00	.00	.08	.08	.18	.23	.50	.70	.56	.29	.09	.05
18. Solids/Liquids (Total)	.39	.53	.09	.18	1.19	3.05	3.97	2.62	2.09	1.86	1.47	1.48	1.96	3.28
19. Motor Vehicle Exhaust	.04	.08	.04	.04	.72	.99	.74	.71	.73	.67	.49	.42	.66	.78
20. Gas/Vapor (Total)	.22	.25	.14	.24	1.31	1.71	1.34	1.18	1.32	1.26	1.20	1.18	1.90	2.10
Falls														
21. Stairs	.09	.10	.03	.01	.03	.09	.13	.19	.40	.83	1.52	2.49	5.51	12.77
22. Ladder/Scaffold	.00	.01	.0C	.01	.08	.19	.25	.23	.33	.55	.82	1.06	1.56	1.61
23. Building/Structure	.11	.37	.11	.10	.33	.64	.59	.40	.54	.67	.70	.96	1.23	1.61
24. Different Level	1.25	.22	.14	.25	.77	.86	.57	.45	.49	.67	.78	1.14	3.56	12.86
25. Same Level	.00	.03	.01	.01	.04	.03	.03	.03	.06	.13	.29	.69	2.27	7.68
26. Other/Unspecified	.57	.34	.14	.23	.57	.67	.68	.97	1.59	2.98	4.67	10.42	40.9	162.67
27. Fall (Total)	2.03	1.06	.44	.61	1.82	2.47	2.26	2.27	3.41	5.83	8.78	16.77	55.1	199.21
Fires and Burns														
28. Housefires	4.21	5.49	2.12	.99	1.04	1.75	1.74	1.59	1.94	2.80	3.47	4.53	7.35	11.54
29. Clothing Ignition	.02	.03	.01	.01	.01	.02	.02	.03	.04	.11	.20	.50	1.52	3.42
30. Fires/Burns Excl. Scalds	4.45	5.96	2.32	1.16	1.27	2.22	2.26	2.21	2.69	3.94	4.87	6.91	12.00	20.98
31. Fires/Burns (Total)	4.67	6.13	2.32	1.17	1.28	2.26	2.32	2.30	2.75	4.08	5.01	7.07	12.55	22.21
Other Unintentional														
32. Firearm	.04	.55	.77	2.11	2.97	2.31	1.69	1.41	1.32	1.23	1.03	.96	.85	.73
33. Excessive Heat	.18	.05	.01	.01	.08	.08	.06	.10	.16	.27	.31	.27	.42	.93
34. Excessive Cold	.07	.02	.01	.05	.15	.20	.18	.16	.36	.70	.99	1.37	2.46	3.77
35. Exposure, Neglect	.15	.01	.00	.01	.02	.06	.09	.09	.16	.20	.32	.57	1.15	3.23
36. Lightning	.00	.01	.04	.11	.16	.08	.08	.12	.10	.08	.05	.04	.01	.00
37. Natural Disaster	.09	.08	.08	.05	.07	.13	.11	.09	.09	.12	.13	.13	.14	.15
38. Aspiration-Food	5.19	.91	.13	.13	.34	.48	.49	.55	.86	1.27	1.87	2.95	4.92	9.73
39. Aspiration-Nonfood	3.52	.65	.12	.08	.12	.15	.15	.14	.28	.44	.79	1.47	3.63	9.44
40. Suffocation	6.88	.80	.54	1.18	.70	.70	.59	.42	.45	.33	.28	.23	.26	.39
41. Struck by Falling Object	.17	.40	.21	.18	.71	1.30	1.16	1.16	1.38	1.55	1.38	1.11	1.03	.49
42. Collision with Obj or Pers	.33	.08	.09	.11	.29	.38	.28	.25	.24	.31	.33	.27	.21	1.03
43. Caught/Crushed	.33	.14	.04	.04	.18	.18	.14	.10	.14	.22	.16	.06	.10	.00
44. Machinery	.00	.37	.46	.46	1.13	1.65	1.29	1.31	1.66	1.87	2.48	2.60	1.81	.59
45. Cutting/Piercing	.04	.04	.08	.06	.08	.11	.07	.11	.13	.10	.13	.16	.24	.10
46. Explosion	.02	.07	.03	.11	.22	.38	.47	.43	.37	.46	.41	.23	.34	.34
47. Electric Current	.15	.19	.23	.42	1.32	1.82	1.50	1.17	1.15	.97	.62	.29	.29	.20
48. Unint Excl. Traffic	29.75	21.99	11.31	13.65	27.09	32.99	29.55	25.62	28.69	34.90	40.45	55.19	116.43	303.88
49. Unintentional (Total)	36.46	30.78	21.59	24.71	90.24	102.77	75.94	59.17	57.06	61.73	66.09	83.56	160.36	351.12
Suicide														
50. Firearm	.00	.00	.00	.72	8.77	16.52	14.96	12.57	13.19	15.63	17.59	22.28	29.64	28.27
51. Poison Solids/Liquids	.00	.00	.00	.03	.55	1.90	2.51	2.08	1.75	1.96	1.50	1.47	1.64	1.96
52. Motor Vehicle Exhaust	.00	.00	.00	.01	.68	1.50	1.86	1.66	1.81	1.93	1.70	1.74	1.69	1.52
53. Hanging	.00	.00	.00	.56	2.51	4.32	3.91	2.72	2.38	2.73	3.30	3.95	6.07	9.34
54. Drowning	.00	.00	.01	.00	.14	.38	.41	.35	.31	.32	.37	.48	.85	1.76
55. Cutting/Piercing	.00	.00	.00	.00	.07	.27	.35	.33	.33	.43	.51	.58	.69	.73
56. Jumping	.00	.00	.00	.02	.31	.74	.82	.78	.54	.60	.58	.71	1.35	2.20
57. Non-Firearm (Total)	.00	.00	.02	.63	4.68	10.18	10.96	8.81	7.98	8.78	8.74	9.53	13.06	18.39
58. Suicide (Total)	.00	.00	.02	1.35	13.45	26.70	25.92	21.38	21.18	24.41	26.32	31.82	42.69	46.66
Homicide														
59. Firearm	.17	.36	.47	1.05	9.94	19.39	20.76	17.41	15.89	11.40	6.86	4.38	2.66	2.05
60. Cutting/Stabbing	.26	.12	.11	.19	2.79	5.12	4.93	4.15	3.83	3.15	2.05	1.33	.99	.68
61. Strangulation	.55	.17	.13	.09	.15	.22	.30	.21	.22	.32	.30	.24	.37	.59
62. Other	4.23	1.95	.37	.25	.70	1.37	1.56	1.51	1.83	2.17	1.99	1.85	2.33	3.62
63. Non-Firearm (Total)	5.04	2.24	.61	.54	3.63	6.70	6.78	5.86	5.88	5.64	4.33	3.41	3.69	4.89
64. Homicide (Total)	5.20	2.60	1.09	1.59	13.57	26.09	27.55	23.27	21.77	17.04	11.19	7.79	6.35	6.95
65. Legal Intervention-Firearm	.00	.00	.00	.01	.37	.61	.63	.42	.33	.18	.10	.08	.03	.05
66. Undetermined-Firearm	.07	.06	.02	.20	.83	1.05	.88	.68	.62	.54	.55	.53	.53	.44
67. Undet.-Poison Sol/Liq	.06	.06	.01	.03	.36	.93	1.30	.87	.59	.55	.34	.30	.22	.24
68. Undetermined (Total)	2.80	1.06	.25	.64	2.14	3.66	3.88	3.27	3.09	3.32	2.87	2.68	3.27	5.28
69. Injuries (Total)	44.45	34.43	22.93	28.27	119.77	159.16	133.90	107.55	103.42	106.73	106.60	125.96	212.74	410.16

Table 5
Number of Deaths of Females by Age, 69 Causes, 1979

Cause	0	1–	5–	10–	15–	20–	25–	30–	35–	45–	55–	65–	75–	85+
Transportation														
1. Motor Vehicle-Train	2	8	17	8	37	22	22	21	21	22	28	19	9	1
2. Motor Vehicle Occupant	95	268	221	278	2079	1682	1063	739	1105	927	924	836	548	114
3. Motorcyclist	0	1	3	16	97	107	51	15	32	10	9	1	2	1
4. Bicyclist	0	3	38	49	30	13	7	4	4	5	2	3	1	0
5. Pedestrian	3	180	241	151	218	158	139	99	188	218	236	307	304	77
6. Motor Vehicle-Traffic (Total)	98	452	503	494	2425	1962	1260	857	1329	1161	1171	1147	856	192
7. Pedestrian-Nontraffic	2	97	11	2	2	0	4	5	7	5	9	14	14	12
8. Pedestrian-Train	0	3	1	3	3	5	6	2	5	5	5	9	5	2
9. Aircraft	0	4	12	6	28	35	49	40	58	36	27	9	2	0
Drowning														
10. Boat-Related	1	4	10	9	10	8	8	9	14	7	11	4	2	0
11. Non-Boat	38	214	70	87	92	78	68	40	66	68	46	50	53	25
12. Drowning (Total)	39	218	80	96	102	86	76	49	80	75	57	54	55	25
Poisoning														
13. Opiates	0	0	0	0	5	12	23	11	9	4	5	0	0	0
14. Barbiturates	1	1	0	0	1	7	11	7	10	17	18	9	5	0
15. Tranquilizers	0	1	0	0	0	1	2	5	6	12	8	3	2	1
16. Antidepressants	1	6	0	0	3	4	7	11	14	15	8	6	0	0
17. Alcohol	0	1	0	0	0	0	5	4	22	22	35	3	2	0
18. Solids/Liquids (Total)	11	34	2	5	42	113	142	104	178	183	188	97	69	31
19. Motor Vehicle Exhaust	1	0	1	4	40	22	14	10	16	16	14	8	9	3
20. Gas/Vapor (Total)	1	11	7	13	66	44	24	19	34	35	41	33	34	14
Falls														
21. Stairs	1	3	0	1	1	1	3	7	16	38	78	107	187	104
22. Ladder/Scaffold	0	1	0	0	0	0	1	0	3	0	7	1	1	0
23. Building/Structure	0	6	3	0	3	5	4	5	6	5	6	12	13	4
24. Different Level	11	12	8	5	8	7	3	7	4	15	14	40	106	142
25. Same Level	1	0	0	0	2	1	1	0	4	5	17	39	82	71
26. Other/Unspecified	11	15	7	5	10	7	11	11	72	123	244	607	1693	2234
27. Fall (Total)	24	37	18	11	24	21	23	30	105	186	366	806	2082	2555
Fires and Burns														
28. Housefires	61	266	143	91	77	122	61	59	103	147	202	235	198	82
29. Clothing Ignition	0	2	2	0	2	1	0	1	5	8	16	40	50	29
30. Fires/Burns Excl. Scalds	63	285	147	99	88	139	66	71	127	186	255	309	296	147
31. Fires/Burns (Total)	68	293	149	99	88	140	67	73	128	190	260	324	318	161
Other Unintentional														
32. Firearm	3	11	26	25	33	46	25	23	24	37	23	8	2	3
33. Excessive Heat	2	3	0	0	0	3	1	1	2	5	2	8	10	12
34. Excessive Cold	1	1	0	0	2	7	7	0	9	21	27	29	46	34
35. Exposure, Neglect	5	0	0	0	1	1	1	1	3	10	9	34	39	38
36. Lightning	0	0	1	1	2	0	2	1	0	2	1	0	1	0
37. Natural Disaster	0	3	1	9	6	9	4	0	7	8	5	10	5	1
38. Aspiration-Food	63	34	4	5	11	20	24	16	41	74	118	179	146	120
39. Aspiration-Nonfood	41	20	6	3	10	4	5	10	18	30	55	72	101	89
40. Suffocation	77	29	11	5	5	4	5	5	8	5	8	8	6	7
41. Struck by Falling Object	2	11	11	3	5	4	3	2	6	6	4	3	7	3
42. Collision with Obj or Pers	3	7	4	2	4	2	1	1	4	1	4	7	3	7
43. Caught/Crushed	0	4	2	1	0	1	2	0	0	0	1	1	1	4
44. Machinery	0	15	10	7	6	4	6	7	8	11	9	1	2	2
45. Cutting/Piercing	0	2	2	1	0	2	2	1	3	1	2	3	3	1
46. Explosion	1	2	1	1	3	4	1	5	3	7	6	4	6	1
47. Electric Current	0	9	7	4	6	8	11	8	2	5	4	0	2	1
48. Unint Excl. Traffic	368	897	408	352	543	632	565	473	877	1154	1555	2179	3514	3466
49. Unintentional (Total)	466	1349	911	846	2968	2594	1825	1330	2206	2315	2726	3326	4370	3658
Suicide														
50. Firearm	0	0	0	31	171	341	311	255	441	455	380	187	60	6
51. Poison Solids/Liquids	0	0	0	8	78	154	192	205	372	372	290	177	87	25
52. Motor Vehicle Exhaust	0	0	0	1	14	40	52	67	148	168	97	52	12	1
53. Hanging	0	0	0	7	39	54	52	47	88	102	136	115	81	21
54. Drowning	0	0	0	0	8	17	12	20	37	35	51	38	29	7
55. Cutting/Piercing	0	0	0	0	2	5	2	11	18	17	25	14	7	4
56. Jumping	0	0	0	1	14	33	31	31	41	43	36	37	27	7
57. Non-Firearm (Total)	0	0	0	17	165	324	373	413	755	807	683	455	252	66
58. Suicide (Total)	0	0	0	48	336	665	684	668	1196	1262	1063	642	312	72
Homicide														
59. Firearm	5	23	25	28	259	436	382	288	431	279	170	96	37	12
60. Cutting/Stabbing	2	8	14	15	95	170	131	92	118	70	65	50	41	5
61. Strangulation	7	11	6	23	81	111	91	40	49	37	36	41	30	10
62. Other	52	118	29	18	75	105	81	66	86	95	58	96	55	37
63. Non-Firearm (Total)	61	137	49	56	251	386	303	198	253	202	159	187	126	52
64. Homicide (Total)	66	160	74	84	510	822	685	486	684	481	329	283	163	64
65. Legal Intervention-Firearm	0	0	0	0	0	0	2	1	2	1	1	0	1	0
66. Undetermined-Firearm	1	1	0	5	17	24	17	12	25	15	5	7	3	0
67. Undet.-Poison Sol/Liq	2	4	0	5	20	45	60	40	83	79	56	21	7	1
68. Undetermined (Total)	49	38	8	25	75	109	122	101	183	187	135	77	53	23
69. Injuries (Total)	581	1547	993	1003	3889	4190	3318	2586	4271	4246	4254	4328	4899	3817

Table 6
Death Rates per 100,000 Population for Females by Age, 69 Causes, 1977-1979

Cause	0	1–	5–	10–	15–	20–	25–	30–	35–	45–	55–	65–	75–	85+
Transportation														
1. Motor Vehicle-Train	.19	.13	.18	.12	.41	.33	.21	.19	.20	.19	.21	.21	.19	.17
2. Motor Vehicle Occupant	6.50	4.06	2.90	3.42	20.02	15.90	10.24	7.92	7.96	7.91	8.27	9.68	11.26	7.42
3. Motorcyclist	.00	.02	.04	.16	.90	.86	.45	.26	.17	.07	.03	.02	.01	.02
4. Bicyclist	.00	.07	.45	.61	.27	.10	.06	.05	.04	.03	.02	.02	.01	.02
5. Pedestrian	.15	3.09	3.08	1.73	2.11	1.50	1.13	1.10	1.22	1.72	1.98	3.43	6.16	4.88
6. Motor Vehicle-Traffic (Total)	6.66	7.24	6.48	5.95	23.32	18.37	11.89	9.32	9.39	9.73	10.32	13.14	17.46	12.34
7. Pedestrian-Nontraffic	.23	1.43	.15	.02	.02	.01	.04	.05	.04	.07	.10	.20	.31	.32
8. Pedestrian-Train	.00	.07	.03	.05	.05	.05	.05	.04	.04	.05	.05	.07	.14	.26
9. Aircraft	.12	.07	.08	.14	.23	.43	.47	.46	.42	.36	.21	.09	.03	.00
Drowning														
10. Boat-Related	.06	.07	.14	.07	.12	.13	.07	.07	.11	.09	.06	.05	.02	.00
11. Non-Boat	1.87	3.21	1.12	1.06	.93	.72	.60	.47	.47	.61	.49	.62	1.30	1.11
12. Drowning (Total)	1.93	3.28	1.26	1.13	1.05	.85	.68	.54	.59	.70	.56	.67	1.32	1.11
Poisoning														
13. Opiates	.02	.02	.00	.00	.06	.14	.17	.11	.06	.04	.03	.01	.01	.02
14. Barbiturates	.02	.02	.00	.00	.03	.11	.12	.07	.10	.12	.10	.12	.08	.13
15. Tranquilizers	.00	.01	.00	.00	.01	.03	.02	.04	.05	.08	.07	.03	.03	.06
16. Antidepressants	.02	.09	.01	.00	.01	.03	.06	.08	.07	.08	.07	.03	.01	.00
17. Alcohol	.00	.01	.00	.00	.01	.02	.04	.05	.13	.25	.27	.07	.03	.00
18. Solids/Liquids (Total)	.52	.54	.04	.09	.54	1.14	1.32	1.19	1.41	1.78	1.63	1.25	1.41	2.16
19. Motor Vehicle Exhaust	.06	.03	.03	.04	.50	.23	.16	.13	.16	.14	.11	.09	.16	.15
20. Gas/Vapor (Total)	.15	.23	.13	.16	.75	.44	.28	.22	.29	.34	.37	.37	.71	.75
Falls														
21. Stairs	.10	.11	.00	.00	.02	.02	.03	.06	.14	.44	.67	1.25	3.79	6.91
22. Ladder/Scaffold	.00	.01	.00	.00	.00	.01	.00	.00	.02	.01	.05	.06	.05	.06
23. Building/Structure	.04	.19	.04	.01	.04	.04	.06	.05	.04	.07	.06	.11	.26	.30
24. Different Level	.60	.19	.06	.07	.10	.10	.04	.06	.05	.12	.13	.49	2.20	9.37
25. Same Level	.04	.00	.00	.01	.01	.01	.01	.02	.02	.06	.13	.42	1.73	5.82
26. Other/Unspecified	.62	.25	.09	.04	.10	.08	.12	.16	.48	1.11	2.28	6.76	35.96	144.54
27. Fall (Total)	1.39	.73	.20	.13	.27	.26	.27	.35	.74	1.80	3.32	9.08	43.99	166.99
Fires and Burns														
28. Housefires	3.78	4.29	1.78	1.08	.77	.93	.64	.64	.86	1.34	1.71	2.54	4.03	5.26
29. Clothing Ignition	.00	.04	.03	.01	.01	.02	.01	.01	.04	.09	.18	.48	1.21	2.07
30. Fires/Burns Excl. Scalds	3.98	4.64	1.88	1.15	.89	1.09	.79	.80	1.10	1.76	2.28	3.68	6.53	9.58
31. Fires/Burns (Total)	4.32	4.85	1.90	1.15	.89	1.10	.80	.82	1.11	1.79	2.35	3.84	6.97	10.39
Other Unintentional														
32. Firearm	.08	.23	.33	.32	.34	.35	.26	.26	.22	.23	.16	.09	.05	.11
33. Excessive Heat	.17	.04	.00	.00	.00	.02	.01	.02	.04	.06	.10	.14	.37	.92
34. Excessive Cold	.06	.02	.00	.00	.04	.06	.03	.03	.08	.18	.23	.31	.86	1.75
35. Exposure, Neglect	.19	.00	.00	.00	.01	.02	.01	.01	.03	.06	.07	.27	.60	1.69
36. Lightning	.00	.00	.01	.03	.02	.01	.02	.01	.02	.02	.01	.00	.01	.00
37. Natural Disaster	.04	.04	.09	.06	.04	.08	.06	.04	.07	.07	.07	.09	.10	.06
38. Aspiration-Food	4.15	.57	.11	.08	.14	.18	.24	.17	.46	.68	1.02	1.72	2.95	5.88
39. Aspiration-Nonfood	2.70	.40	.11	.09	.07	.09	.07	.09	.16	.24	.43	.74	1.79	5.20
40. Suffocation	4.94	.50	.13	.07	.04	.05	.06	.04	.05	.05	.08	.13	.17	.68
41. Struck by Falling Object	.10	.22	.16	.03	.04	.04	.03	.02	.04	.03	.03	.03	.09	.09
42. Collision with Obj or Pers	.17	.11	.05	.02	.04	.02	.01	.01	.03	.01	.03	.08	.06	.45
43. Caught/Crushed	.00	.06	.02	.01	.00	.01	.02	.00	.00	.00	.01	.01	.02	.26
44. Machinery	.00	.24	.12	.08	.06	.04	.06	.08	.06	.09	.08	.01	.04	.13
45. Cutting/Piercing	.02	.03	.01	.01	.00	.01	.01	.01	.01	.03	.03	.03	.08	.13
46. Explosion	.02	.04	.03	.01	.03	.03	.03	.03	.03	.05	.08	.06	.12	.15
47. Electric Current	.06	.12	.06	.06	.07	.07	.08	.06	.03	.04	.04	.00	.05	.09
48. Unint Excl. Traffic	23.04	14.58	5.47	4.32	5.54	6.05	5.68	5.29	7.15	10.73	14.30	25.22	73.71	220.78
49. Unintentional (Total)	29.70	21.82	11.94	10.27	28.86	24.42	17.56	14.61	16.55	20.46	24.62	38.36	91.17	233.12
Suicide														
50. Firearm	.00	.00	.00	.24	1.72	3.05	3.05	3.05	3.56	4.12	3.09	2.02	1.15	.41
51. Poison Solids/Liquids	.00	.00	.00	.10	.71	1.73	2.24	2.34	2.98	3.44	2.77	2.33	2.02	1.50
52. Motor Vehicle Exhaust	.00	.00	.00	.00	.12	.36	.59	.77	1.09	1.49	.87	.60	.27	.11
53. Hanging	.00	.00	.00	.06	.33	.50	.55	.57	.72	1.05	1.26	1.38	1.59	1.33
54. Drowning	.00	.00	.00	.00	.06	.11	.14	.20	.28	.41	.45	.46	.58	.43
55. Cutting/Piercing	.00	.00	.00	.00	.02	.04	.04	.10	.11	.16	.19	.16	.15	.17
56. Jumping	.00	.00	.00	.01	.15	.33	.39	.36	.30	.44	.37	.40	.48	.38
57. Non-Firearm (Total)	.00	.00	.00	.18	1.49	3.34	4.27	4.71	5.87	7.53	6.29	5.62	5.28	4.09
58. Suicide (Total)	.00	.00	.00	.42	3.22	6.38	7.31	7.76	9.43	11.65	9.38	7.65	6.43	4.49
Homicide														
59. Firearm	.27	.31	.31	.42	2.25	3.99	3.70	3.16	3.40	2.26	1.40	1.09	.71	.51
60. Cutting/Stabbing	.14	.14	.18	.22	.90	1.36	1.26	.94	.79	.66	.55	.51	.67	.36
61. Strangulation	.48	.19	.10	.28	.79	.96	.79	.42	.31	.33	.32	.39	.67	.81
62. Other	3.47	1.74	.41	.27	.73	.87	.79	.70	.71	.66	.51	.80	1.19	1.78
63. Non-Firearm (Total)	4.09	2.07	.69	.76	2.41	3.19	2.84	2.06	1.81	1.65	1.38	1.70	2.52	2.95
64. Homicide (Total)	4.36	2.38	1.00	1.18	4.66	7.18	6.54	5.22	5.21	3.91	2.78	2.79	3.23	3.46
65. Legal Intervention-Firearm	.00	.00	.00	.00	.00	.00	.02	.01	.01	.01	.00	.00	.01	.00
66. Undetermined-Firearm	.04	.01	.02	.04	.19	.24	.23	.18	.22	.16	.08	.06	.03	.00
67. Undet.-Poison Sol/Liq	.06	.06	.00	.06	.25	.47	.65	.53	.66	.75	.58	.31	.19	.09
68. Undetermined (Total)	2.35	.71	.16	.21	.76	1.18	1.39	1.25	1.47	1.64	1.37	1.05	1.18	1.48
69. Injuries (Total)	36.36	24.86	13.07	12.07	37.48	39.13	32.82	28.79	32.61	37.64	38.15	49.83	102.00	242.56

Table 7
Number of Deaths by Age, 69 Causes, 1979

Cause	0	1–	5–	10–	15–	20–	25–	30–	35–	45–	55–	65–	75–	85+
Transportation														
1. Motor Vehicle-Train	7	17	26	22	139	124	103	69	84	67	86	54	20	8
2. Motor Vehicle Occupant	209	519	495	714	7541	7724	4859	3245	4144	3229	2903	2205	1339	280
3. Motorcyclist	0	1	17	92	882	1126	639	363	285	100	54	26	6	1
4. Bicyclist	0	14	165	264	152	53	39	34	26	23	26	24	17	5
5. Pedestrian	7	468	709	380	786	810	609	420	719	789	830	834	753	228
6. Motor Vehicle-Traffic (Total)	216	1002	1391	1453	9366	9720	6148	4064	5177	4145	3815	3091	2116	514
7. Pedestrian-Nontraffic	3	207	32	8	11	21	28	21	34	41	36	44	35	17
8. Pedestrian-Train	0	3	9	18	43	59	45	35	54	36	38	32	16	9
9. Aircraft	0	10	26	27	84	189	271	253	394	290	159	35	5	0
Drowning														
10. Boat-Related	1	10	36	49	129	160	146	134	176	145	126	61	20	1
11. Non-Boat	76	680	383	440	932	790	514	294	461	326	297	220	150	66
12. Drowning (Total)	77	690	419	489	1061	950	660	428	637	471	423	281	170	67
Poisoning														
13. Opiates	0	4	0	0	15	69	107	72	42	17	12	1	1	0
14. Barbiturates	1	1	1	0	9	27	30	17	20	26	25	13	8	0
15. Tranquilizers	0	1	0	0	0	7	17	13	24	21	13	6	2	2
16. Antidepressants	1	7	0	0	3	8	13	16	20	17	12	8	0	0
17. Alcohol	0	2	0	0	13	14	29	33	83	112	97	27	4	0
18. Solids/Liquids (Total)	19	59	11	20	162	441	528	361	434	393	353	203	121	54
19. Motor Vehicle Exhaust	2	2	1	7	101	120	96	72	100	80	60	38	31	7
20. Gas/Vapor (Total)	7	20	14	30	179	219	160	117	189	165	147	106	92	27
Falls														
21. Stairs	3	8	4	2	4	12	20	28	57	133	233	269	352	190
22. Ladder/Scaffold	0	2	1	1	8	14	21	19	42	64	79	66	41	13
23. Building/Structure	0	36	14	8	40	71	77	43	77	67	77	85	45	13
24. Different Level	30	22	18	25	87	89	60	40	58	80	96	111	207	222
25. Same Level	1	0	0	0	4	6	4	4	10	18	43	98	148	118
26. Other/Unspecified	23	36	19	29	68	86	73	86	273	459	689	1327	2819	3288
27. Fall (Total)	57	104	56	65	211	278	255	220	517	821	1217	1956	3612	3844
Fires and Burns														
28. Housefires	130	648	331	179	190	312	235	200	356	431	563	534	430	173
29. Clothing Ignition	1	3	2	1	4	3	3	2	12	22	32	64	85	55
30. Fires/Burns Excl. Scalds	134	693	348	204	222	381	290	255	457	580	736	743	642	296
31. Fires/Burns (Total)	141	710	350	205	224	388	297	266	467	597	760	770	679	319
Other Unintentional														
32. Firearm	4	53	87	228	354	314	207	151	189	172	128	78	30	9
33. Excessive Heat	4	6	1	2	2	11	7	4	12	18	28	17	15	18
34. Excessive Cold	2	3	2	3	23	31	24	11	68	91	122	130	131	67
35. Exposure, Neglect	6	0	0	1	3	9	12	9	24	37	40	83	82	67
36. Lightning	0	0	4	8	13	3	13	14	17	9	2	2	2	0
37. Natural Disaster	1	5	3	14	13	22	16	5	15	20	19	17	7	1
38. Aspiration-Food	153	97	15	14	40	59	66	63	152	213	307	414	310	189
39. Aspiration-Nonfood	103	58	12	10	24	19	10	26	53	82	144	205	230	174
40. Suffocation	181	75	44	108	78	74	67	48	61	43	34	24	14	12
41. Struck by Falling Object	7	36	24	20	84	151	121	115	164	177	142	74	43	5
42. Collision with Obj or Pers	9	12	12	12	35	43	28	23	34	35	37	25	9	14
43. Caught/Crushed	6	13	5	5	19	20	16	9	18	24	17	5	4	4
44. Machinery	0	39	49	50	127	180	131	121	217	217	261	177	54	6
45. Cutting/Piercing	2	3	11	2	5	14	13	12	20	13	19	11	10	1
46. Explosion	2	7	3	9	29	47	45	36	44	44	43	18	17	1
47. Electric Current	6	22	24	31	133	216	143	114	133	107	66	17	8	4
48. Unint Excl. Traffic	864	2347	1316	1529	3323	4165	3491	2749	4468	4881	5505	5922	6839	5550
49. Unintentional (Total)	1080	3349	2707	2982	12689	13885	9639	6813	9645	9026	9320	9013	8955	6064
Suicide														
50. Firearm	0	0	0	84	1137	2084	1789	1396	2138	2060	2065	1677	937	186
51. Poison Solids/Liquids	0	0	0	9	134	323	442	383	599	583	429	264	136	41
52. Motor Vehicle Exhaust	0	0	0	1	78	189	233	205	344	381	264	158	59	17
53. Hanging	0	0	0	56	294	512	440	306	381	375	424	372	276	84
54. Drowning	0	0	1	0	21	66	61	45	88	74	84	67	51	24
55. Cutting/Piercing	0	0	0	0	10	36	40	37	60	64	86	47	25	10
56. Jumping	0	0	0	1	47	125	116	107	113	105	94	87	66	25
57. Non-Firearm (Total)	0	0	1	67	651	1374	1482	1190	1738	1729	1503	1053	640	208
58. Suicide (Total)	0	0	1	151	1788	3458	3271	2586	3876	3789	3568	2730	1577	394
Homicide														
59. Firearm	7	43	68	119	1416	2710	2586	1995	2475	1620	894	401	116	24
60. Cutting/Stabbing	5	16	26	30	476	778	676	499	657	401	276	141	66	8
61. Strangulation	19	17	19	31	104	134	121	61	75	77	73	53	42	15
62. Other	139	238	52	49	148	262	254	224	336	363	261	231	136	62
63. Non-Firearm (Total)	163	271	97	110	728	1174	1051	784	1068	841	610	425	244	85
64. Homicide (Total)	170	314	165	229	2144	3884	3637	2779	3543	2461	1504	826	360	109
65. Legal Intervention-Firearm	0	0	0	0	47	80	78	50	40	25	8	8	4	1
66. Undetermined-Firearm	1	2	3	16	91	135	85	64	90	54	48	32	18	1
67. Undet.-Poison Sol/Liq	3	8	0	7	55	140	199	109	159	132	89	44	14	1
68. Undetermined (Total)	85	95	28	72	283	495	492	375	548	528	408	242	134	57
69. Injuries (Total)	1335	3758	2901	3434	16951	21803	17117	12607	17656	15834	14813	12822	11032	6625

Table 8
Death Rates per 100,000 Population by Age, 69 Causes, 1977-1979

Cause	0	1–	5–	10–	15–	20–	25–	30–	35–	45–	55–	65–	75–	85+
Transportation														
1. Motor Vehicle-Train	.23	.17	.15	.12	.76	.69	.52	.39	.32	.38	.38	.37	.40	.33
2. Motor Vehicle Occupant	6.47	4.00	2.95	4.28	35.44	35.51	23.21	17.14	15.12	14.13	13.29	14.14	17.29	12.99
3. Motorcyclist	.00	.03	.09	.58	3.96	5.00	2.92	1.67	.92	.41	.20	.13	.06	.09
4. Bicyclist	.00	.12	.95	1.42	.68	.23	.17	.14	.09	.09	.10	.16	.19	.16
5. Pedestrian	.22	3.88	4.42	2.23	3.44	3.33	2.72	2.33	2.56	3.34	3.86	5.31	9.73	9.72
6. Motor Vehicle-Traffic (Total)	6.69	8.03	8.43	8.56	43.56	44.08	29.04	21.29	18.70	17.99	17.49	19.74	27.27	22.96
7. Pedestrian-Nontraffic	.20	1.47	.19	.05	.09	.10	.12	.11	.14	.18	.19	.27	.46	.48
8. Pedestrian-Train	.00	.06	.05	.11	.22	.26	.25	.18	.20	.22	.21	.21	.23	.49
9. Aircraft	.09	.08	.12	.16	.40	1.01	1.46	1.46	1.45	1.28	.69	.21	.07	.00
Drowning														
10. Boat-Related	.03	.10	.22	.24	.64	.84	.77	.72	.67	.62	.56	.41	.21	.04
11. Non-Boat	1.95	5.03	2.61	2.71	4.72	3.76	2.52	1.78	1.73	1.50	1.42	1.46	2.01	1.99
12. Drowning (Total)	1.98	5.12	2.83	2.95	5.35	4.60	3.29	2.50	2.41	2.12	1.98	1.87	2.22	2.04
Poisoning														
13. Opiates	.01	.02	.00	.00	.08	.38	.51	.33	.13	.07	.03	.01	.01	.03
14. Barbiturates	.01	.01	.00	.00	.05	.13	.14	.09	.08	.10	.09	.10	.07	.09
15. Tranquilizers	.07	.05	.08	.13	.25	.58	.78	.80	.91	.84	.47	.12	.04	.00
16. Antidepressants	.07	.05	.08	.13	.25	.58	.78	.80	.91	.84	.47	.12	.04	.00
17. Alcohol	.00	.01	.00	.00	.05	.05	.11	.14	.31	.47	.40	.17	.05	.01
18. Solids/Liquids (Total)	.45	.53	.07	.14	.87	2.09	2.64	1.89	1.74	1.82	1.56	1.35	1.62	2.50
19. Motor Vehicle Exhaust	.05	.05	.03	.04	.61	.61	.45	.42	.44	.39	.29	.23	.35	.34
20. Gas/Vapor (Total)	.19	.24	.14	.20	1.04	1.08	.81	.70	.79	.79	.76	.72	1.15	1.16
Falls														
21. Stairs	.09	.10	.02	.01	.03	.05	.08	.13	.27	.63	1.07	1.79	4.43	8.69
22. Ladder/Scaffold	.00	.01	.00	.01	.04	.10	.13	.12	.17	.27	.41	.49	.61	.54
23. Building/Structure	.08	.28	.08	.05	.19	.34	.32	.22	.29	.36	.36	.48	.62	.70
24. Different Level	.93	.20	.10	.16	.44	.48	.31	.25	.26	.38	.44	.77	2.70	10.43
25. Same Level	.02	.02	.01	.01	.03	.02	.02	.02	.04	.10	.20	.53	1.93	6.38
26. Other/Unspecified	.59	.29	.12	.14	.34	.38	.40	.56	1.02	2.01	3.40	8.35	37.82	150.06
27. Fall (Total)	1.72	.90	.32	.38	1.06	1.36	1.26	1.30	2.05	3.74	5.87	12.42	48.11	176.80
Fires and Burns														
28. Housefires	4.00	4.90	1.95	1.03	.91	1.34	1.19	1.11	1.39	2.05	2.53	3.41	5.26	7.17
29. Clothing Ignition	.01	.03	.02	.01	.01	.02	.02	.02	.04	.10	.19	.49	1.32	2.49
30. Fires/Burns Excl. Scalds	4.22	5.31	2.11	1.16	1.08	1.66	1.52	1.50	1.88	2.81	3.49	5.08	8.56	13.05
31. Fires/Burns (Total)	4.50	5.50	2.11	1.16	1.09	1.68	1.56	1.55	1.92	2.89	3.59	5.24	9.04	13.99
Other Unintentional														
32. Firearm	.06	.39	.55	1.24	1.68	1.33	.97	.83	.76	.71	.57	.46	.35	.30
33. Excessive Heat	.18	.04	.01	.01	.04	.05	.04	.06	.09	.16	.20	.19	.39	.92
34. Excessive Cold	.07	.02	.01	.03	.10	.13	.10	.09	.22	.43	.59	.77	1.46	2.37
35. Exposure, Neglect	.17	.01	.00	.00	.02	.04	.05	.05	.09	.13	.18	.40	.81	2.16
36. Lightning	.00	.00	.03	.07	.09	.04	.05	.06	.05	.05	.03	.02	.01	.00
37. Natural Disaster	.07	.06	.08	.05	.05	.10	.09	.06	.08	.09	.10	.11	.11	.09
38. Aspiration-Food	4.68	.74	.12	.11	.24	.33	.36	.36	.66	.96	1.42	2.25	3.68	7.05
39. Aspiration-Nonfood	3.12	.53	.12	.08	.10	.12	.11	.12	.22	.34	.60	1.06	2.47	6.49
40. Suffocation	5.93	.66	.34	.64	.37	.37	.33	.23	.25	.18	.17	.18	.20	.60
41. Struck by Falling Object	.13	.31	.19	.11	.38	.67	.59	.58	.70	.76	.66	.50	.44	.21
42. Collision with Obj or Pers	.25	.09	.07	.07	.17	.20	.14	.13	.13	.15	.17	.16	.12	.62
43. Caught/Crushed	.17	.10	.03	.03	.09	.09	.08	.05	.07	.11	.08	.03	.05	.18
44. Machinery	.07	.05	.08	.13	.25	.58	.78	.80	.91	.84	.47	.12	.04	.00
45. Cutting/Piercing	.03	.03	.05	.04	.04	.06	.04	.06	.07	.06	.08	.09	.14	.12
46. Explosion	.02	.06	.03	.06	.13	.20	.25	.23	.20	.25	.23	.13	.20	.21
47. Electric Current	.10	.16	.15	.24	.70	.94	.79	.61	.58	.49	.31	.13	.14	.12
48. Unint Excl. Traffic	26.47	18.37	8.45	9.08	16.49	19.52	17.55	15.34	17.71	22.40	26.53	38.21	89.56	246.06
49. Unintentional (Total)	33.16	26.40	16.88	17.64	60.05	63.28	46.59	36.63	36.41	40.39	44.02	57.96	116.83	269.02
Suicide														
50. Firearm	.00	.00	.00	.48	5.30	9.78	8.97	7.75	8.28	9.68	9.87	10.81	11.72	8.88
51. Poison Solids/Liquids	.00	.00	.00	.06	.63	1.82	2.38	2.21	2.38	2.73	2.18	1.96	1.88	1.64
52. Motor Vehicle Exhaust	.00	.00	.00	.01	.41	.93	1.22	1.21	1.45	1.70	1.26	1.09	.79	.54
53. Hanging	.00	.00	.00	.31	1.44	2.41	2.22	1.6[illegible]	1.53	1.86	2.22	2.49	3.25	3.76
54. Drowning	.00	.00	.00	.00	.10	.25	.27	.28	.29	.37	.41	.47	.68	.83
55. Cutting/Piercing	.00	.00	.00	.00	.04	.15	.20	.21	.22	.29	.34	.34	.35	.34
56. Jumping	.00	.00	.00	.01	.23	.54	.60	.56	.42	.51	.47	.53	.80	.94
57. Non-Firearm (Total)	.00	.00	.01	.41	3.11	6.76	7.60	6.73	6.91	8.13	7.43	7.32	8.16	8.44
58. Suicide (Total)	.00	.00	.01	.90	8.42	16.54	16.57	14.49	15.19	17.81	17.30	18.13	19.88	17.32
Homicide														
59. Firearm	.22	.33	.40	.74	6.16	11.69	12.18	10.20	9.52	6.67	3.95	2.52	1.43	.98
60. Cutting/Stabbing	.20	.13	.15	.20	1.86	3.24	3.08	2.52	2.28	1.86	1.25	.86	.78	.46
61. Strangulation	.52	.18	.11	.18	.46	.59	.54	.32	.27	.32	.31	.32	.56	.74
62. Other	3.86	1.85	.39	.26	.71	1.12	1.17	1.10	1.26	1.39	1.20	1.26	1.61	2.34
63. Non-Firearm (Total)	4.58	2.16	.65	.65	3.03	4.95	4.80	3.94	3.80	3.58	2.76	2.44	2.95	3.54
64. Homicide (Total)	4.79	2.49	1.04	1.39	9.19	16.64	16.98	14.14	13.33	10.25	6.71	4.96	4.39	4.52
65. Legal Intervention-Firearm	.00	.00	.00	.00	.19	.30	.32	.21	.17	.09	.05	.04	.02	.01
66. Undetermined-Firearm	.06	.03	.02	.13	.51	.64	.55	.43	.41	.34	.30	.27	.22	.13
67. Undet.-Poison Sol/Liq	.06	.06	.00	.04	.30	.70	.97	.70	.63	.66	.47	.31	.20	.13
68. Undetermined (Total)	2.58	.89	.21	.43	1.46	2.42	2.62	2.25	2.26	2.45	2.07	1.76	1.95	2.63
69. Injuries (Total)	40.59	29.79	18.13	20.38	77.86	71.45	83.06	67.77	67.35	71.02	70.17	82.85	143.08	293.56

Table 9

Death Rates per 100,000 Population by Per Capita Income of Area of Residence, 69 Causes, 1977-1979

Cause	< $3,000	$3,000–	$4,000–	5,000–	6,000+	Total
Transportation						
1. Motor Vehicle-Train	.73	.61	.40	.20	.18	.40
2. Motor Vehicle Occupant	29.58	22.75	15.81	13.01	11.08	16.97
3. Motorcyclist	.98	1.32	1.40	1.87	1.19	1.45
4. Bicyclist	.38	.35	.35	.36	.31	.35
5. Pedestrian	4.89	3.66	3.53	3.50	2.98	3.58
6. Motor Vehicle-Traffic (Total)	35.85	28.12	21.11	18.75	15.58	22.37
7. Pedestrian-Nontraffic	.40	.31	.21	.19	.14	.23
8. Pedestrian-Train	.34	.20	.19	.14	.21	.19
9. Aircraft	.56	.74	.70	.91	1.09	.78
Drowning						
10. Boat-Related	1.01	.68	.49	.37	.44	.53
11. Non-Boat	4.56	3.05	2.39	2.28	1.75	2.56
12. Drowning (Total)	5.57	3.72	2.88	2.65	2.19	3.09
Poisoning						
13. Opiates	.04	.05	.11	.30	.20	.14
14. Barbiturates	.03	.04	.06	.16	.06	.08
15. Tranquilizers	.03	.03	.04	.06	.03	.04
16. Antidepressants	.03	.03	.03	.05	.02	.04
17. Alcohol	.22	.23	.15	.14	.11	.16
18. Solids/Liquids (Total)	1.34	1.20	1.28	1.93	1.30	1.41
19. Motor Vehicle Exhaust	.45	.36	.37	.24	.38	.34
20. Gas/Vapor (Total)	.98	.83	.73	.49	.64	.71
Falls						
21. Stairs	.21	.45	.68	.56	.76	.59
22. Ladder/Scaffold	.15	.18	.19	.16	.19	.18
23. Building/Structure	.28	.28	.31	.27	.23	.29
24. Different Level	.46	.53	.54	.58	.47	.54
25. Same Level	.11	.25	.21	.19	.21	.21
26. Other/Unspecified	4.42	4.37	4.37	3.77	3.57	4.18
27. Fall (Total)	5.64	6.06	6.29	5.54	5.43	5.99
Fires and Burns						
28. Housefires	4.06	2.72	2.01	1.40	1.08	2.06
29. Clothing Ignition	.29	.22	.13	.10	.06	.15
30. Fires/Burns Excl. Scalds	5.39	3.61	2.66	1.83	1.45	2.72
31. Fires/Burns (Total)	5.50	3.68	2.74	1.92	1.54	2.81
Other Unintentional						
32. Firearm	2.68	1.35	.67	.53	.30	.85
33. Excessive Heat	.17	.13	.11	.09	.05	.11
34. Excessive Cold	.73	.41	.29	.16	.12	.29
35. Exposure, Neglect	.43	.20	.11	.07	.07	.14
36. Lightning	.11	.07	.04	.03	.02	.04
37. Natural Disaster	.09	.11	.09	.04	.05	.08
38. Aspiration-Food	1.06	1.07	.89	.79	.72	.90
39. Aspiration-Nonfood	.84	.58	.46	.35	.29	.47
40. Suffocation	.68	.46	.39	.36	.33	.41
41. Struck by Falling Object	1.29	.83	.44	.27	.23	.51
42. Collision with Obj or Pers	.19	.19	.13	.12	.14	.14
43. Caught/Crushed	.04	.08	.08	.07	.05	.07
44. Machinery	1.69	1.21	.62	.38	.30	.72
45. Cutting/Piercing	.11	.08	.05	.05	.03	.06
46. Explosion	.29	.23	.16	.13	.08	.17
47. Electric Current	.87	.68	.42	.34	.28	.47
48. Unint Excl. Traffic	35.64	28.01	23.11	20.58	18.04	23.84
49. Unintentional (Total)	71.49	56.13	44.22	39.32	33.62	46.21
Suicide						
50. Firearm	9.03	8.44	6.53	6.49	4.72	6.92
51. Poison Solids/Liquids	.63	.91	1.48	2.54	1.85	1.58
52. Motor Vehicle Exhaust	.14	.57	.92	1.07	1.60	.89
53. Hanging	.81	1.25	1.67	1.85	1.91	1.60
54. Drowning	.17	.22	.27	.28	.21	.25
55. Cutting/Piercing	.10	.12	.18	.22	.24	.18
56. Jumping	.07	.12	.47	.52	.44	.39
57. Non-Firearm (Total)	2.11	3.54	5.45	6.97	6.82	5.32
58. Suicide (Total)	11.15	11.97	11.99	13.46	11.53	12.24
Homicide						
59. Firearm	8.37	5.44	6.51	5.90	2.92	6.00
60. Cutting/Stabbing	1.46	1.13	1.90	1.84	.89	1.64
61. Strangulation	.22	.22	.40	.46	.24	36
62. Other	1.15	.94	1.26	1.20	.72	1.14
63. Non-Firearm (Total)	2.82	2.29	3.57	3.50	1.85	3.13
64. Homicide (Total)	11.20	7.73	10.07	9.40	4.76	9.13
65. Legal Intervention-Firearm	.15	.11	.14	.12	.10	.13
66. Undetermined-Firearm	.86	.44	.32	.23	.18	.34
67. Undet.-Poison Sol/Liq	.21	.25	.54	.49	.53	.45
68. Undetermined (Total)	1.66	1.25	2.24	1.54	1.93	1.83
69. Injuries (Total)	95.66	78.69	67.98	63.86	51.96	69.51

Table 10
Death Rates per 100,000 Population by Place of Residence, 69 Causes, 1977-1979

Cause	6 Largest Cities	Other Large SMSA	Other SMSA	Rural Non-Remote	Rural Remote	Total
Transportation						
1. Motor Vehicle-Train	10	.20	.35	.69	.64	.40
2. Motor Vehicle Occupant	7.89	12.30	15.35	24.94	31.90	16.97
3. Motorcyclist	1.03	1.67	1.53	1.29	1.41	1.45
4. Bicyclist	.28	.33	.36	.37	.32	.35
5. Pedestrian	4.94	4.53	3.25	3.49	3.56	3.58
6. Motor Vehicle-Traffic (Total)	14.16	18.83	20.51	30.12	37.26	22.37
7. Pedestrian-Nontraffic	.09	.20	.21	.32	.47	.23
8. Pedestrian-Train	.29	.16	.17	.22	.17	.19
9. Aircraft	.40	.73	.80	.84	.97	.78
Drowning						
10. Boat-Related	.20	.46	.47	.77	1.02	.53
11. Non-Boat	2.28	2.88	2.25	3.17	3.77	2.56
12. Drowning (Total)	2.48	3.34	2.72	3.94	4.79	3.09
Poisoning						
13. Opiates	.43	.27	.12	.04	.02	.14
14. Barbiturates	.16	.11	.07	.04	.04	.08
15. Tranquilizers	.07	.07	.03	.03	.02	.04
16. Antidepressants	.06	.06	.03	.02	.02	.04
17. Alcohol	.10	.24	.14	.21	.20	.16
18. Solids/Liquids (Total)	2.14	2.15	1.29	1.15	1.06	1.41
19. Motor Vehicle Exhaust	.33	.31	.31	.43	.56	.34
20. Gas/Vapor (Total)	.58	.65	.62	.95	1.14	.71
Falls						
21. Stairs	.95	.91	.54	.43	.54	.59
22. Ladder/Scaffold	.15	.22	.18	.17	.19	.18
23. Building/Structure	.59	.35	.24	.28	.28	.29
24. Different Level	.53	.67	.49	.58	.65	.54
25. Same Level	.11	.26	.20	.24	.32	.21
26. Other/Unspecified	4.53	5.55	3.63	4.71	5.57	4.18
27. Fall (Total)	6.86	7.96	5.28	6.42	7.55	5.99
Fires and Burns						
28. Housefires	2.49	2.57	1.57	2.80	3.09	2.06
29. Clothing Ignition	.10	.20	.11	.21	.24	.15
30. Fires/Burns Excl. Scalds	3.11	3.36	2.10	3.73	4.03	2.72
31. Fires/Burns (Total)	3.24	3.51	2.17	3.81	4.13	2.81
Other Unintentional						
32. Firearm	.34	.68	.63	1.52	2.27	.85
33. Excessive Heat	.13	.21	.07	.13	.10	.11
34. Excessive Cold	.23	.34	.19	.48	1.20	.29
35. Exposure, Neglect	.05	.11	.10	.23	.49	.14
36. Lightning	.01	.03	.04	.07	.10	.04
37. Natural Disaster	.03	.06	.08	.12	.23	.08
38. Aspiration-Food	.87	1.04	.82	1.04	1.16	.90
39. Aspiration-Nonfood	.33	.71	.38	.61	.68	.47
40. Suffocation	.23	.42	.37	.52	.94	.41
41. Struck by Falling Object	.23	.27	.36	.99	1.39	.51
42. Collision with Obj or Pers	.13	.16	.12	.21	.20	.14
43. Caught/Crushed	.10	.07	.06	.09	.18	.07
44. Machinery	.25	.35	.50	1.46	2.35	.72
45. Cutting/Piercing	.07	.04	.05	.08	.10	.06
46. Explosion	.10	.14	.15	.24	.32	.17
47. Electric Current	.23	.34	.39	.77	.82	.47
48. Unint Excl. Traffic	22.70	27.52	20.44	29.79	37.33	23.84
49. Unintentional (Total)	36.86	46.36	40.95	59.91	74.59	46.21
Suicide						
50. Firearm	4.55	7.87	6.38	8.37	9.76	6.92
51. Poison Solids/Liquids	2.41	2.66	1.58	.88	.75	1.58
52. Motor Vehicle Exhaust	.38	.92	1.07	.64	.42	.89
53. Hanging	2.24	1.94	1.60	1.26	1.19	1.60
54. Drowning	.34	.35	.24	.22	.18	.25
55. Cutting/Piercing	.32	.25	.17	.12	.14	.18
56. Jumping	1.69	.85	.26	.09	.08	.39
57. Non-Firearm (Total)	7.95	7.39	5.38	3.55	3.09	5.32
58. Suicide (Total)	12.50	15.26	11.76	11.93	12.84	12.24
Homicide						
59. Firearm	16.55	11.40	4.16	4.62	4.85	6.00
60. Cutting/Stabbing	5.98	3.24	1.09	.88	.84	1.64
61. Strangulation	1.10	.73	.26	.18	.11	.36
62. Other	2.84	2.16	.87	.81	.84	1.14
63. Non-Firearm (Total)	9.92	6.13	2.21	1.87	1.78	3.13
64. Homicide (Total)	26.47	17.53	6.38	6.49	6.63	9.13
65. Legal Intervention-Firearm	.20	.30	.10	.09	.08	.13
66. Undetermined-Firearm	.36	.26	.26	.54	.75	.34
67. Undet.-Poison Sol/Liq	1.06	.91	.37	.24	.29	.45
68. Undetermined (Total)	5.94	2.68	1.31	1.36	1.57	1.83
69. Injuries (Total)	81.98	82.15	60.51	79.79	95.72	69.51

Table 11
Death Rates per 100,000 Population by State of Residence, 69 Causes, 1977-1979

Cause	AL	AK	AZ	AR	CA	CO	CN	DE	DC	FL
Transportation										
1. Motor Vehicle-Train	.52	.17	.15	.89	.18	.52	.03	.22	.16	.39
2. Motor Vehicle Occupant	25.76	20.24	25.43	21.12	16.09	19.69	11.26	14.97	6.06	14.54
3. Motorcyclist	1.28	1.82	1.73	.48	2.76	.91	2.07	1.29	.21	1.99
4. Bicyclist	.22	.33	.49	.19	.42	.29	.34	.45	.26	.61
5. Pedestrian	3.63	3.98	6.32	2.86	3.89	2.96	2.72	3.48	4.65	5.33
6. Motor Vehicle-Traffic (Total)	30.90	26.46	33.99	24.67	23.17	23.86	16.41	20.19	11.17	22.49
7. Pedestrian-Nontraffic	.33	.08	.48	.29	.31	.13	.04	.17	.05	.24
8. Pedestrian-Train	.25	.00	.36	.17	.15	.10	.13	.22	.10	.13
9. Aircraft	.76	15.84	1.70	.93	1.39	1.85	.39	.22	.31	1.01
Drowning										
10. Boat-Related	.70	9.54	.18	.95	.38	.38	.32	.67	.26	.80
11. Non-Boat	3.73	10.04	3.88	3.24	2.76	1.83	1.42	3.03	2.87	3.99
12. Drowning (Total)	4.43	19.58	4.06	4.18	3.15	2.21	1.74	3.70	3.13	4.79
Poisoning										
13. Opiates	.03	.17	.13	.01	.62	.13	.04	.00	.21	.06
14. Barbiturates	.03	.08	.00	.06	.34	.10	.04	.06	.00	.05
15. Tranquilizers	.00	.00	.02	.03	.10	.05	.01	.06	.00	.04
16. Antidepressants	.01	.17	.01	.03	.10	.02	.00	.00	.05	.01
17. Alcohol	.05	.33	.10	.16	.17	.17	.03	.00	.05	.07
18. Solids/Liquids (Total)	.93	2.49	.90	.90	3.35	1.76	.58	.50	1.31	1.23
19. Motor Vehicle Exhaust	.21	.50	.06	.26	.08	.57	.19	.22	.10	.15
20. Gas/Vapor (Total)	.60	1.82	.49	1.02	.32	.88	.51	.34	.52	.45
Falls										
21. Stairs	.25	.66	.11	.22	.27	.53	.86	.39	1.31	.27
22. Ladder/Scaffold	.15	.17	.21	.07	.15	.18	.15	.00	.16	.18
23. Building/Structure	.32	.41	.18	.35	.32	.24	.12	.17	.26	.25
24. Different Level	.47	1.00	1.01	.38	.59	1.04	.50	.39	.47	.46
25. Same Level	.11	.00	.10	.04	.19	.35	.12	.06	.16	.26
26. Other/Unspecified	4.19	1.74	5.04	4.29	2.93	4.37	4.63	2.75	8.56	4.06
27. Fall (Total)	5.49	3.98	6.65	5.35	4.44	6.71	6.38	3.76	10.91	5.47
Fires and Burns										
28. Housefires	3.89	5.14	1.53	3.28	1.17	.78	1.10	2.86	4.96	1.52
29. Clothing Ignition	.33	.08	.17	.22	.11	.05	.12	.22	.16	.09
30. Fires/Burns Excl. Scalds	5.16	6.30	1.90	4.32	1.61	1.13	1.51	3.42	5.80	2.02
31. Fires/Burns (Total)	5.31	6.39	1.94	4.36	1.69	1.20	1.53	3.53	6.01	2.09
Other Unintentional										
32. Firearm	2.17	4.65	.94	1.73	.69	.97	.38	.56	.16	.55
33. Excessive Heat	.15	.00	.74	.07	.12	.02	.14	.00	.10	.05
34. Excessive Cold	.30	2.65	.52	.28	.07	.42	.12	.17	1.15	.06
35. Exposure, Neglect	.22	.58	.39	.26	.06	.15	.05	.06	.21	.07
36. Lightning	.09	.00	.06	.10	.00	.15	.03	.00	.00	.09
37. Natural Disaster	.25	.50	.13	.26	.04	.23	.03	.00	.00	.02
38. Aspiration-Food	.70	.66	.74	.86	1.03	.88	.58	.50	1.15	.89
39. Aspiration-Nonfood	.62	.83	.45	.69	.24	.54	.54	.28	1.20	.43
40. Suffocation	.51	1.33	.36	.51	.38	.62	.20	.34	.78	.36
41. Struck by Falling Object	1.04	.91	.40	.74	.27	.58	.25	.28	.21	.30
42. Collision with Obj or Pers	.13	.50	.22	.09	.11	.14	.03	.34	.16	.12
43. Caught/Crushed	.00	.00	.04	.04	.02	.07	.03	.17	.31	.02
44. Machinery	.87	.50	.77	1.27	.49	.76	.26	.50	.31	.47
45. Cutting/Piercing	.12	.00	.04	.09	.06	.02	.08	.11	.16	.06
46. Explosion	.23	.25	.15	.16	.10	.30	.08	.34	.10	.11
47. Electric Current	.63	.25	.56	.61	.27	.50	.27	.56	.05	.54
48. Unint Excl. Traffic	30.47	70.92	26.43	29.04	22.78	24.26	17.14	20.08	33.52	22.56
49. Unintentional (Total)	61.37	97.38	60.42	53.71	45.96	48.12	33.55	40.27	44.70	45.05
Suicide										
50. Firearm	8.31	13.02	11.38	8.48	7.47	10.53	3.61	6.11	3.39	9.05
51. Poison Solids/Liquids	.31	1.33	2.55	.71	3.85	1.93	.63	1.91	.99	2.77
52. Motor Vehicle Exhaust	.21	.50	.86	.20	.69	2.34	1.23	1.07	.26	.81
53. Hanging	.82	.83	1.52	.67	1.97	1.73	2.18	2.02	2.09	1.57
54. Drowning	.21	.08	.16	.10	.21	.07	.18	.50	.84	.61
55. Cutting/Piercing	.11	.00	.10	.07	.27	.15	.25	.22	.00	.24
56. Jumping	.08	.17	.21	.07	.62	.22	.34	.67	1.93	.33
57. Non-Firearm (Total)	2.01	2.99	5.90	2.13	8.08	6.90	5.57	6.56	6.37	6.70
58. Suicide (Total)	10.32	16.01	17.28	10.61	15.55	17.43	9.18	12.68	9.77	15.75
Homicide										
59. Firearm	9.93	7.96	5.29	6.97	6.85	3.54	2.49	3.59	15.61	6.81
60. Cutting/Stabbing	1.98	2.07	1.64	.96	2.45	1.02	.97	1.29	6.37	1.74
61. Strangulation	.26	.50	.50	.25	.64	.32	.24	.11	.99	.45
62. Other	1.20	1.99	1.32	.82	1.51	.80	.57	1.35	4.44	1.61
63. Non-Firearm (Total)	3.43	4.56	3.47	2.03	4.60	2.13	1.77	2.75	11.80	3.81
64. Homicide (Total)	13.36	12.53	8.76	9.00	11.45	5.67	4.26	6.34	27.42	10.62
65. Legal Intervention-Firearm	.10	.08	.17	.16	.13	.09	.12	.11	.94	.11
66. Undetermined-Firearm	1.22	3.32	.32	1.20	.18	.24	.25	.39	.37	.47
67. Undet.-Poison Sol/Liq	.21	.41	.65	.41	.53	.76	.23	.56	1.46	.56
68. Undetermined (Total)	2.17	4.73	1.78	2.49	1.36	1.72	1.63	1.51	7.78	1.96
69. Injuries (Total)	87.34	130.73	88.42	75.98	74.46	73.06	48.74	60.91	90.60	73.51

Table 11 *(continued)*

Cause	GA	HI	ID	IL	IN	IA	KS	KY	LA	ME	MD	MA	MI	MN	MS	MO
Transportation																
1.	.52	.00	.78	.61	1.14	.61	.97	.37	.58	.21	.13	.03	.38	.65	.54	.48
2.	22.37	13.13	29.24	15.14	20.02	18.03	20.32	19.95	21.49	14.49	11.86	10.50	15.86	16.90	27.00	19.26
3.	.90	1.80	.32	.76	.81	2.46	1.42	1.07	.86	1.99	1.28	1.61	1.36	2.01	.44	1.39
4.	.32	.10	.25	.29	.28	.26	.21	.33	.48	.56	.25	.28	.49	.45	.36	.23
5.	3.93	3.56	3.85	3.21	2.53	1.89	1.99	3.19	3.80	2.61	3.30	3.47	3.83	3.05	3.60	3.02
6.	27.53	18.59	33.65	19.41	23.65	22.71	23.99	24.54	26.65	19.65	16.69	15.87	21.63	22.43	31.42	23.91
7.	.24	.24	.81	.11	.22	.19	.41	.32	.29	.15	.05	.13	.22	.23	.26	.28
8.	.34	.03	.18	.34	.22	.07	.14	.31	.16	.00	.11	.16	.06	.06	.19	.20
9.	.62	.86	3.43	.70	.73	.69	.97	.38	.74	.77	.46	.30	.50	.65	.63	.50
Drowning																
10.	.68	.24	.74	.41	.27	.62	.45	.70	1.96	1.13	.58	.35	.38	.52	1.16	.43
11.	3.41	3.52	3.96	2.14	2.11	1.93	2.02	2.73	4.97	2.25	2.30	1.83	2.21	1.97	4.42	2.30
12.	4.09	3.77	4.70	2.56	2.37	2.55	2.47	3.43	6.93	3.38	2.88	2.18	2.59	2.49	5.58	2.73
Poisoning																
13.	.07	.17	.00	.29	.06	.01	.03	.06	.07	.00	.11	.16	.04	.06	.01	.03
14.	.05	.00	.07	.06	.05	.02	.03	.05	.10	.06	.03	.09	.01	.02	.01	.03
15.	.01	.00	.11	.04	.03	.01	.01	.06	.03	.00	.02	.03	.03	.02	.04	.05
16.	.05	.00	.04	.04	.03	.01	.06	.04	.04	.00	.01	.02	.01	.02	.07	.05
17.	.41	.07	.07	.14	.07	.07	.04	.18	.02	.03	.02	.06	.05	.08	.07	.09
18.	1.65	.52	1.31	1.65	.94	.51	1.06	1.41	1.29	.77	1.09	1.25	.89	.65	1.22	.92
19.	.27	.00	.18	.83	.76	.49	.52	.65	.25	.12	.17	.41	.44	.74	.40	.35
20.	.59	.00	.42	1.24	1.29	.71	1.10	1.03	.52	.41	.38	.68	.81	1.19	.85	.71
Falls																
21.	.35	.28	.39	.63	.43	.71	.47	.60	.17	1.13	.92	1.03	.75	.93	.11	.84
22.	.13	.03	.42	.17	.24	.13	.18	.19	.17	.27	.21	.17	.14	.16	.09	.15
23.	.27	.31	.14	.34	.21	.39	.38	.33	.22	.36	.21	.31	.23	.16	.20	.31
24.	.62	1.04	.85	.36	.38	.80	.55	.62	.36	.50	.47	.83	.41	.38	.29	.71
25.	.24	.07	.25	.11	.16	.47	.34	.24	.10	.50	.24	.40	.14	.22	.05	.31
26.	3.93	1.42	3.67	3.63	4.98	5.50	5.44	4.87	3.66	3.79	3.47	6.89	4.26	5.59	4.11	5.28
27.	5.55	3.14	5.72	5.25	6.40	8.00	7.36	6.85	4.68	6.55	5.50	9.63	5.94	7.43	4.85	7.60
Fires and Burns																
28.	3.05	.55	1.70	2.52	2.40	1.75	1.99	2.68	2.80	3.26	1.93	1.71	2.36	1.55	4.24	2.53
29.	.27	.03	.18	.11	.13	.08	.18	.18	.18	.21	.11	.19	.07	.11	.28	.14
30.	4.01	.83	2.37	3.01	3.02	2.25	2.71	4.11	3.89	3.82	2.45	2.31	2.88	2.09	5.83	3.51
31.	4.12	.86	2.47	3.12	3.11	2.30	2.76	4.20	3.99	3.97	2.50	2.38	2.96	2.15	5.92	3.65
Other Unintentional																
32.	1.67	.10	1.70	.51	.90	.72	.86	1.61	2.10	.53	.32	.20	.57	.61	2.80	.94
33.	.21	.00	.00	.06	.05	.06	.11	.11	.07	.09	.03	.14	.05	.04	.12	.35
34.	.40	.00	.42	.32	.35	.34	.48	.56	.13	.21	.23	.16	.27	.52	.37	.42
35.	.10	.00	.42	.07	.15	.09	.14	.17	.10	.15	.09	.12	.19	.19	.28	.12
36.	.08	.00	.04	.03	.05	.06	.03	.03	.09	.06	.04	.03	.01	.06	.09	.06
37.	.26	.03	.00	.03	.02	.11	.31	.05	.05	.03	.02	.00	.03	.08	.17	.16
38.	1.28	.59	.99	1.01	.91	.82	1.16	1.03	1.17	.50	.76	.95	.82	.67	1.60	.98
39.	.57	.55	.39	.27	.41	.42	.66	.75	.80	.27	.57	.71	.59	.42	1.18	.66
40.	.62	.21	.92	.38	.53	.57	.39	.39	.39	.36	.28	.26	.40	.56	.69	.52
41.	.82	.24	1.34	.35	.55	.69	.65	1.00	.72	.83	.38	.19	.45	.56	.99	.62
42.	.16	.00	.53	.16	.04	.10	.04	.16	.21	.09	.12	.03	.08	.17	.24	.16
43.	.04	.10	.11	.05	.09	.07	.08	.11	.12	.09	.14	.05	.06	.07	.00	.04
44.	.53	.52	1.27	.58	.93	2.20	1.35	1.17	.88	1.07	.43	.23	.41	1.18	1.55	1.34
45.	.09	.07	.14	.06	.07	.02	.04	.05	.03	.06	.04	.03	.04	.05	.16	.06
46.	.17	.10	.18	.13	.19	.17	.23	.17	.59	.24	.14	.09	.15	.26	.30	.16
47.	.57	.14	.88	.49	.59	.64	.78	.83	.84	.47	.34	.17	.41	.38	.82	.66
48.	27.73	14.44	32.24	22.22	23.85	24.15	27.13	29.53	30.66	23.86	20.16	23.33	20.82	23.95	34.45	27.02
49.	55.26	33.03	65.89	41.63	47.50	46.86	51.12	54.07	57.31	43.51	36.85	39.20	42.44	46.39	65.87	50.94
Suicide																
50.	9.62	4.35	9.78	4.47	7.10	6.19	7.88	9.25	9.21	7.29	5.87	2.46	6.79	5.39	7.78	7.64
51.	1.06	2.07	1.20	.92	.84	1.00	.86	.76	.93	1.87	1.58	1.33	1.48	.86	.50	1.34
52.	.40	.35	.74	1.39	1.15	1.75	.72	.47	.12	1.36	.79	.96	1.35	1.61	.15	.96
53.	.89	3.18	.78	1.76	1.65	1.86	1.21	1.11	.71	1.51	1.52	2.42	1.85	1.61	.61	1.11
54.	.16	.14	.14	.18	.16	.19	.14	.40	.22	.68	.33	.46	.21	.17	.09	.22
55.	.07	.28	.14	.20	.16	.19	.04	.19	.08	.21	.25	.20	.17	.14	.03	.20
56.	.07	1.59	.21	.33	.10	.08	.18	.16	.14	.06	.40	.52	.25	.30	.15	.19
57.	2.94	7.81	3.78	5.24	4.62	5.23	3.93	3.34	2.40	6.02	5.21	6.73	6.00	5.14	1.64	4.42
58.	12.56	12.16	13.56	9.71	11.72	11.42	11.82	12.59	11.61	13.31	11.08	9.19	12.80	10.53	9.42	12.06
Homicide																
59.	10.45	2.90	3.43	7.51	4.91	1.42	4.06	6.98	11.86	1.45	5.40	1.56	6.48	1.38	9.67	7.80
60.	1.89	1.28	.88	2.28	.73	.30	.80	.64	2.03	.36	2.26	1.08	1.59	.41	1.80	1.36
61.	.33	.45	.21	.46	.26	.15	.25	.25	.37	.21	.33	.24	.45	.16	.28	.34
62.	1.46	1.31	.78	1.29	.88	.46	.78	.84	1.33	.59	.81	.59	1.23	.48	1.34	1.14
63.	3.68	3.04	1.87	4.03	1.88	.90	1.83	1.73	3.73	1.16	3.40	1.91	3.27	1.05	3.41	2.83
64.	14.13	5.94	5.30	11.53	6.79	2.32	5.89	8.71	15.60	2.61	8.80	3.47	9.75	2.43	13.08	10.64
65.	.16	.00	.07	.08	.15	.07	.13	.11	.36	.06	.25	.05	.23	.04	.19	.13
66.	.16	.14	.46	.51	.40	.25	.58	.73	.25	.12	.24	.08	.20	.14	.86	.66
67.	.20	1.38	.32	.68	.32	.16	.47	.17	.12	.24	.49	.41	.50	.39	.20	.73
68.	.63	3.39	1.38	3.97	1.41	1.03	1.93	1.44	.59	.68	1.59	1.00	1.36	1.61	1.49	2.36
69.	82.75	54.53	86.20	66.93	67.59	61.71	70.89	76.95	85.48	60.20	58.58	52.92	66.58	61.01	90.04	76.13

Table 11 *(continued)*

Cause	MT	NB	NV	NH	NJ	NM	NY	NC	ND	OH
Transportation										
1. Motor Vehicle-Train	.51	1.27	.21	.22	.10	.46	.05	.52	1.43	.57
2. Motor Vehicle Occupant	30.80	18.43	26.69	12.67	10.37	33.67	9.38	18.82	21.50	14.90
3. Motorcyclist	2.08	2.12	2.75	2.32	1.04	2.56	.82	1.36	2.04	1.07
4. Bicyclist	.42	.19	.42	.14	.32	.28	.33	.43	.26	.28
5. Pedestrian	2.42	1.89	3.79	2.43	3.76	7.93	3.90	4.31	1.84	2.61
6. Motor Vehicle-Traffic (Total)	35.72	22.66	33.65	17.56	15.50	44.47	14.46	24.95	25.69	18.87
7. Pedestrian-Nontraffic	.55	.42	.21	.04	.19	.38	.10	.26	.56	.25
8. Pedestrian-Train	.42	.36	.21	.04	.24	.43	.26	.29	.15	.15
9. Aircraft	1.91	1.19	2.00	.83	.31	1.54	.29	.75	.97	.42
Drowning										
10. Boat-Related	1.23	.42	.25	.58	.30	.33	.27	.64	.56	.34
11. Non-Boat	3.47	1.93	3.29	1.67	1.70	3.20	1.43	3.26	2.55	1.68
12. Drowning (Total)	4.70	2.36	3.54	2.24	2.00	3.53	1.70	3.90	3.12	2.03
Poisoning										
13. Opiates	.04	.04	.21	.04	.09	.13	.15	.06	.05	.04
14. Barbiturates	.08	.06	.25	.00	.05	.10	.04	.03	.05	.04
15. Tranquilizers	.08	.02	.12	.00	.01	.03	.02	.05	.10	.02
16. Antidepressants	.00	.06	.04	.00	.01	.08	.02	.03	.00	.04
17. Alcohol	.13	.04	.42	.04	.02	.08	.02	1.81	.05	.03
18. Solids/Liquids (Total)	.93	1.02	2.42	.47	.99	1.94	.94	2.86	.51	.90
19. Motor Vehicle Exhaust	.59	.76	.17	.22	.12	.38	.27	.31	.51	.70
20. Gas/Vapor (Total)	1.53	1.17	.62	.47	.45	1.43	.53	.70	1.33	1.10
Falls										
21. Stairs	.97	.66	.37	.58	.91	.03	.85	.30	1.23	.84
22. Ladder/Scaffold	.08	.15	.21	.11	.24	.08	.17	.14	.15	.23
23. Building/Structure	.21	.34	.33	.36	.33	.23	.41	.18	.20	.24
24. Different Level	.93	.81	.67	.72	.49	1.05	.46	.37	.71	.54
25. Same Level	.47	.57	.21	.29	.17	.10	.14	.04	.31	.31
26. Other/Unspecified	6.53	5.80	2.71	3.95	4.25	3.89	4.16	3.71	4.90	4.76
27. Fall (Total)	9.19	8.32	4.50	6.01	6.40	5.37	6.20	4.74	7.51	6.92
Fires and Burns										
28. Housefires	1.95	1.44	1.37	1.70	1.96	1.28	1.64	3.05	.97	1.98
29. Clothing Ignition	.25	.21	.04	.14	.06	.18	.10	.16	.10	.13
30. Fires/Burns Excl. Scalds	3.01	2.00	1.83	2.14	2.58	2.12	2.12	3.98	1.89	2.75
31. Fires/Burns (Total)	3.09	2.02	1.92	2.24	2.64	2.25	2.20	4.06	2.04	2.85
Other Unintentional										
32. Firearm	2.25	1.02	1.17	.43	.34	1.13	.33	1.28	1.63	.61
33. Excessive Heat	.08	.13	.21	.11	.07	.13	.07	.18	.00	.06
34. Excessive Cold	.93	.42	.54	.18	.17	.90	.19	.49	1.43	.31
35. Exposure, Neglect	.30	.19	.08	.11	.12	1.02	.03	.31	.10	.12
36. Lightning	.08	.06	.04	.04	.04	.08	.02	.07	.00	.06
37. Natural Disaster	.00	.06	.00	.11	.00	.26	.02	.07	.36	.01
38. Aspiration-Food	1.36	.87	1.08	.87	.83	.84	.95	.79	1.07	.87
39. Aspiration-Nonfood	.51	.38	.25	.54	.37	64	.31	.69	.20	.39
40. Suffocation	.89	.76	.92	.25	.29	.49	.24	.28	.66	.36
41. Struck by Falling Object	1.27	.51	.50	.65	.18	.84	.27	.56	.92	.49
42. Collision with Obj or Pers	.38	.13	.12	.11	.12	.46	.09	.19	.00	.19
43. Caught/Crushed	.13	.13	.37	.00	.07	.23	.07	.05	.15	.11
44. Machinery	1.78	1.85	.25	.33	.26	.61	.37	.94	1.99	.50
45. Cutting/Piercing	.21	.04	.00	.07	.03	.03	.05	.05	.05	.03
46. Explosion	.47	.32	.17	.07	.09	.23	.08	.18	.31	.15
47. Electric Current	.72	.57	.50	.18	.24	.59	.17	.61	.71	.46
48. Unint Excl. Traffic	37.08	26.44	25.86	19.19	18.97	30.32	18.49	27.76	29.57	22.29
49. Unintentional (Total)	72.79	49.09	59.50	36.75	34.47	74.78	32.95	52.71	55.26	41.16
Suicide										
50. Firearm	11.40	5.90	14.99	6.48	2.54	12.02	2.75	8.60	6.28	6.80
51. Poison Solids/Liquids	1.19	.62	3.12	1.52	.71	2.00	1.39	1.18	.77	1.43
52. Motor Vehicle Exhaust	1.57	1.02	1.21	1.59	.74	.77	.73	.33	1.28	1.54
53. Hanging	1.48	1.61	1.96	2.06	2.23	2.05	2.13	.78	1.69	1.80
54. Drowning	.08	.15	.00	.29	.14	.00	.35	.29	.20	.19
55. Cutting/Piercing	.13	.11	.17	.22	.21	.15	.23	.14	.15	.14
56. Jumping	.04	.11	.33	.18	.43	.10	1.38	.11	.05	.36
57. Non-Firearm (Total)	4.66	3.99	7.20	6.19	5.05	5.22	6.72	3.21	4.39	5.94
58. Suicide (Total)	16.06	9.89	22.19	12.67	7.59	17.24	9.48	11.81	10.67	12.73
Homicide										
59. Firearm	3.01	2.34	7.54	.69	2.89	7.47	6.23	8.04	.97	5.04
60. Cutting/Stabbing	1.02	.57	2.25	.43	1.53	1.94	2.91	1.45	.05	.91
61. Strangulation	.25	.17	.62	.18	.20	.28	.56	.27	.20	.25
62. Other	.89	.53	2.29	.40	1.15	2.07	1.36	1.20	.36	.97
63. Non-Firearm (Total)	2.16	1.27	5.16	1.01	2.88	4.30	4.83	2.92	.61	2.13
64. Homicide (Total)	5.17	3.61	12.70	1.70	5.77	11.77	11.05	10.96	1.58	7.17
65. Legal Intervention-Firearm	.21	.00	.33	.04	.07	.18	.09	.10	.10	.17
66. Undetermined-Firearm	.76	.57	.42	.36	.15	.51	.23	.23	.46	.27
67. Undet.-Poison Sol/Liq	.25	.19	.79	.36	.19	.59	.69	.39	.51	.33
68. Undetermined (Total)	1.91	2.06	1.50	1.67	1.29	2.25	4.55	1.20	1.43	1.28
69. Injuries (Total)	96.18	64.66	96.32	52.86	49.20	106.25	58.13	76.79	69.04	62.54

Table 11 *(continued)*

Cause	OK	OR	PA	RI	SC	SD	TN	TX	UT	VT	VA	WA	WV	WI	WY
Transportation															
1.	.97	.42	.13	.07	.50	.24	.54	.58	.46	.46	.22	.47	.41	.53	.35
2.	24.43	20.69	14.17	9.92	22.38	23.84	22.06	20.53	16.88	19.68	16.38	19.66	21.76	15.41	35.85
3.	2.29	1.96	.63	1.48	1.27	2.22	1.39	1.89	1.69	.85	.30	1.82	.89	1.94	1.28
4.	.25	.47	.28	.25	.49	.68	.22	.40	.34	.07	.20	.27	.24	.48	.14
5.	3.23	3.37	3.32	3.24	4.87	2.70	3.33	4.09	3.97	2.93	3.12	2.88	3.09	2.65	3.90
6.	30.21	26.48	18.41	14.92	29.01	29.48	27.00	26.94	22.93	23.59	20.04	24.64	25.99	20.56	41.24
7.	.33	.34	.16	.11	.36	.43	.27	.26	.71	.00	.17	.29	.22	.13	.35
8.	.22	.22	.17	.07	.26	.05	.18	.16	.11	.07	.19	.15	.31	.10	.28
9.	.94	1.46	.43	14	.38	.97	.49	.68	1.92	.39	.55	1.52	.44	.39	2.27
Drowning															
10.	.53	1.28	.19	.84	.89	.48	.67	.52	.34	.33	.52	1.16	.26	.51	.07
11.	2.70	3.39	1.46	1.76	3.63	2.56	2.87	3.51	2.10	2.22	2.56	2.93	3.18	2.05	1.92
12.	3.23	4.67	1.65	2.60	4.52	3.04	3.54	4.03	2.44	2.54	3.08	4.09	3.44	2.56	1.99
Poisoning															
13.	.02	.06	.05	.14	.02	.00	.03	.10	.02	.07	.09	.02	.09	.04	.00
14.	.04	.03	.04	.07	.05	.00	.04	.06	.00	.00	.03	.06	.00	.06	.00
15.	.01	.01	.02	.00	.05	.00	.01	.07	.02	.07	.04	.04	.02	.06	.00
16.	.06	.05	.01	.07	.04	.00	.03	.05	.00	.00	.01	.02	.03	.04	.00
17.	.32	.03	.04	.18	.30	.00	.09	.08	.07	.20	1.18	.04	.10	.05	.21
18.	1.20	1.35	.79	.95	1.72	.58	1.23	1.19	1.10	.85	2.08	1.47	1.08	1.05	.78
19.	.10	.28	.45	.35	.25	.58	.33	.10	.07	.20	.16	.19	.68	.80	.50
20.	.75	.59	.87	.46	.47	1.45	1.02	.46	.55	.39	.41	.35	1.27	1.26	1.63
Falls															
21.	.22	.39	1.42	.60	.29	.97	.33	.13	.57	1.11	.55	.56	.53	1.01	.50
22.	.18	.15	.22	.21	.15	.10	.15	.17	.18	.20	.16	.17	.92	.24	.14
23.	.22	.19	.36	.21	.27	.29	.22	.26	.25	.33	.25	.34	.32	.28	.43
24.	.51	.94	.47	.53	.35	.87	.60	.41	.75	.52	.43	.94	.51	.60	.78
25.	.28	.37	.15	.32	.06	.58	.25	.17	.50	.13	.12	.23	.22	.53	.64
26.	4.31	4.14	4.53	4.36	3.15	5.16	4.28	3.62	4.43	5.21	5.01	3.69	4.68	3.40	3.48
27.	5.71	6.18	7.15	6.23	4.27	7.96	5.82	4.76	6.68	7.49	6.52	5.93	7.20	6.06	5.96
Fires and Burns															
28.	2.44	1.91	2.03	1.76	3.79	1.93	2.76	1.82	1.05	2.28	2.31	1.64	3.18	1.93	1.77
29.	.19	.16	.17	.07	.15	.19	.24	.21	.05	.13	.21	.20	.32	.14	.00
30.	3.33	2.35	2.70	2.08	4.75	2.99	3.65	2.61	1.46	3.13	3.17	2.04	4.10	2.30	2.41
31.	3.38	2.39	2.77	2.22	4.83	3.04	3.73	2.72	1.53	3.19	3.29	2.17	4.12	2.39	2.41
Other Unintentional															
32.	1.31	.85	.50	.07	1.73	2.12	1.43	1.29	.59	.65	.87	.54	.85	.61	2.20
33.	.22	.03	.09	.07	.27	.00	.04	.19	.00	.07	.07	.04	.05	.05	.07
34.	.40	.42	.26	.39	.56	1.40	.44	.13	.18	.46	.56	.23	.56	.38	.99
35.	.26	.05	.15	.00	.23	.29	.12	.10	.14	.07	.22	.18	.17	.14	.43
36.	.08	.04	.03	.00	.11	.10	.06	.05	.14	.00	.04	.01	.05	.04	.14
37.	.18	.04	.21	.00	.02	.19	.05	.18	.11	.00	.14	.06	.07	.04	.14
38.	.68	.63	.75	.81	1.07	.87	.87	.94	.41	.98	.77	.71	.92	.81	1.77
39.	.61	.46	.52	.35	.77	.53	.52	.50	.48	.59	.58	.34	.46	.23	.50
40.	.46	.62	.28	.39	.37	.92	.37	.48	.78	.39	.44	.56	.24	.43	.92
41.	.64	1.27	.44	.25	.73	1.06	.78	.51	.55	.72	.65	.61	1.50	.62	1.21
42.	.43	.42	.12	.11	.10	.14	.13	.14	.07	.00	.15	.34	.10	.32	.21
43.	.13	.11	.11	.00	.00	.43	.00	.08	.21	.00	.06	.29	.10	.00	.64
44.	.89	1.29	.56	.11	.86	1.74	1.13	.82	.89	.78	.80	.56	1.33	1.21	1.92
45.	.07	.09	.05	.07	.14	.10	.11	.07	.05	.07	.06	.09	.09	.08	.00
46.	.34	.13	.12	.04	.13	.34	.17	.31	.21	.00	.15	.17	.39	.11	.35
47.	.99	.42	.31	.21	.56	.68	.58	.77	.55	.46	.55	.41	.65	.45	.64
48.	27.33	27.04	22.24	19.07	27.65	31.70	26.25	23.77	23.52	24.11	25.01	24.47	28.86	21.24	32.16
49.	57.54	53.52	40.65	34.00	56.67	61.19	53.25	50.70	46.45	47.71	45.05	49.12	54.85	41.79	73.40
Suicide															
50.	9.50	8.79	5.73	3.45	8.17	6.42	9.50	8.41	7.67	8.80	9.99	6.95	9.28	6.00	11.29
51.	1.42	1.84	1.51	3.10	.62	.68	.83	1.19	1.71	1.76	1.66	1.97	1.04	1.25	1.06
52.	.55	1.24	.93	1.44	.33	1.16	.45	.43	1.10	.65	.48	1.61	.41	1.98	.99
53.	1.06	1.23	1.90	2.46	.93	2.07	.97	1.11	.89	1.56	1.22	1.24	.92	2.05	2.20
54.	.10	.28	.36	1.09	.13	.10	.31	.09	.00	.26	.35	.36	.31	.33	.00
55.	.11	.16	.17	.39	.06	.19	.11	.15	.07	.39	.12	.18	.14	.26	.00
56.	.11	.38	.46	.53	.07	.00	.17	.11	.18	.20	.21	.52	.10	.23	.14
57.	3.86	5.47	5.87	9.22	2.34	4.34	3.06	3.44	4.20	5.87	4.42	6.15	3.18	6.55	4.54
58.	13.35	14.25	11.60	12.67	10.51	10.76	12.55	11.85	11.86	14.66	14.41	13.11	12.46	12.54	15.83
Homicide															
59.	6.25	2.67	3.49	1.94	8.35	1.50	7.94	10.05	2.28	1.89	6.46	2.63	4.94	1.81	4.26
60.	1.15	.84	1.27	.77	1.47	.63	1.26	2.52	.46	.26	1.17	.88	.75	.55	.78
61.	.32	.22	.22	.18	.25	.05	.23	.33	.25	.26	.25	.29	.34	.18	.14
62.	1.45	.71	.99	1.20	1.32	1.50	.68	1.26	1.03	.46	1.13	.71	1.03	.52	.57
63.	2.92	1.76	2.49	2.15	3.04	2.17	2.17	4.10	1.73	.98	2.55	1.88	2.12	1.25	1.49
64.	9.17	4.43	5.98	4.08	11.39	3.67	10.11	14.16	4.02	2.87	9.01	4.51	7.06	3.06	5.75
65.	.31	.13	.07	.14	.09	.19	.10	.11	.09	.00	.13	.12	.14	.06	.07
66.	.37	.44	.30	.14	.45	.77	.82	.25	.27	.13	.09	.19	.72	.14	1.49
67.	.28	.95	.75	.49	.17	.29	.36	.16	.89	.33	.17	.41	.63	.28	.78
68.	1.08	2.34	2.12	1.06	1.04	1.69	1.79	.70	1.78	1.17	.58	1.59	2.05	.91	2.98
69.	81.47	74.70	60.43	51.95	79.70	77.50	77.84	76.00	64.20	66.41	69.19	68.46	76.58	58.38	98.04

Index of Authors

Index of Subjects

Italicized page numbers refer to figures or tables without relevant text on the same page.

About the Authors

Susan Pardee Baker is professor of Health Policy and Management and of Environmental Health Sciences at The Johns Hopkins School of Hygiene and Public Health. She holds a joint appointment in Pediatrics at The Johns Hopkins School of Medicine. An epidemiologist specializing in injury control, she is the author of four textbook chapters and more than forty major articles in medical and public health journals. A recipient of the American Trauma Society's Distinguished Achievement Award for her work in injury severity scoring, Professor Baker is internationally recognized for her research in the areas of highway, home, and occupational injuries. She is a graduate of Cornell University and received her M.P.H. from The Johns Hopkins University.

Brian O'Neill is senior vice president of the Insurance Institute for Highway Safety and the Highway Loss Data Institute, where he is responsible for developing and implementing research programs related to highway loss reduction. Mr. O'Neill's own research includes the development of an index for measuring the overall severity of multiple injuries, studies of motor vehicle occupant and pedestrian deaths and injuries, studies of the effectiveness of automobile occupant restraints, and an evaluation of breath alcohol testing devices. He has served on two executive committees of the National Safety Council, as well as the editorial boards of *Accident Analysis and Prevention* and *Traffic Safety Evaluation Research Review.* Mr. O'Neill received his B.Sc. in mathematics and statistics from the Bath University of Technology in Bath, England.

Ronald Steven Karpf is a mathematical statistician with the Insurance Institute for Highway Safety. He specializes in statistical computing and research in the field of motor vehicle injuries and deaths. Dr. Karpf received his Ph.D. from the American University in Washington, D.C.

Insurance Institute for Highway Safety: List of Books

The Insurance Institute for Highway Safety is an independent, non-profit, scientific and educational organization dedicated to reducing the losses—deaths, injuries, and property damage—resulting from crashes on the nation's highways. The institute is supported by the nation's insurance companies, independently and through their trade organizations.

Insurance Institute for Highway Safety books:

The Incidence and Economic Costs of Major Health Impairments: A Comparative Analysis of Cancer, Motor Vehicle Injuries, Coronary Heart Disease, and Stroke, Nelson S. Hartunian, Charles N. Smart, and Mark S. Thompson (1981)

Deterring the Drinking Driver: Legal Policy and Social Control, H. Laurence Ross (1982)

Injuries: Causes, Control Strategies, and Public Policy, Leon S. Robertson (1983)